Spine Trauma

Vikas V. Patel
Evalina Burger
Courtney W. Brown (Editors)

Spine Trauma

Surgical Techniques

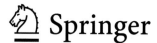 Springer

Vikas V. Patel, M.D.
Associate Professor
Department of Orthopaedics
University of Colorado, Denver
School of Medicine
12631 East 17th Avenue
Aurora, CO 80045
USA
vikas.patel@ucdenver.edu

Courtney W. Brown, M.D.
Panorama Orthopaedics and Spine Center
660 Golden Ridge Road, Suite 250
Golden, CO 80401
USA
cbrown@panoramaortho.com

Evalina Burger, M.D., B.Med.Sc., M.B.Ch.B.
Associate Professor
Senior Orthopaedic Surgeon
Vice Chair, Department of Orthopaedics
University of Colorado, Denver
School of Medicine
12631 East 17th Avenue
Aurora, CO 80045
USA
evalina.burger@ucdenver.edu

ISBN: 978-3-642-03693-4   e-ISBN: 978-3-642-03694-1

DOI: 10.1007/978-3-642-03694-1

Springer Heidelberg Dordrecht London New York

Library of Congress Control Number: 2010925788

Cover design: eStudio Calamar, Figueres/Berlin

Printed on acid-free paper

Springer is part of Springer Science+Business Media (www.springer.com)

To Sir Ludwig Gutman, who personally changed medicine's attitude and approach toward catastrophic spine injuries, thus opening the door for innovative concepts of reconstructing traumatic spine injuries. Sir Gutman was knighted for his work with injured soldiers during World War II.

The editors also dedicate this book to their families for their continuous support and understanding of the time and energy involved in treating spine injury patients.

Preface

Many textbooks already exist in the ever-changing world of spine surgery, few, however, focus on spine trauma. The spine trauma books that are available provide comprehensive historical and mechanistic perspectives on spine trauma with excellent reviews on the thought process and recommendations of treatment. They do not, however, provide the technical information that is often needed in the trauma setting when surgeons must make quick decisions and quick plans for surgical treatment. This is especially important for the junior attending surgeon and, perhaps, for those who do not cover spine trauma on a daily basis. Thus, the focus of this text is exactly that situation. It is meant to be used as a quick reference when planning surgical treatment for spine trauma victims. Internationally renowned authors have been assembled to provide details on the basic steps of trauma care including preoperative planning, patient positioning, equipment needed, surgical steps, postoperative care, and avoidance and treatment of complications. This is a book that every spine surgeon should have as a reference and refresher when covering spine trauma call.

Denver, Colorado, USA   Vikas V. Patel
Aurora, Colorado, USA   Evalina Burger
Golden, Colorado, USA   Courtney W. Brown

Acknowledgment

To Heidi Armbruster for her tireless efforts in the organization and logistics of this endeavor.

Contents

Cervical Spinal Stability and Decision Making

1

Alpesh A. Patel

1.1 Introduction

Cervical spine injuries occur commonly around the world and across socioeconomic classes [7, 12]. Traumatic injury to the cervical spine, especially when associated with spinal cord injury, can have a profound impact on the patient, his or her family, and society. Despite the frequency and implications of cervical spine trauma, there is little consensus in surgical decision making [1, 6, 8]. Significant variances are seen across nations, geographic regions, institutions, and individual surgeons.

Surgical decision making in cervical spinal trauma is influenced by a number of factors, cervical stability being a key component. While some injury patterns mandate surgical stabilization (Fig. 1.1), in a larger number of injuries, spinal stability remains in question. Although a large number of classification systems have been reported in an attempt to define cervical stability, unfortunately, an accurate and reliable method remains elusive. No single system has demonstrated superior reliability or widespread acceptance. Instead of improving our understanding of cervical trauma, these systems have often created the opposite effect by adding inconsistent terminology and confusion.

The purpose of this chapter is to review pertinent issues regarding cervical spinal stability after trauma and surgical decision making. This will review prior classification systems, identify critical clinical variables, and update current concepts in the classification and treatment of subaxial spine injuries.

A.A. Patel
Department of Orthopaedic Surgery,
Department of Neurosurgery, University of Utah,
590 Wakara Way, Salt Lake City, UT 84124, USA
e-mail: alpesh.patel@hsc.utah.edu

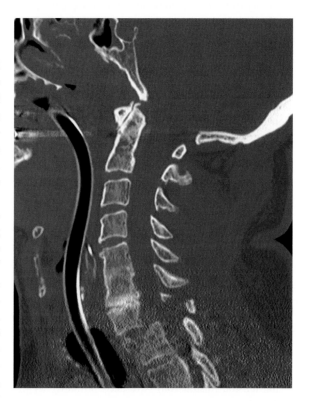

Fig. 1.1 Sagittal CT image of C7-T1 bilateral facet dislocation with >50% anterior translation and canal impingement

1.2 Cervical Stability

Cervical stability is one of the most important factors affecting medical decision making after traumatic injury. An "unstable" cervical injury is commonly treated with operative stabilization, while a "stable" injury may be managed through nonoperative measures such as immobilization, bracing, or observation. The difficulty lies in defining stability and instability based upon clinical and radiographic parameters.

V.V. Patel et al. (eds.), *Spine Trauma*,
DOI: 10.1007/978-3-642-03694-1_1, © Springer-Verlag Berlin Heidelberg 2010

One commonly accepted definition of spinal stability, as defined by White and Panjabi, is the "ability of the spine under physiologic loads to limit patterns of displacement so as not to damage or irritate the spinal cord or nerve roots and, in addition, to prevent incapacitating deformity or pain due to structural changes" [17]. While this definition does not provide clinical or radiographic specifics, it does incorporate many of the critical determinants of medical decision making: has traumatic injury led to spinal cord or nerve root injury? Will the injury lead to deformity? Will the deformity lead to long-term disability from either pain or further neurological injury?

While it is common to interpret spinal stability as a Boolean variable ("yes" or "no"), spinal stability more likely exists on a continuum. The degree of spinal instability will depend upon the anatomic constraints that have been disrupted. Normal cervical anatomy provides constraints to motion from both bony relationships as well as the intervertebral disk and ligamentous structures (anterior longitudinal ligament, posterior longitudinal ligament, annulus, facet capsules, interspinous and supraspinous ligaments).

Work by White and Panjabi has demonstrated that bony articulations of the cervical spine are significantly supported by the anterior and posterior ligamentous structures, as well as the intervertebral disk, to provide stability [17]. The bony articulation and facet capsules are the primary restraints against forward subluxation with the posterior ligaments and muscle tension providing additional support. The anterior longitudinal ligament (ALL), anterior annulus, and facet joints resist extension while the posterior bony and ligamentous structures resist flexion. Compression is resisted by the vertebral bodies, intervertebral disk, and facet joints, while tension (distraction) is resisted primarily by the disk and ligamentous structures.

Disruption of these supporting structures, commonly occurring along a spectrum of severity, contributes to the potential for cervical instability. A number of cervical spine injury classification systems have been developed in an attempt to categorize and quantify the degree of disruption and, thereby, define spinal instability.

1.3 Classification Systems

Classification systems have traditionally been focused upon descriptive radiographic findings and mechanisms of injury. The mechanistic systems are formed by synthesizing radiographic findings with biomechanical modes of failure to produce an inferred injury mechanism (ex; flexion, distraction injury). These subjective systems lack any firm injury descriptors and lead to ambiguity – a single fracture pattern may be described as a fracture-dislocation, compression flexion injury, or facet dislocation to others. The addition of purely descriptive terms (e.g., "tear drop" pattern) to the trauma vernacular brings more confusion to injury classification. Despite these shortcomings, the evolution of cervical classification systems has increased our understanding of subaxial cervical trauma.

1.3.1 Holdsworth

Holdsworth provided the earliest comprehensive classification system for spinal column injuries through a retrospective review of over two thousand patients [10]. His was one of the first attempts to classify spinal trauma according to the mechanism of injury. He identified categories of (a) Simple wedge fracture, (b) dislocation, (c) rotational fracture-dislocation, (d) extension injury, (e) burst injury, and (f) shear fracture. While his system encompassed all regions of the spine (cervical, thoracic, and lumbar), it was the first to highlight the posterior ligamentous structures as a crucial determinant of spinal stability.

1.3.2 Mechanistic Systems

Subsequently, two other classification systems specific to the subaxial cervical spine evolved. Allen and Ferguson proposed a mechanistic classification system of subaxial cervical spine injuries based on the retrospective review of radiographs of 165 patients [2]. The authors identified six distinct mechanisms: (1) compressive flexion; (2) vertical compression; (3) distractive flexion; (4) compressive extension; (5) distractive extension, and (6) lateral flexion. Increasing numerical values were assigned to each category to account for progressive degrees of spinal instability. Subsequently, Harris identified six mechanisms of injury: (1) flexion; (2) flexion and rotation; (3) hyperextension and rotation; (4) vertical compression; (5) extension; and (6) lateral flexion [9]. Though the terminology introduced by the two systems remains widely used, they neither account for neurological injury nor guide surgical decision making.

1.3.3 White and Panjabi

White and Panjabi defined cervical instability, through cadaveric studies, as 3.5 mm horizontal displacement of one vertebra in relation to an adjacent vertebra or greater than 11° of angulation difference between adjacent vertebrae on a lateral X-ray [17]. The authors, using these findings along with clinical data, created a point-based classification system for subaxial cervical spine injuries [4]. Unfortunately, the descriptors are either too subjective (anterior/posterior element "destruction," dangerous anticipated loads) or are impractical to obtain clinically (the stretch test). Despite this, the system is the first classification to acknowledge the importance of neurological status, to account for differences between the cord and nerve root level injuries, and to incorporate these into medical decision making. It is also the first stress objective findings rather than inferred injury mechanisms.

1.3.4 AO (Arbeitsgemeinschaft für Osteosynthesefragen) System

The AO Classification for thoracolumbar spine injuries is often applied to cervical spine injuries [13]. This system was developed through a retrospective review of 1,445 thoracolumbar injuries, assessing the level of the injury, frequency of fracture types/groups, and incidence of neurological deficits. Categories in this system are based on the mechanism of injury and injury pattern and are classified into three large groups with subgroup options (Table 1.1) The system categorizes injuries in increasing amount of spinal instability. Group A (focuses on compressive injuries of the vertebral body), group B (involves distractive disruption of either anterior or posterior elements), and group C (involves axial rotation/torque). Despite its excellent organization, the AO system has demonstrated poor interobserver reliability [18]. Additionally, it does not provide thorough guidelines for optimal treatment of different injury types.

These classification systems have contributed to cervical trauma care, but have also demonstrated limitations. Identifying a unique mechanism of injury can be

Table 1.1 AO classification system for spinal injuries

A. Compression injury
A1: Impaction fracture
A1.1 Endplate impaction
A1.2 Wedge Impaction
A1.3 Vertebral body collapse
A2: Split fracture
A2.1 Sagittal split fracture
A2.2 Coronal split fracture
A2.3 Pincer fracture
A3: Burst fracture
A3.1 Incomplete burst fracture
A3.2 Burst-split fracture
A3.3 Complete burst fracture
B. Distraction injury
B1: Posterior ligamentary lesion
B1.1 With disk rupture
B1.2 With type A fracture
B2: Posterior osseous lesion
B2.1 Transverse bicolumn
B2.2 With disk rupture
B2.3 With type A fracture
B3: Anterior disk rupture
B3.1 With subluxation
B3.2 With spondylolysis
B3.3 With posterior dislocation
C. Rotation injury
C1: Type A with rotation
C1.1 Rotational wedge fracture
C1.2 Rotational split fracture
C1.3 Rotational burst fracture
C2: Type B with rotation
C2.1 B1 Lesion with rotation
C2.2 B2 Lesion with rotation
C2.3 B3 Lesion with rotation

difficult. Agreement on the ideal injury classification remains. These systems, excluding that of White and Panjabi, do not account for the neurological status of the patient – a critical determinant of spinal stability and medical decision making. Additionally, these systems are based almost exclusively upon plain radiographs only and do not account for diagnostic information from advanced imaging modalities (CT, MRI) [19].

1.4 Advances in Cervical Trauma Classification

To address the limitations of the other systems, two novel cervical classifications have recently been validated and reported: (1) Cervical spine injury severity score; (2) Subaxial Cervical Spine Injury Classification (SLIC). Both the systems attempt to define cervical stability and instability and, in turn, guide surgical decision making.

1.4.1 Cervical Spine Injury Severity Score

Anderson et al. have developed a point-based system on the basis of fracture displacement and ligamentous injury to each of the four spinal columns (anterior, posterior, right lateral, left lateral) [3]. The four column approach is a modification of the three-column system described by Louis [11]. This system avoids subjective criteria and utilizes advanced imaging to define injuries based upon measured amounts of fracture or ligamentous displacement. The system showed good-to-excellent intra- and interobserver reliability and a strong association between cumulative score, clinical status, and treatment choice, with all patients with a score of ≥7 treated surgically. It remains to be seen if this system can be effectively applied prospectively in a clinical setting. Given its objective measurements and excellent reliability, it may serve ultimately as a better tool for clinical research.

1.4.2 Subaxial Cervical Spine Injury Classification (SLIC)

The SLIC proposed by Vaccaro et. al defines subaxial trauma according to six clinical criteria: (1) spinal level, (2) injury morphology, (3) bony injury description, (4) discoligamentous complex (DLC) injury, (5) neurological status, and (6) confounders (ex; diffuse idiopathic skeletal hyperostosis (DISH), cervical stenosis, osteoporosis, prior surgery, etc.) 5, 15]. The system identifies three of these – injury morphology, DLC, and neurologic status – as the most influential

criteria in determining cervical stability and guiding surgical decision making (Table 1.2).

Injury morphology defines the relationship of the vertebrae to each other in terms of anterior anatomical support, soft tissue structures, facet relationships, and overall alignment based upon plain radiographs and advanced imaging. In an increasing order of severity, injury morphology is categorized as compression, distraction, or rotation/translation. Inferred descriptive terms of "flexion" and "extension" are not included in this system. By doing so, the SLIC system distinguishes injury morphology from injury mechanism.

The DLC refers to the intervertebral disk, the anterior and posterior longitudinal ligaments, interspinous ligaments, facet capsules, and ligamentum flavum. This is a unique descriptor to the SLIC system and is categorized as disrupted, intact, or indeterminate.

Table 1.2 Subaxial injury classification (SLIC) and severity scale

Morphology	Points
No Abnormality	0
Compression Burst	1 +1 = 2
Distraction (e.g., facet perch, hyperextension)	3
Rotation/translation (e.g., facet dislocation, unstable teardrop or advanced staged flexion compression injury)	4
Discoligomentous complex (DLC)	
Intact	0
Indeterminate (e.g., isolated interspinous widening, MRI signal change only)	1
Disrupted (e.g., widening of anterior disk space, facet perch or dislocation, kyphotic deformity)	2
Neurological status	
Intact	0
Root injury	1
Complete cord injury	2
Incomplete cord injury	3
Ongoing cord compression (in the setting of a neurologic deficit)	+1
Treatment	*Total score*
Nonoperative (rigid orthoses, halo-vest, etc...)	<4
Operative (surgical decompression/ stabilization)	>4

Disruption of the DLC is suggested by abnormal facet alignment (articular apposition <50% or diastasis >2 mm through the facet joint), abnormal widening of the anterior disk space, translation or rotation of the vertebral bodies, or kyphotic spinal alignment. The additional finding of high signal intensity on T2 fat suppressed sagittal MRI involving the nucleus, annulus, or posterior ligaments may infer the disruption of the DLC. The "disrupted" designation should be used only with convincing evidence of DLC compromise (Fig. 1.2). Indeterminate injury is defined when radiographic disruption of the DLC is not otherwise obvious on radiographic or CT imaging, but a hyperintense signal is found through the posterior ligamentous regions on T2 weighted MRI images, suggesting edema and injury. Intact DLC is defined

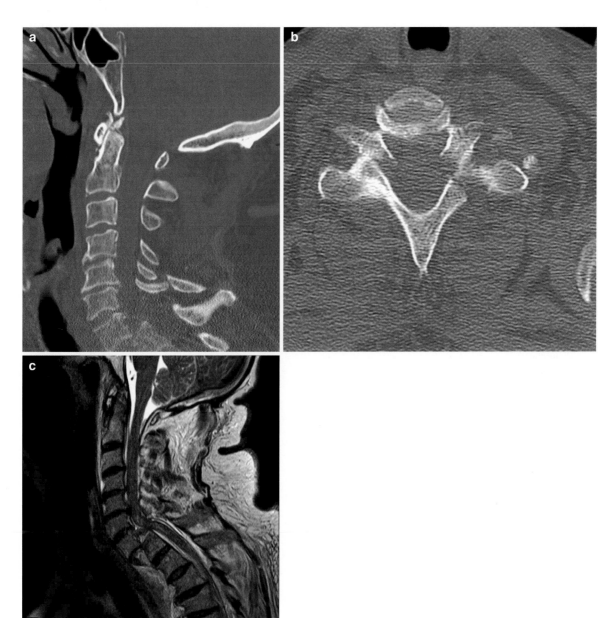

Fig. 1.2 Seventy-one-year-old male presents with neck pain and a complete spinal cord injury after a motor vehicle accident. (**a**) Sagittal CT and (**b**) axial CT images demonstrate bilateral C7-T1 dislocation with anterior translation and canal impingement. (**c**) Sagittal T2 weighted image demonstrates disruption of the discoligamentous complex as well as spinal cord signal change. *SLIC classification:* Injury morphology – translation (4 points), DLC – disrupted (2 points), neurological status – complete spinal cord injury (2 points). *Total score = 8 (operative treatment)*

by normal spinal alignment, disk space characteristics, and appearance of the ligamentous structures.

The presence of neurological injury is often a critical factor in surgical decision making. Additionally, that neurologic injury is a strong indicator of spinal instability. The neurologic status is categorized as: intact (normal), root injury, complete spinal cord injury, or incomplete spinal cord injury. An additional modifier, continuous cord compression, is also described in the setting of either complete or incomplete spinal cord injury with spinal cord compression due to disk, bone,

ligamentum, hematoma, or other structures. With translation or rotation injuries, assessment of cord compression should be made after an attempted reduction of the injury (Fig. 1.3).

Weighted scores are assigned to each major injury characteristic (Table 1.2). The scores are then added to produce an injury severity score. This score, a quantification of the degree of spinal instability, is used to guide surgical decision making. Scores <4 are treated nonoperatively, scores ≥4 surgically. The SLIC system has demonstrated greater reliability than the

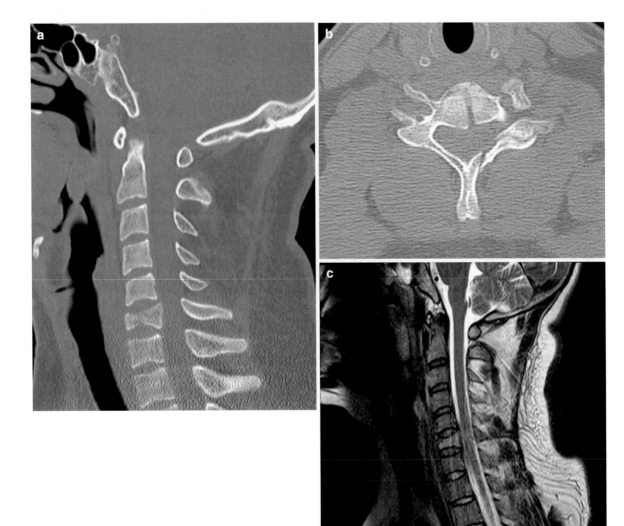

Fig. 1.3 Thirty-four-year-old male presents with neck pain and no neurological deficit after a diving accident. (**a**) Sagittal CT and (**b**) axial CT images reveal a C6 burst fracture with well-maintained alignment of the spine. (**c**) Sagittal T2 weighted image shows normal signal intensity in the disk, liga-mentous structures, and spinal cord. *SLIC classification*: Injury morphology – burst (2 points), DLC – intact (0 points), neurological status – intact (0 points). *Total score = 2 (nonoperative treatment)*

Allen–Ferguson or Harris classification systems and has produced >90% interobserver agreement on treatment choice [15].

Though concise, objective, and promising, the SLIC system is yet to be prospectively applied. It is similar in construct and content, however, to a thoracolumbar injury classification system that has demonstrated widespread use, rapid learning, and easy incorporation into the clinical setting [14, 16]. Future investigations may reveal its clinical usefulness better. Nevertheless, the SLIC system has helped by clearly identifying the critical components of posttraumatic cervical stability and surgical decision making.

1.5 Summary: Critical Clinical Variables

Critical clinical factors in assessing the cervical spine after spinal trauma include:

- Bony injury pattern or morphology
- Neurological injury
- Disruption of the intervertebral disk and ligamentous structures

1.6 Conclusions

Cervical stability remains the most critical determinant of surgical decision making. Defining posttraumatic stability accurately and reproducibly has proved to be difficult. This has contributed to wide variations in the treatment of cervical trauma. Recent advances in cervical classification systems have attempted to define cervical stability more objectively by identifying critical clinical variables – injury morphology, neurological injury, and disruption of the discoligamentous complex. A more accepted clinical diagnosis of cervical stability may provide physicians with better guidelines for surgical decision making and, thereby, improve patient care.

References

1. Aebi M, Zuber K, Marchesi D (1991) Treatment of cervical spine injuries with anterior plating. Indications, techniques, and results. Spine 16(3 suppl):S38–S45

2. Allen BL Jr, Ferguson RL, Lehmann T (1982) A mechanistic classification of closed, indirect fractures and dislocations of the lower cervical spine. Spine 7(1):1–27
3. Anderson PA et al (2007) Cervical spine injury severity score. Assessment of reliability. J Bone Joint Surg Am 89(5):1057–1065
4. Bernhardt M, White AA, Panjabi MM (1999) Biomechanical considerations of spinal stability. In: Herkowitz HN (ed). WB Saunders, Philadelphia, pp 1071–1096
5. Dvorak MF, Fisher CG, Fehlings MG, Rampersaud YR, Oner FC, Aarabi B, Vaccaro AR (2007) The surgical approach to subaxial cervical spine injuries: an evidence-based algorithm based on the SLIC classification system. Spine 32(23):2620–2629
6. Glaser JA, Jaworski BA, Cuddy BG, Albert TJ, Hollowell JP, McLain RF, Bozzette S (1998) Variation in surgical opinion regarding management of selected cervical spine injuries. A preliminary study. Spine 23(9):975–982
7. Goldberg W, Mueller C, Panacek E, Tigges S, Hoffman JR, Mower WR (2001) Distribution and patterns of blunt traumatic cervical spine injury. Ann Emerg Med 38(1):17–21
8. Hadley MN (2002) Guidelines for management of acute cervical injuries. Neurosurgery 50(3):S1–S6
9. Harris JH, Edeiken-Monroe B, Kopansiky DR (1986) A practical classification of acute cervical spine injuries. Orthop Clin North Am 1(15):15–30
10. Holdsworth F (1970) Fractures, dislocations, and fracture-dislocations of the spine. J Bone Joint Surg 52(8):1534–1551
11. Louis R (1985) Spinal stability as defined by the three-column concept. Anatomia Clinica 7(1):33–42
12. Lowery DW, Wald MM, Browne BJ, Tigges S, Hoffman JR, Mower WR (2001) Epidemiology of cervical spine injury victims. Ann Emerg Med 38(1):12–16
13. Moore TA, Vaccaro AR, Anderson PA (2006) Classification of lower cervical spine injuries. Spine 31(11 suppl):S37–S43; discussion S61
14. Patel AA et al (2007) The adoption of a new classification system: time-dependent variation in interobserver reliability of the thoracolumbar injury severity score classification system. Spine 32(3):E105–E110
15. Vaccaro AR et al (2007) The subaxial cervical spine injury classification system: a novel approach to recognize the importance of morphology, neurology, and integrity of the disco-ligamentous complex. Spine 32(21):2365–2374
16. Vaccaro AR et al (2005) A new classification of thoracolumbar injuries: the importance of injury morphology, the integrity of the posterior ligamentous complex, and neurologic status. Spine 30(20):2325–2333
17. White AA, Panjabi MM (1990) (eds) Physical properties and functional biomechanics of the spine. In: Clinical biomechanics of the spine. Lippincott Willam and Wilkins, Philadelphia, pp 22
18. Wood KB, Khanna G, Vaccaro AR, Arnold PM, Harris MB, Mehbod AA (2005) Assessment of two thoracolumbar fracture classification systems as used by multiple surgeons. J Bone Joint Surg 87-A(7):1423–1429
19. Woodring JH, Lee C (1993) Limitations of cervical radiography in the evaluation of acute cervical trauma. J Trauma 34(1):32–39

Clearing the Cervical Spine

2

Ronald W. Lindsey and Zbigniew Gugala

2.1 Introduction

Clearing the cervical spine is among the highest priorities in the early assessment of trauma patients in emergency centers. Annually, more than ten million patients present to trauma centers in the USA, and in all of these patients, the possibility of cervical spine injury must be considered [34, 43, 60]. The actual incidence of cervical spine injury among blunt trauma patients is only 1–3% [77, 80, 81, 96]. Therefore, the need for a concise, yet thorough, approach to cervical spine clearance mandates that efficacious clearing guidelines are established and adhered to.

Traditionally, most physicians have considered imaging as the principal, if not the sole, method by which the cervical spine should be cleared. This opinion resulted in the tendency for many physicians to ignore the merits of the history and physical examination in the clearance process, and impeded the development of dependable clinical indicators of cervical injury. Subsequently, most initially developed cervical spine clearance protocols relied almost entirely on indiscriminate imaging [72]. The liberal use of imaging produces a large number of predominately normal or inadequate cervical spine X-rays, creates frequent delays in the patient's emergency workup and subsequent treatment, and results in enormous costs for both personnel time and institutional resources [13, 86, 97].

Despite the numerous problems associated with indiscriminate cervical spine plain radiography in the trauma setting, this practice has been difficult to restrict. Although the history and physical examination are integral components of the cervical spine evaluation, there is no consensus among physicians on how to prioritize the impact of these clinical components on the diagnostic process. When cervical spine injury is missed and/or its treatment delayed, resultant patient morbidity can be devastating, and the cost to society is enormous. Finally, for many physicians, the potential liability of a missed cervical spine injury more than justifies routine X-ray imaging.

More than two decades ago, Jacobs and Schwartz [49] reported that the ability of emergency physician to clinically predict the presence of cervical spine injury in trauma patients was only 50%. However, the same physicians were able to successfully identify 94% of trauma patients without cervical spine injury. Inadvertently, this study not only emphasized the true focus of cervical spine clearance, that is, accurately determining the absence of cervical spine injury, but also affirmed that the clinical designation of absence of cervical spine injury was more feasible than the clinical detection on injury.

Because of the very low incidence of positive imaging findings, clearing the cervical spine solely dependent on imaging is extremely inefficient. In a retrospective series of 1,686 consecutive trauma patients subjected to cervical spine clearing, Lindsey et al. [57] questioned the efficacy of routine cervical spine imaging. These authors identified only 1.9% of patients with cervical spine injuries. Moreover, most of the detected cervical spine injuries were nonthreatening to the patient's spinal stability or neurologic integrity. These findings suggest that the concept of a specific clinical protocol to better select patients who warrant imaging has enormous merit.

R.W. Lindsey (✉) and Z. Gugala
Department of Orthopaedic Surgery and Rehabilitation,
Rebecca Sealy Hospital, University of Texas Medical Branch,
301 University Boulevard, Galveston,
TX 77555-0165, USA
e-mail: rlindsey@utmb.edu

V.V. Patel et al. (eds.), *Spine Trauma*,
DOI: 10.1007/978-3-642-03694-1_2, © Springer-Verlag Berlin Heidelberg 2010

The objective of this chapter is to explore the complex issue of clearing the cervical spine in trauma patients. Among the topics addressed are: (1) defining cervical spine clearance, its rationale, and objectives; (2) identifying the trauma patient groups that determine the most appropriate clearing process; (3) establishing the clinical and imaging components of clearance; (4) reviewing the currently available guidelines for clearing the cervical spine; and (5) devising a new comprehensive algorithm for clearing of the cervical spine in the emergency setting.

2.2 Cervical Spine Clearance: Definition, Rationale, Objectives

The overwhelming majority of blunt trauma victims presenting to the emergency center do not have a cervical spine injury [42]. In order to reliably and effectively identify the patients who are injury-free, the term "clearance" of the cervical spine has recently been introduced to emergency medicine [59].

Cervical spine clearance in the trauma setting is defined as reliably ruling out the presence of cervical spine injury in a patient who indeed does not have a cervical spine injury. Contrary to the common misconception, cervical clearance is not intended to detect or classify an injury, or determine its most appropriate treatment. Clearance simply declares that injury is not present. The clearing process always requires a complete clinical evaluation, and occasionally warrants adjunctive imaging. Ideally, clearing should occur at the earliest point in the trauma assessment process so that it can be accomplished reliably. However, the clearance process does not place its major emphasis on how quickly it is accomplished, but on its accuracy.

The fundamental objective of cervical spine clearance is to improve the efficiency and accuracy of the entire trauma assessment process. When cervical spine injury can reliably be ruled out, neck immobilization precautions can be discontinued, additional neck diagnostic or therapeutic modalities are not warranted, and the trauma evaluation can focus on the other areas of the patient's assessment. Considerable pressure may be placed on the emergency clinician to expeditiously clear, especially when the index of suspicion for injury is low. However, one must accept the reality that some patients simply cannot be cleared in the acute setting. If cervical spine injury cannot be reliably excluded, vigilant cervical spine precautions are maintained and efforts to establish a definitive position based on the status of the cervical spine must continue.

2.3 Cervical Spine Clearance: Patient Groups

Two basic principles are applied to all blunt trauma patients in regard to the cervical spine clearance process. First, a meaningful clinical examination is imperative before cervical spine clearance can be considered. The fundamental requirement is a lucid patient. Therefore, the initial step in the clearance process is to determine the patient's level of alertness (Tables 2.1 and 2.2). Although all patients should be thoroughly evaluated, only fully alert patients (Ransohoff Class 1, Glasgow Coma Scale >14) are capable of undergoing a dependable physical examination, and constitute the only type of patients in whom cervical injury can reliably be ruled out, with or without supplemental imaging. Secondarily, alert, oriented patients should be assessed in respect to the presence or absence of symptoms that can either be attributed to or possibly mask cervical spine injury. These include intoxication and distracting injuries. On the basis of these principles, all blunt trauma patients can be acutely categorized into three cervical spine patient clearance groups [59] (Table 2.3).

Table 2.1 Ransohoff classification of consciousness levels

Class	Description
1	Alert; responds immediately to questions; may be disoriented and confused; follows complex commands
2	Drowsy, confused, uninterested; does not lapse into sleep when undisturbed; follows simple commands only
3	Stuporous; sleeps when not disturbed; responds briskly and appropriately to noxious stimuli
4	Deep stupor; responds defensively to prolonged noxious stimuli
5	Coma; no appropriate response to any stimuli; includes decorticate and decerebrate responses
6	Deep coma; flaccidity; no response to any stimuli

Adapted from Ransohoff and Fleischer [75]

Table 2.2 Glasgow coma scale

Feature	Response	Score
Eye opening	Spontaneous	4
	To speech	3
	To pain	2
	None	1
Verbal response	Oriented	5
	Confused conversation	4
	Words inappropriate	3
	Sounds incomprehensible	2
	None	1
Best motor response	Obeys commands	6
	Localizes pain	5
	Flexion normal	4
	Flexion abnormal	3
	Extended	2
	None	1
Total coma score		3–15

Table 2.3 Cervical spine clearance patient group designation

Group	Designation		Patient characteristics
I	Asymptomatic		Awake, alert
			No neck pain/tenderness
			Normal neurologic function
			No intoxication
			No distracting injuries
II	Symptomatic		Neck pain and/or tenderness
			Neurologic deficits
III	Nonevaluable	Temporarily	Intoxicated (alcohol, drugs)
			Presence of distracting injury
		Indefinitely	Obtunded (brain injury)
			Intubated
			Pharmacological coma

2.3.1 Group I (Asymptomatic)

Patients who can be reliably cleared by clinical examination alone without imaging (i.e., no plain radiography, computed tomography (CT), magnetic resonance imaging (MRI), etc.) constitute *Group I*. Patients in this group must satisfy all of the following five criteria [44]: (1) full alertness; (2) no intoxication; (3) no midline tenderness; (4) no focal neurologic deficit, and (5) no distracting painful injury (Table 2.4). A randomized, prospective study of 34,069 patients by the National Emergency X-Radiography Utilization Study (NEXUS) group [42] demonstrated that significant cervical spine injury could be reliably excluded by physical examination alone when applying these criteria. The reliability of cervical spine clearance by physical examination of the alert patient has been corroborated by other studies [4, 27, 57]. Successfully clinically cleared patients do not require further diagnostic measures, and cervical spine precautions can be discontinued.

2.3.2 Group II (Symptomatic)

Fully oriented and alert patients who demonstrate symptoms of neck pain, tenderness, neurologic deficit, and decreased mobility on physical examination require additional diagnostic assessment to effectively clear the cervical spine comprise *Group II*. This group also includes patients with a distracting injury or past history of cervical spine pathology. Additional diagnostic studies typically consist of three-view radiography (anteroposterior, lateral, open-mouth odontoid) and may also require adjunctive CT or MRI [59]. Voluntary lateral flexion–extension radiography is indicated only after symptomatic treatment has failed over a brief period of time (typically 2 weeks), and is not generally recommended in the acute setting. An alert patient who presents with a partial or complete neurologic deficit is assumed to have a spine injury, and thereby always requires imaging. Whether the deficit is due to spinal cord, spinal root, or peripheral nerve injury, an exhaustive diagnostic effort must be made to rule out spine instability and/or injury. Throughout this process, the physician must strictly adhere to all precautionary spine immobilization techniques, even if the initial examination suggests a complete neurologic deficit. Plain radiography and/or sophisticated imaging are always indicated

Table 2.4 Clinical cervical spine clearance criteria as defined by the NEXUS group

Altered neurologic function is present if any of the following is present: (a) Glasgow Coma Scale score of 14 or less; (b) disorientation to person, place, time, or events; (c) inability to remember 3 objects at 5 min; (d) delayed or inappropriate response to external stimuli; or (e) any focal deficit on motor or sensory examination. Patients with none of these individual findings should be classified as having normal neurologic function

Patients should be considered intoxicated if they have either of the following: (a) a recent history of intoxication or intoxicating substance ingestion; or (b) evidence of intoxication on physical examination. Patients may also be considered to be intoxicated if tests of bodily secretions are positive for drugs that affect the level of alertness, including a blood alcohol level greater than 0.08 mg/dL

Midline posterior bony cervical spine tenderness is present if the patient complains of pain on palpation of the posterior midline neck from the nuchal ridge to the prominence of the first thoracic vertebra, or if the patient evinces pain with direct palpation of any cervical spinous process

Patients should be considered to have a distracting painful injury if they have any of the following: (a) a long bone fracture; (b) a visceral injury requiring surgical consultation; (c) a large laceration, degloving injury, or crush injury; (d) large burns; or (e) any other injury producing acute functional impairment. Physicians may also classify any injury as distracting if it is thought to have the potential to impair the patient's ability to appreciate other injuries

Adapted from Hoffman et al. [44]

to diagnose and categorize the injury. Prophylactic treatment modalities such as high dose steroids administration, when indicated, must be instituted emergently. Serial examinations to document neurologic progression or improvement, ideally performed by the same physician, are recommended, irrespective of whether the patient's neurologic deficit is partial or complete.

2.3.3 Group III (Nonevaluable)

Patients who cannot be cleared at the time of the emergency center presentation constitute *Group III* [59]. Definitive clearance is not feasible in this group because of the patient's medical instability, the patient's inability to undergo a reliable clinical examination, or inconclusive results of the initially performed diagnostic studies. The majority of patients in this group present with an impaired level of consciousness due to head injury or intoxication, and this alone inhibits the clearance process. The adjunctive imaging in this group can detect obvious cervical injury, but it cannot definitively rule it out, even if it is negative. This group typically consists of two subgroups: patients who are *temporarily nonevaluable* and those who are *indefinitely nonevaluable*. The temporarily nonevaluable patients include those who are intoxicated or present with a distracting injury. These patients may be asymptomatic, but the presence of intoxication and/or distracting injury renders their clinical examination unreliable. The expectation is that these temporary conditions will resolve in 24–48 h, and these

patients can subsequently be reclassified to enter either patient *Group I* or *II*, or will remain in *Group III*. The subgroup of indefinitely nonevaluable patients includes those who are obtunded, intubated, and/or pharmacologically compromised, and therefore they cannot submit to a meaningful clinical examination. For all *Group III* patients, strict adherence to basic principles of cervical spine external support and/or stabilizing precautions is recommended. Imaging is indicated for these patients to detect but not to definitively exclude cervical spine injury. Even if the cervical spine imaging is negative, the prudent physician is obliged to maintain all neck precautions until the patient becomes more alert and receptive to supplemental clinical assessment. Although some reports [19, 39, 89, 98] suggest that negative sophisticated imaging (CT and/or MRI) may adequately clear the cervical spine of these patients, the authors submit that definitive clearance cannot be reliably established until the patient is alert and a valid physical examination can be performed.

The efficiency of cervical spine clearance can be greatly enhanced by assigning patients to one of these three groups. Although one of the primary clinical objectives will always be to increase the sensitivity of cervical injury detection, the emergency clinicians must recognize that the greater challenge is to be proficient in cervical spine injury exclusion. Indeed, the inability to clinically clear a patient is not equivalent to the presence of injury, and always requires the use of adjunctive imaging. However, most imaging modalities are more sensitive for injury detection than being specific for its exclusion. Therefore, cervical spine imaging alone cannot substitute for a thorough clinical evaluation in establishing clearance. Furthermore, the effectiveness of imaging in cervical spine clearance is enhanced when combined with a meaningful clinical examination.

2.4 Patient Management Before and During Cervical Spine Clearance

Cervical spine injury should be assumed to be present in all patients during pre-hospital trauma management. Cervical spine immobilization is uniformly applied and typically consists of a cervical collar and/or securing the head to the backboard with sandbags and/or tape [1, 24]. Although neck immobilization in trauma patients has been questioned because of reported elevations in intracranial pressure and an increased risk for respiratory problems [70], routine rigid neck immobilization is still the standard recommended for all trauma patients [36].

After arrival at the hospital, all external neck support should be maintained. These principles apply even during the assessment of the airway; the head and neck should not be excessively flexed, extended, or rotated at this juncture. If external neck support must be temporarily removed (e.g., neck wound inspection), a member of the trauma team should manually maintain control of the head and neck using in-line immobilization techniques [1]. The physician's adherence to these precautions cannot be overstated because a significant subset of cervical trauma patients can experience the onset or progression of neurologic deficit after arrival at the hospital [9]. The first premise in clearing trauma patients for cervical injury is the assumption that a cervical spine injury exists, and all patients should be managed accordingly until it can be definitely excluded [97].

If other injuries warrant more immediate or greater attention, the cervical spine evaluation can be safely deferred as long as cervical immobilization is diligently maintained. The only aspects of the initial trauma patient assessment that are of greater priority than the cervical spine are the patient's airway, breathing, circulation, and head/brain. A patent airway should be expeditiously identified or established immediately after the trauma patient's arrival to the hospital. Breathing must then be documented or external ventilation initiated. Hemorrhage, the most prevalent cause of preventable deaths posttrauma, must be quickly

controlled to ensure hemodynamic stability [1]. Finally, a neurologic evaluation is performed to establish the patient's level of consciousness, and if a brain injury exists, it must also be managed emergently. Cervical spine clearance becomes the focus of the evaluation, only after these "ABCs" have been addressed.

The cervical spine screening begins with each patient being assigned to one of the three patient groups following a brief clinical examination. The majority of the published clearance guidelines address the oriented and alert patient (*Group I*, *Group II*) [26, 42, 65, 68, 79, 92, 100], whereas in the indefinitely non-evaluable (obtunded) patients (*Group III*), the initial evaluation protocols are controversial [5, 10, 11, 14, 30, 67]. In *Group I*, reliable clinical clearance of the cervical spine can be achieved for those patients who present without symptoms or a history suggestive of cervical spine injury [57, 79, 96]. In an alert patient who presents with symptoms of possible cervical spine injury (*Group II*), clearance will require adjunctive imaging.

2.5 Clinical Clearance of the Cervical Spine

2.5.1 History

A detailed history is essential in the cervical spine assessment of trauma patients. The initial priority in obtaining a valid history is an early, accurate determination of the patient's level of alertness. Although the ideal history is the one obtained from an alert, oriented trauma victim, significant information is also available from a host of other individuals who may have experienced the same mishap, or are simply familiar with the scene of the accident (e.g., police, emergency medical technicians, other passengers, witnesses). In addition to documenting the mechanism of injury, the history should provide a detailed account of the events and patient's condition from immediately postinjury up to the time of presentation to a medical facility. Information regarding the victim's past medical history, especially as it pertains to previous cervical spine conditions, is especially helpful. Special attention should be given to the elderly patient who has sustained a fall or minor trauma; these individuals are particularly susceptible to cervical spine injury [27, 56].

The risk for cervical spine injury and its severity can be directly correlated with the energy associated with the traumatic insult [4, 47, 49]. Therefore, the level of energy (i.e., high vs. low) and the manner by which injury is sustained (direct vs. indirect) are crucial information. The clinician should determine if the accident is the result of a high-speed motor vehicle accident (MVA), or a fall from a considerable height vs. an altercation. If due to a fall, the approximate height of the fall should be calculated; if due to an MVA, the record should reflect if the patient was restrained or ejected from the vehicle. The possibility of direct vs. indirect whiplash injury should also be established.

The previously noted study by Jacobs and Schwartz [49] not only established the feasibility of clinical clearance of the cervical spine, but also identified a number of subjective variables that seemed to correlate with an increased risk for the cervical spine injury (Table 2.5). In a recent study, Stiell et al. [92] have also calculated

Table 2.5 Variables positively correlating with cervical spine injury

Variable	P value
Motor vehicle accident	0.052
Fall > 10 ft.	0.007
Neck tenderness	0.002
Numbness	0.001
Loss of sensation	0.001
Weakness	0.001
Neck spasm	0.001
Loss of muscle power (0–5)	0.001
Decreased sensation	0.001
Loss of anal tone/wink	0.001
Fall <10 ft.	0.083
Low-energy injury	0.700
Drug/alcohol intoxication	0.400
Flexion/extension	0.400
Compression/torsion	0.960
Head trauma	0.370
Neck pain	0.140
Headache	0.140
Loss of consciousness	0.382
Bradycardic hypotension	0.760

Adapted from Jacobs and Schwartz [49]

Table 2.6 Odds ratios of a clinical variable predicting clinically significant cervical spine injury

Variable	OR (95% CI)[a]
Dangerous mechanism[b]	5.2 (3.7–7.3)
Age ≥65 years	3.7 (2.4–5.6)
Paresthesis in extremities	2.2 (1.4–3.3)
Ambulatory at any time after injury	1.0 (0.7–1.5)
Sitting position in EC	0.61 (0.3–1.2)
Delayed onset of neck pain	0.4 (0.3–0.7)
Absence of midline neck tenderness	0.5 (0.3–0.8)
Able to rotate neck 45° left and right	0.04 (0.01–0.3)
Simple rear-end MVA[c]	0.08 (0.03–0.2)

Adapted from Stiell et al. [92]

[a]OR odds ratio; CI confidence interval; MVA motor vehicle accident

[b]Fall from ≥1 m; axial load to the head; high-speed MVA, rollover, or ejection; bicycle collision; recreational motorized vehicle collision

[c]Excludes vehicle pushed into oncoming traffic, hit by bus or large truck, rollover, or hit by high-speed vehicle; collision

the odds ratio of several clinical variables that could predict a significant cervical spine injury (Table 2.6). Although these variables may serve to heighten one's awareness of the risk for cervical spine injury in a particular patient, ruling out the presence of these variables alone does not establish cervical clearance.

2.5.2 Physical Examination

The physical examination, albeit challenging in the acute posttraumatic environment, is essential for valid clearance of the cervical spine. This principle exists regardless of whether adjunctive imaging is also deemed necessary to complete the process. The physical examination can be accomplished only in patients who demonstrate a Glasgow Coma Scale score >14, and therefore, it is feasible only for patients from *Groups I* and *II*. Unlike the obtunded patients in *Group III*, the *Group I* and *II* patients are alert and oriented to participate in a physical examination, which must demonstrate their ability to respond to complex commands, voluntarily mobilize their neck, indicate symptomatic anatomic regions, and undergo a comprehensive neurologic evaluation. *Group II* patients, although suitable for physical examination, are not candidates for clinical clearance and must undergo appropriate imaging to complete a valid clearing process. Only *Group I* patients can undergo physical examination and have the cervical spine definitively cleared by clinical assessment alone if that examination is normal.

The initial cervical spine examination in the trauma patient should consist of a static assessment. At this stage, the physical examination is performed while the external cervical support remains in place, the neck is not manipulated, and the patient is maintained in a supine posture. The static stage components of the physical examination that have positively correlated with cervical spine injury include the presence of neck pain, focal neck tenderness or spasm, and/or neurologic deficits [49, 78]. Neurologic deficit of any degree precludes the ability to achieve clinical clearance, and adjunctive cervical spine imaging is mandatory [59]. Many clinicians suggest that cervical spine injury should be assumed to be present in the neurologically compromised patient until further workup can conclusively establish its absence. Particular attention must be given to patients who sustain direct face, head, or neck trauma [3, 6, 35, 41, 87]. Although neck injury usually occurs through an indirect injury mechanism (e.g., whiplash), patients who sustain direct trauma above the shoulders are at particularly significant risk for cervical spine injury.

The second phase of the physical examination consists of a dynamic evaluation. External neck support should be removed and, while still supine, the patient should be asked to voluntarily perform neck flexion–extension, rotation, and lateral bending. If these maneuvers are successfully performed without pain or a change in the patient's neurologic status, the examiner should apply gentle axial load to the cervical spine by way of compressing or distracting the skull. If the neck/patient remains asymptomatic after these maneuvers, the patient may be permitted to sit or stand upright. The components of the static assessment should be reviewed as needed to ensure that they are unchanged. At this juncture, the clinician must also determine if the patient projects any degree of apprehension related to his neck or neurologic status that would warrant further evaluation. If the patient is nonapprehensive, and conclusively demonstrates a normal physical examination in both the static and dynamic phases of assessment, the cervical spine can be clinically cleared without adjunctive diagnostic modalities.

The physical examination alone can be unreliable in select patients even if they appear lucid. Major distracting injuries to the chest, abdomen, pelvis, or even the extremities (e.g., open fractures) may alter the patient's perception of subtle neck or neurologic symptoms and, thereby, negate the feasibility of clinical clearance. As previously noted, a patient's history of past neck pathology would do likewise. The most frequently encountered setting that threatens reliable clinical clearance is the unruly intoxicated or drugged patient in whom accurate imaging is not possible. These patients are often briefly admitted to the hospital for observation and/or until they become detoxicated. Although a later physical examination may suggest that cervical spine injury is unlikely, the clinician must still consider supplemental imaging if any degree of the patient's behavior appears altered.

2.6 Imaging Clearance of the Cervical Spine

Cervical spine clearance of the *Group II* patients who present with neck pain, tenderness, or neurologic symptoms require radiographic imaging as an adjunct to physical examination to evaluate their cervical spine. Imaging options include plain radiography, flexion–extension radiography, CT, and MRI.

2.6.1 Plain Radiography

Given its availability and relatively low cost, plain radiography is usually the first imaging modality for patients who cannot be cleared solely by clinical assessment [23, 37, 51, 57, 61, 62, 75, 85]. However, there are currently no validated guidelines for the use of plain radiography in trauma patients [32, 92]. The overall sensitivity of plain radiography is rather low, ranging from 52 to 85%, although many missed injuries have little significance [29, 46]. The clearance effectiveness of plain radiography is dependent on the number and/or type of views obtained [61] technical adequacy of the study [21], and the interpretive skills of the clinician. It has been suggested that cervical X-rays are not very specific for cervical spine injury and some clinicians advocate a variety of views, or more sophisticated adjunctive imaging. However, Mower et al. [68] from the NEXUS group demonstrated that plain radiography in conjunction with a thorough clinical examination in alert and nonintoxicated patients can result in a very small (0.07%)

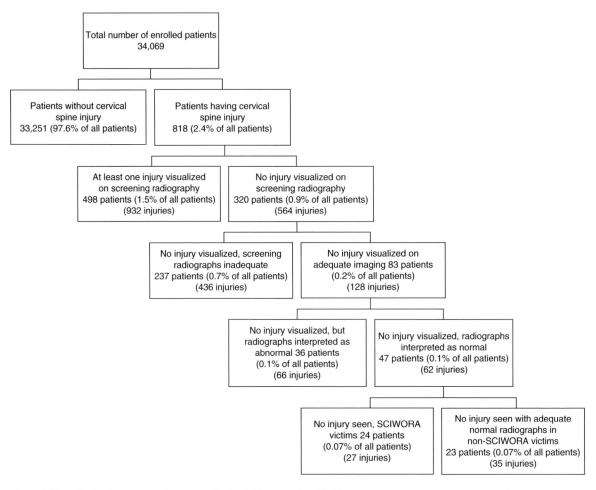

Fig. 2.1 The distribution of the patients from the NEXUS study classified by the injury status and radiographic findings

incidence of false-negative results (Fig. 2.1). The major limitation of plain radiography is its inability to reliably delineate injuries at the occipitocervical and cervicothoracic junctions in many patients.

The first radiograph to obtain is a single lateral view [23, 39, 51, 61, 62, 80, 85]. The lateral view alone is typically considered to be insufficient [51, 61, 99]. The sensitivity of the single lateral view among patients with cervical spine injury ranges from 74 to 86% [8, 51, 62, 99]. In a retrospective study, Shaffer and Doris [85] reported that 21% of all cervical spine injuries were missed with a lateral view alone. MacDonald et al. [61] found that the lateral view missed 16 of 92 cervical spine injuries; moreover in 18 cases, it was falsely read as positive. The accepted standard currently consists of a full cervical series (FCS), which includes anteroposterior, lateral, and open-mouth

odontoid views as the minimum projections necessary for maximum specificity and sensitivity.

The efficacy of cervical X-rays is highly dependent on the quality of the views obtained. The emergency cervical radiographs are frequently inadequate. In a study by Davis et al. [21], 94% of the errors leading to missed or delayed diagnosis of cervical spine injuries were the result of the failure to obtain adequate cervical spine radiographs. Ross et al. [80] reported that a technically adequate FCS could significantly increase the diagnostic accuracy of plain radiography. However, misinterpretation errors by trauma surgeons and emergency physicians can be frequent [31, 76]. Even when FCS is of adequate quality and properly interpreted, significant cervical spine injuries may occasionally go undetected. Some authors recommend the addition of two oblique views to better delineate spinal alignment and the integrity of the facets and pedicles [25, 94]. The swimmer's view, which provides better visualization of the cervicothoracic junction, has also been recommended [50]. However, the practice of using additional X-ray views in the trauma setting usually leads to escalation of costs in time and resources. Freemyer et al. [28] prospectively compared the three-view vs. the five-view cervical spine series and noted that the latter did not increase injury detection but allowed only more specific diagnosis. Therefore, for the purposes of screening, the three-view FCS should suffice. If further imaging is still required, more sophisticated modalities (e.g., CT, MRI) are preferred.

2.6.2 Flexion–Extension Radiography

Despite the adequacy of the studies obtained, static cervical spine radiographs may fail to detect an unstable cervical spine injury [53], Lateral flexion–extension views should be considered only in alert patients with a negative FCS and persistent pain, who can voluntarily perform the study. The efficacy of lateral flexion–extension views in the acute setting is controversial. In a retrospective review, Lewis et al. [55] reported that flexion–extension views in the emergency setting detected cervical spine instability in approximately 8% of patients otherwise cleared by FCS. None of these patients experienced adverse neurologic sequelae and the authors recommended their use in the acute setting. On the other hand, the NEXUS group [53, 74] reported that flexion–extension films obtained acutely added little to the screening process for the risk involved. Anglen et al. [2] included flexion–extension films in the acute evaluation of 837 trauma patients and concluded that they were not cost effective since they did not detect significant injury that was not detected by other modalities. These authors recommended that other modalities (e.g., MRI, CT) be used in the acute setting, and flexion–extension films be reserved for the delayed setting.

2.6.3 Dynamic Fluoroscopy

Lateral flexion–extension views are indicated in the alert patient with persistent pain and negative static X-rays. Dynamic views, however, are thought to be hazardous in the obtunded patient who is without the normal protective reflexes. In obtunded patients, Cox et al. [17] reported that dynamic fluoroscopy was an effective modality that did not miss injuries, nor did it compromise the patient's neurologic status. This was further supported by Brooks and Willet [11], who noted that dynamic fluoroscopy was a quick way to identify more subtle cases of cervical spine instability without reported neurologic complications. Sees et al. [84] also reported that fluoroscopy was both safe and effective in the assessment of the cervical spine.

In the acute setting, dynamic fluoroscopy also has its detractors. Davis et al. [20] reported that isolated ligamentous injuries of the cervical spine without fractures are rare, and in their reported series, such patients accounted for only 0.04% of all trauma patients. In the two patients identified with isolated ligamentous injury without fracture, the cervical spine was stable and did not require surgical consideration. These authors concluded that routine dynamic lateral flexion–extension imaging was not indicated to clear obtunded trauma patients because its potential risks exceeded any potential benefits.

2.6.4 Computed Tomography

CT is indicated in patients who have negative X-rays but continue to have symptoms, in those with questionable radiographic abnormalities, and those with plain radiography depicting prevertebral swelling that can be suggestive of cervical spine trauma.

Plain radiographs, static or dynamic, may fail to detect many cervical spine injuries and/or accurately depict the full extent of a cervical spine injury [10, 11, 80]. In a retrospective review Woodring and Lee [100] analyzed consecutive patients with cervical spine injury and determined that FCS failed to identify 61% of the fractures and 36% of the subluxations/dislocations. Barba et al. [5] studied patients who underwent head CT following a lateral view plain radiography and demonstrated that the combination of FCS with CT increased the accuracy of injury detection from 54 to 100%. Schenarts et al. [82] reported that CT can be especially effective in the evaluation of the upper cervical spine (occiput through C3). In obtunded patients, plain radiography identified only 55% of these injuries compared with 95.7% identified by CT. Berne et al. [7] found CT to be efficacious in imaging intensive care patients as the sensitivity of X-rays was only 60% in comparison to 90% with CT scans. In a study of 120 patients, 93% could be cleared within 24 hours by CT without missing a single injury [10, 11].

Recently, CT with reformations has gradually replaced plain radiography for cervical spine clearance. Helical, multidetector CT (MDCT) offers volume imaging, provides quick and efficient imaging in all planes and is becoming the primary method for the detection of spinal injury in many trauma centers. MDCT has equal sensitivity in all planes so that there is less risk for missing nondisplaced transverse fractures such as a type II dens fracture. CT alone identified 99.3% of all cervical spine fractures; the missed fractures required minimal or no treatment [12]. Recent studies have recognized the cost effectiveness of helical CT to complement its superior sensitivity [64]. The cost effectiveness of cervical spine CT is even greater when applied as an extension of a primary CT of other organs (head, thorax, abdomen). Some authors advocate CT as the preferred initial imaging modality for patients with moderate to high risk for cervical spine injury [33].

The disadvantages of CT include its greater expense, increased radiation exposure, and limited availability (compared with plain radiography). Additionally, CT is ineffective in detecting some ligamentous injuries. CT is best utilized in conjunction with plain radiography to increase both the accuracy and the sensitivity of the clearance process [7].

2.6.5 Magnetic Resonance Imaging

MRI is an effective noninvasive imaging tool for the detection of neural, ligamentous, or disk injury. MRI is primarily indicated for those patients who present with neurologic deficit. In this setting, MRI is an effective and safe method for evaluating the spinal cord because it can depict (a) epidural hematoma; (b) spinal cord edema; and (c) spinal cord compression. Additional MRI is indicated when ligamentous injury is suspected. This includes clinical findings of focal tenderness or gaps present between spinous processes on examination or where kyphosis or inter-spinous widening is seen on CT or plain radiographs.

However, MRI is not indicated for primary cervical spine clearance imaging. MRI requires extensive time to perform, interferes with the patient's monitoring equipment, and is expensive. MRI is most useful in patients for whom other imaging modalities are not consistent with the patient's neurologic presentation. It has been reported that 25% of patients with cervicothoracic injuries and a neurologic deficit on presentation had their preliminary treatment plan altered after MRI, while it had no effect on neurologically intact patients [95]. Although MRI can have a negative predictive value approaching 100%, its positive predictive value has been less gratifying [69].

MRI provides valuable information regarding cervical ligaments, disks, and joint capsules without placing the spinal cord and/or neural elements at risk. Currently, however, no consensus exists on the imaging criteria for establishing a significant ligamentous injury. Fat suppression sequences including T2 and STIR are most sensitive to fluid and hemorrhage, whereas T1 sagittal images can depict the anterior and posterior longitudinal as well as the supraspinous ligaments. A disruption of the black stripe on T1 and increased signal that extends through normal ligamentous structures on fat-suppressed images can be indicative of ligamentous injury. Delays that allow resolution of edema and hemorrhage can decrease MRI sensitivity in cervical spine clearance; although 48–72 h has been suggested as an optimal time interval, no data exist to substantiate this notion [69].

2.7 Current Cervical Spine Clearance Guidelines

2.7.1 ATLS Recommendations

The ATLS protocol [1] was developed by the American College of Surgeons with the intent of creating a reproducible approach to rapidly identify injuries and initiate intervention for life- and limb-threatening injuries. In addition, the ATLS recommendations seek to reduce the incidence of missed injuries and delayed diagnosis and are applicable to any patient in any trauma situation. The initial vital steps in the ATLS evaluation include assessment of the airway, breathing, and circulation while maintaining strict vigilance toward spinal precautions.

The ATLS recommendations [1] for screening patients for cervical spine injury are listed in Table 2.7. Their recommendations for clinical clearance are applicable only to the adult patient who is fully awake, alert, and sober. When these criteria are met, the next priority is to establish the patient's neurologic status. Any degree of neurologic deficit would suggest that clinical clearance alone is not feasible and appropriate imaging is mandatory. In the alert, neurologically intact patient, the external cervical support (collar) can be removed, and the neck assessed for pain while the patient remains supine. During this assessment, the clinician should determine if the neck is symptomatic while at rest, voluntarily mobilized, or upon palpation. The absence of neck pain without neurologic deficit in these alert patients achieves clinical clearance of the cervical spine, and the focus of the trauma workup can be directed elsewhere. However, if focal neck symptoms can be solicited, and/or neurologic deficit exists, clinical assessment alone is insufficient, and further diagnostic modalities are warranted before clearance can be accomplished. For patients with midline cervical tenderness with palpation or neck pain with active range of motion, a screening cervical spine CT scan performed with an MDCT scanner is indicated. A similar protocol is initiated in patients who exhibit altered levels of consciousness, or who have distracting injuries. For patients who are unable to undergo CT imaging, a lateral cervical plain film is warranted to provide initial information on the status of the cervical spine. In the event of significant malalignment, cranial tongs can be placed and traction applied during the resuscitation period. Further definitive radiographs can be obtained once the patient is stabilized. If the cervical spine cannot be cleared clinically, the patient's status reverts to the ATLS category of "suspected unstable cervical injury" and the collar is left in place.

Table 2.7 ATLS guidelines for clearing cervical spine

The presence of paraplegia or quadriplegia is a presumptive evidence of spinal instability
Patients who are awake, alert, sober, and neurologically intact, have no neck pain or midline tenderness: These patients are extremely unlikely to have an acute C-spine fracture or instability. With the patient in a supine position, remove the collar. If there is no significant tenderness, ask the patient to voluntarily move his neck from side to side. Never force the patient's neck. If there is no pain, C-spine radiography is not necessary
Patients who are awake, alert, neurologically intact, cooperative, but do have neck pain or midline tenderness: All such patients should undergo three-view radiography (lateral, AP, open-mouth odontoid) of the C-spine with axial CT images of suspicious areas or of the lower cervical spine, if not adequately visualized on the plain films. If these films are normal, remove the collar. Under the care of a knowledgeable doctor, obtain flexion and extension, lateral cervical spine films with the patient voluntarily flexing and extending the patient's neck. If the films show no subluxation, the patient's C-spine can be cleared and the collar removed. However, if any of these films are suspicious or unclear, replace the collar and obtain consultation from a spine specialist
Patients who have an altered level of consciousness or cannot describe their symptoms: Lateral, AP, and open-mouth odontoid films with CT supplementation through suspicious areas should be obtained on all such patients. If the entire C-spine can be visualized and is found to be normal, the collar can be removed after appropriate evaluation by a doctor skilled in the management of spine-injured patients. Clearance of the C-spine is particularly important if the pulmonary or other care of the patient is compromised by the inability to mobilize the patient
When there is doubt leave the collar on
Consult: doctors who are skilled in the evaluation and management of the spine-injured patient should be consulted in all cases in which a spine injury is detected or suspected
Backboards: patients who have neurologic deficits (quadriplegia or paraplegia) should be evaluated quickly and taken off the backboard as soon as possible. A paralyzed patient who is allowed to lie on a hard board for more than 2 h is at high risk for developing serious decubiti
Emergency situations: trauma patients who require emergent surgery before a complete workup of the spine can be accomplished should be transported and moved carefully with the assumption than an unstable spine injury is present. The collar should be left on and the patient log-rolled

The ATLS recommendations also provide a number of recommendations on how to optimally protect the cervical spine throughout the entire trauma diagnostic and therapeutic process [1]. First, external neck support should be maintained until a conclusive position on the cervical spine has been established. Second, ATLS suggests that the backboard, a necessity in the acute phase, should be eliminated by 2 hours to avoid decubiti. Next, if the patient requires surgery to thwart a life-threatening condition prior to cervical spine clearance, the clinician should assume that an unstable neck injury exists and the entire surgical team should approach the patient accordingly. Finally, the ATLS recommendations recognize that a thorough cervical spine evaluation may occasionally exceed the capabilities of the trauma physician, and it suggests that a physician with spine expertise be consulted not simply for detected injuries, but when cervical clearance cannot be decisively established.

It must be emphasized that the ATLS cervical spine recommendations were developed for the physician providing initial care for the traumatized patient. These recommendations provide a basic diagnostic and therapeutic algorithm designed to assist the nonspecialized physician in maintaining a rational, generalized approach to cervical spine clearance [15, 39]. Therefore, the ATLS recommendations are not intended to be the authoritative treatise on cervical spine injury detection or treatment; their intent is to minimize the risk for overall patient morbidity/mortality in the trauma patient due to an early inadequate suspicion of or external support for neck injuries. Furthermore, although the ATLS recommendations were compiled by knowledgeable specialists, they have been advocated without scientific validation.

2.7.2 EAST Guidelines

The Eastern Association for Surgery of Trauma (EAST) recognized the merits of an evidenced-based protocol and endeavored to establish a number of trauma national consensus-based clinical guidelines that included screening recommendations for cervical clearance [71]. These clinical guidelines were formulated by a panel of trauma surgeons who were instructed to assess the scientific quality of the available evidence on the topic. The panel then rendered criteria for cervical spine clearance based on the extent to which they could be supported by the evidence that existed at the time. The final recommendations were abridged after presentation to the EAST National Meeting in 1997, and these revisions were adopted. Subsequently, an update to EAST guidelines [63] has been available online in the EAST website for download (http://www.east.org/tpg/chap3.pdf).

The EAST group recognized cervical spine instability as a frequent, challenging problem confronting physicians providing acute trauma care. The complexity of this problem not only encompasses a number of serious medical concerns (e.g., missed or inappropriately treated cervical spine injury), but also represented major economic and legal issues. The clinical question initially addressed by this group was simply which trauma patients require cervical spine radiography? This suggests that there is a core group of trauma patients in whom X-rays are not warranted. Furthermore, EAST noted that although there was a plethora of literature on cervical spine instability and trauma, a Level I (prospective, randomized, and controlled) clinical trial did not exist at that time. Therefore, their recommendations were made from Level II evidence, and were deemed only reasonably justifiable [71].

Although the EAST cervical clearance recommendations for high-risk trauma patients (i.e., with neck symptoms, neurologic compromise, or an altered mental state) remain controversial, clinicians' support for the feasibility of select cervical spine clearance solely by clinical evaluation has been sustained.

The EAST guidelines incorporated clinical criteria for excluding imaging [31], specified the minimum number and type of radiographs to be obtained in the indicated patients, established specific criteria for obtaining CT, and recognized the benefit of voluntary lateral flexion–extension stress views in select patients. The consensus EAST recommendation identified that there were select trauma patients who could be successfully cleared for cervical spine injury without radiography. Their indications for clinical screening included patients who are awake; have no mental status changes; are without neck pain; have no distracting injuries, and have no neurologic deficit. By their selective criteria, all other patients required imaging. The EAST guidelines also encouraged the prompt use of MRI in all trauma patients in whom neurologic deficit could be documented [63, 71]. The principal disadvantage of these guidelines was their lack of clinical validation.

2.7.3 NEXUS Guidelines

The NEXUS guidelines constitute the largest study to date designed to validate clinical criteria that could reliably clear the cervical spine in trauma patients [42]. In this multicenter, prospective, observational study, five clinical criteria were used to exclude the need for cervical spine radiography in the trauma setting. These criteria were: (1) normal alertness; (2) the absence of intoxication; (3) the absence of cervical tenderness; (4) the absence of focal neurologic deficit; and (5) the absence of a painful distracting injury (Table 2.4) [44]. Standard trauma three-view radiography was obtained for all patients and was correlated with clinical criteria.

The NEXUS study reviewed 34,069 patients; cervical spine injury was determined in 818 patients, and the clinical criteria failed to suggest injury (false negative) in only eight patients (Fig. 2.1). Among the false-negative patients, only two had injuries that were considered clinically significant. Although this decision instrument was 99.6% sensitive for the presence of injury, it was only 12.9% specific. These clinical cervical clearance criteria would have eliminated radiography in 4,309 (12.6%) patients. The authors concluded that these clinical assessment criteria were reliable in excluding injury and effective in decreasing the need for routine cervical spine imaging.

The NEXUS study could be criticized for its low 12.9% specificity. Furthermore, two of the clinical parameters, intoxication and painful distracting injuries, were found to be poorly reproducible [92]. In this large, well-controlled study, the low incidence of cervical spine injury further emphasized the need for a more efficient clinical instrument to clear cervical spine without imaging.

2.7.4 Canadian C-Spine Rule

Stiell et al. [92] performed a prospective cohort study of alert, stable trauma patients to determine the clinical parameters that would exclude the need for imaging to clear the cervical spine (Fig. 2.2). The top priority of

neck clearance was readily accepted by these authors who also recognized that 98% of acute trauma patients present without cervical spine injury. The indiscriminate use of radiology as a screening tool was viewed not only as increasing costs, but also as prohibiting an expeditious acute trauma workup. The study assessed trauma patients for 20 standardized clinical parameters in a multicenter effort to determine whether cervical clearance could be reliably achieved without radiography.

The study possessed several unique features. First, its primary outcome measure was not simply the absence of injury, but the absence of clinically significant injury. Clinically significant injury was defined as a fracture, dislocation, neurologic deficit, or soft tissue injury that would require stabilization or specialized follow-up. Clinically insignificant cervical injuries included osteophyte avulsions, isolated transverse process fractures, isolated posterior spinous process fractures, and vertebral body compression fractures with <25% collapse. Clinically insignificant injuries were confirmed after 14 days by the following criteria: (1) no/mild neck pain; (2) no/mild restriction of neck mobility; (3) no cervical collar requirement; and (4) the patient being able to return to full/normal employment.

The Canadian C-Spine Rule study prospectively applied its clinical variable to 8,424 patients. The study was able to successfully exclude the necessity for cervical spine clearance radiography for patients who could satisfactorily respond to three simple questions related to presence of high-risk factors (increased age, dangerous mechanism, parathesia), low-risk factors that would prohibit the safe assessment of neck range of motion, and the patient's ability to voluntarily rotate the neck (Table 2.6). The initial multicenter study utilizing this instrument demonstrated that only 58% of trauma patients warranted radiography, with a sensitivity of 95% for cervical spine injury detection, and a specificity of 42.5% for cervical spine injury exclusion. Moreover, the Canadian C-Spine Rule proved to be relatively favorable with regard to intraobserver reliability.

However, this study has several limitations. Although all patients were followed up clinically, only selected patients received confirmatory radiography. The distinction between important and unimportant cervical spine injury can be biased, and, therefore is controversial. Furthermore, the study's cohort did not constitute a consecutive series of patients. Despite this, the Canadian C-Spine Rule added credence to the merits of

Fig. 2.2 The Canadian
C-Spine Rule study design

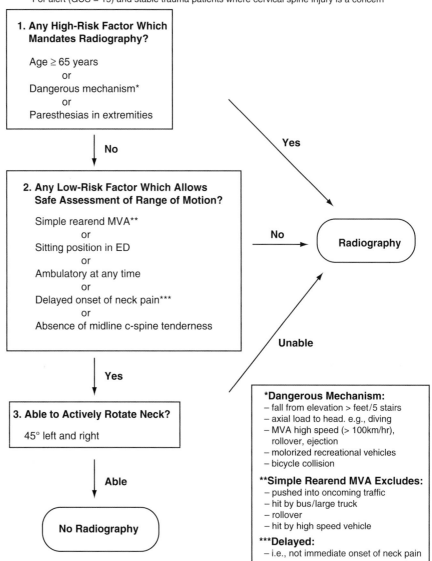

The Canadian C-Spine Rule

For alert (GCS = 15) and stable trauma patients where cervical spine injury is a concern

1. Any High-Risk Factor Which Mandates Radiography?

Age ≥ 65 years
or
Dangerous mechanism*
or
Paresthesias in extremities

No

Yes

2. Any Low-Risk Factor Which Allows Safe Assessment of Range of Motion?

Simple rearend MVA**
or
Sitting position in ED
or
Ambulatory at any time
or
Delayed onset of neck pain***
or
Absence of midline c-spine tenderness

No → **Radiography**

Unable

Yes

3. Able to Actively Rotate Neck?

45° left and right

Able

No Radiography

*Dangerous Mechanism:
– fall from elevation > feet/5 stairs
– axial load to head. e.g., diving
– MVA high speed (> 100km/hr), rollover, ejection
– molorized recreational vehicles
– bicycle collision

**Simple Rearend MVA Excludes:
– pushed into oncoming traffic
– hit by bus/large truck
– rollover
– hit by high speed vehicle

***Delayed:
– i.e., not immediate onset of neck pain

clinical cervical spine clearance criteria in select alert trauma patients [52].

2.7.5 Obtunded Patient Clearance Protocols

Clearance of the cervical spine in patients with impaired consciousness is controversial and unresolved. The decision to discontinue the cervical collar for these patients is not synonymous with determining that the cervical spine has been cleared as in *Groups I* and *II*. In each of these patients, the risks of an occult cervical spine injury must be weighed against the morbidities of continued cervical immobilization. The concern is that cervical injuries resulting from high-energy trauma may have soft tissue damage that may not be readily identifiable on plain radiographs or CT. Chiu et al. [14] estimated a 0.6% incidence of isolated ligamentous cervical spine injuries in all blunt trauma patients. These isolated soft tissue injuries are difficult to detect, and may result in neural injury, ranging from minor sensory deficits to complete tetraplegia [73, 88, 89]. Neurologic sequelae associated with a spinal injury are ten times more likely to occur in the event of a missed injury [22].

There is consensus that patients who have altered mentation require imaging of their cervical spine [1, 18, 38, 40]. A variety of methods have been recommended, but no "gold standard" currently exists. Numerous algorithms have been advocated that incorporate clinical examination (often unreliable), plain radiographs, dynamic fluoroscopy, CT, and MRI. In the last decade, CT and MRI have largely replaced these other imaging modalities and the current debate revolves around the extent to which an MDCT can direct clearance of the cervical spine.

Several recent investigations have advocated CT as a single modality capable of detecting all clinically significant cervical spine injuries [7, 16, 38, 45, 54, 93]. Harris et al. [38] analyzed obtunded trauma patients by using CT and reported that all clinically significant cervical spine injuries were identified. Furthermore, CT failed to detect minor injury in only one patient. Tomycz et al. [93] analyzed 180 obtunded blunt trauma patients with no neurologic deficit and GCS score <13 by CT and normal by MRI. In 21% of patients with a negative CT, MRI was able to identify acute abnormalities; however, none of the injuries identified by MRI were deemed clinically significant. This led the authors to conclude that the use of MRI is obviated by a negative MDCT [16, 83]. CT was found to have a 98.9% negative predictive value for ligament injury and a 100% negative predictive value for cervical instability. In this investigation, four of the 366 patients with negative CT had isolated ligamentous injuries on MRI, none of which were felt to be unstable. Comparison of the results of a clinical examination CT and MRI demonstrated that CT alone had equal sensitivity to MRI, but was faster and resulted in 67% fewer adverse events such as decubiti, delirium, and hospital-acquired pneumonia while awaiting imaging [90].

While CT is sensitive in the identification of osseous abnormalities, it has not been shown to have the same level of accuracy in detecting an isolated ligamentous injury. Analysis of obtunded trauma patients who had negative CT demonstrated an 8.9% incidence of abnormality identified by MRI [66]. In this study, two patients found to have a normal cervical spine by CT interpretation required surgical intervention for ligamentous injury while 14 others required immobilization in an orthosis. These researchers concluded that CT imaging cannot reliably detect all clinically significant cervical injuries and MRI remains a necessary adjunct in the evaluation of obtunded patients with suspected cervical trauma. Similarly, Diaz et al. [22] reported 32% sensitivity for CT for cervical spine ligamentous injuries. This group found that the negative predictive value of CT for ligamentous injury was only 78%. On the basis of these findings, it was concluded that CT imaging was not effective in evaluating ligamentous injuries and recommended that obtunded patients undergo MRI.

Recently, Muchow et al. [69] published a meta-analysis involving five Level I studies, representing 464 trauma patients evaluated using MRI and plain radiographs or CT. Comparable to other reports in the literature, these authors found a 20.9% incidence of abnormalities on MRI that were not detected by plain radiographs or CT. They found that MRI demonstrated a sensitivity of 97.2%, a specificity of 98.5%, and a negative predictive value of 100%. Based on these findings, it was concluded that a negative MRI should be the gold standard for cervical spine clearance in the obtunded patient. However, the high rate of false negatives makes the usefulness of MRI as a screening tool questionable. Stassen et al. [89] advocated an algorithm in which obtunded trauma patients received both CT and MRI to facilitate cervical spine clearance. In this investigation, 30% of the patients with negative CT demonstrated abnormal findings on MRI ($p<0.01$). Furthermore, MRI identified all abnormalities that were indicated by CT. These authors suggested that both CT and MRI be employed in the evaluation of the cervical spine in obtunded trauma patients. Such a recommendation is in accord with the American College of Radiology's (ACR) Appropriateness Criteria on suspected spine trauma [18]. The ACR has stated that CT and MRI are the most appropriate modalities for cervical spine evaluation in the obtunded trauma patient.

2.7.6 Authors' Cervical Spine Clearance Algorithm

Follwoing an exhaustive review the existing literature, the authors have developed their own algorithm for clearing the cervical spine in accordance with specific patient group designation (Figs. 2.3–2.5). The algorithm begins with the assumption that a cervical spine injury is present in all trauma patients. The initial clinical

Fig. 2.3 The authors' algorithm for clinical clearance of the cervical spine without a need for spine imaging. Only a fully awake and alert patient's (Ransohoff Class 1 or Glasgow Coma Scale >14) cervical spine can be reliably cleared with clinical examination alone

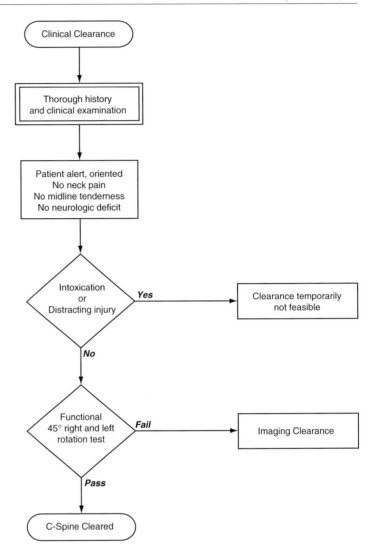

examination should immediately establish the level of patient consciousness and assign patients to one of three clearance groups.

Fully alert (Ransohoff Class 1, Glasgow Coma Scale >14) patients without neurologic deficit, neck pain, or a major distracting injury (*Group I*) constitute the only patients for whom clinical clearance of the cervical spine is appropriate (Fig. 2.3). Cervical spine imaging is not indicated in those *Group I* patients. In these select patients, cervical spine precautions can be discontinued, and the trauma team should direct its focus to the other aspects of the patient's care.

Fully alert patients with neurologic deficit, neck pain (with or without voluntary neck mobilization), or a major distracting injury (*Group II*) cannot be cleared until adjunctive imaging confirms the absence of

cervical spine injury. The authors' algorithm for the imaging clearance of the cervical spine in depicted in (Fig. 2.4).

For *Group III* patients who have impaired consciousness, imaging is indicated to detect cervical spine injury, but not to clear the cervical spine (Fig. 2.5). Even if the imaging is negative, conclusive clearance cannot be achieved until the patient becomes lucid. This management scenario typically occurs in the intoxicated and/or distracting injury (temporally non-evaluable) patient, but should also be applied to obtunded (indefinitely nonevaluable) patients with traumatic brain injury. If the patient becomes alert after detoxication, or distracting injuries are resolved, a reliable and thorough history and physical examination can be performed and clearance becomes feasible.

Fig. 2.4 The authors'
algorithm for imaging
clearance of the cervical
spine. Only in a fully awake
and alert patient (Ransohoff
Class 1 or Glasgow Coma
Scale >14), can the cervical
spine be cleared with a
combination of clinical exam
and supplemental imaging

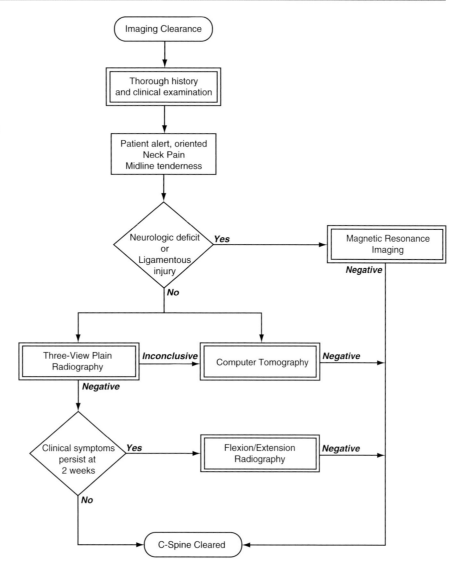

2.8 Summary and Conclusions

Although the modern approach to clearing the cervical
spine in the trauma patient has improved dramatically
in recent years, many aspects of the existing evaluation
protocols are still inadequate. The algorithms that are
currently applied are not sufficiently comprehensive,
forgo ease of application for improved specificity, or
are more often focused on cervical injury detection
than its exclusion.

The absence of penetrating trauma to the neck in
existing cervical spine clearance protocols reflects their
failure to be suitably comprehensive. Epidemiological
studies suggest that gunshot injury has become a leading cause for spinal cord injury in the United States,

and much of this is due to direct neck trauma [48, 58].
The surgical literature has recognized the increased
risk for patient morbidity and mortality with civilian
gunshot injury to the neck; however, current cervical
spine clearance guidelines continue to neglect the
inclusion of this injury mechanism. Clinical cervical
spine clearance is not feasible in trauma patients with a
penetrating injury to the neck. All of these patients
should be assessed by plain cervical spine radiography;
many of these patients may warrant more sophisticated
imaging (e.g., arteriography, barium swallow, CT, etc.)
to rule out the presence of visceral injury [58]. If the
present gunshot injury trends continue, future cervical
spine clearance guidelines must be expanded to include
this mechanism in their evaluation algorithms.

Fig. 2.5 The authors' algorithm for managing patients with suspected cervical spine injury who cannot be cleared at the time of emergency department presentation. These patients are designated as temporarily or indefinitely nonevaluable due to impaired consciousness that renders a meaningful clinical examination unreliable. Imaging for these patients is not to clear their cervical spine, but to detect an obvious injury. The consideration to remove or maintain the spinal precautions in the face of negative sophisticated imaging (MDCT, MRI) is left to the treating physician; however, the present authors recommend that the spinal precautions be maintained until clearance becomes feasible

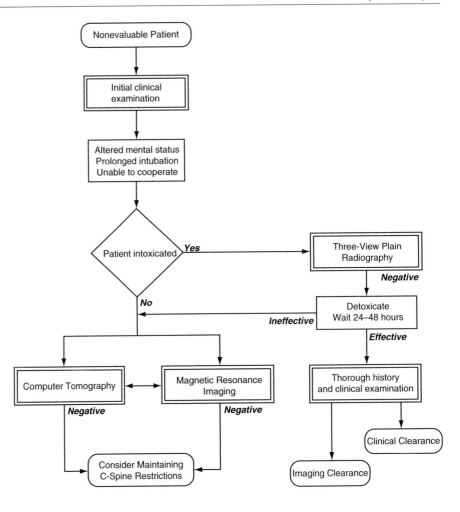

The next major consideration for cervical spine clearance protocol would be the ease by which it can be applied in the hectic, highly stressed emergency center environment. The Canadian C-Spine Rule has the highest reported specificity (42.5%) (Table 2.8) of the currently validated clinical decision-making instruments. However, the physician has to evaluate an exorbitant number of clinical variables with this algorithm [92]. This inherent complexity would require a clinical study to establish its inter- and intrarater reliability. Conversely, the NEXUS algorithm, with its lower specificity (12.6%) consists of only five simple criteria (Table 2.8). The less complex nature of the NEXUS instrument not only ensures its timely application, but also suggests that it would be more readily accepted. Therefore, the optimal clinical cervical spine clearance protocol must not only solely establish high sensitivity and specificity, but also demonstrate *sensibility* to be universally accepted [59, 91, 92].

Table 2.8 Comparison of NEXUS and Canadian C-Spine Rule studies

Variable	NEXUS	C-spine rule
Total patients	34,069	6,185[a]
Positive for cervical injury	818	151
Sensitivity	99.6%	100
Specificity	12.9%	42.5%

[a]Patients who underwent radiographic examination of the cervical spine

Finally, future cervical spine algorithms for trauma patients must address semantics. Cervical spine injury detection, clearance, screening, and evaluation are terms that are commonly confused; moreover, many trauma algorithms offer guidelines that simultaneously attempt to both clear and detect cervical spine injury. Cervical spine injury clearance and detection should form the basis for two very separate algorithms as the information they seek differs. Cervical spine injury detection algorithms are in response to the inquiry, "Is a cervical spine injury present?" It is always the second question to be asked and the answer may require complex and sophisticated diagnostic modalities. However, cervical spine clearance algorithms are in response to the inquiry, "Is a cervical spine injury absent?" This is the first question to be asked when assessing trauma patients, and if it cannot be reliably answered in the affirmative, the second question must be asked. The more adept the future guidelines become at answering the first question, the more proficient we will become in clinically clearing the cervical spine in trauma patients.

References

1. American College of Surgeons Committee on Trauma (2004) Spine and spinal cord trauma. In: Advanced trauma life support for doctors. The student manual, 7th edn. First Impression Publishing, Chicago, pp 177–189
2. Anglen J, Metzler M, Bunn P, Griffiths H (2002) Flexion and extension views are not cost-effective in a cervical spine clearance protocol for obtunded trauma patients. J Trauma 52:54–59
3. Ardekian L, Gaspar R, Peled M, Manor R, Laufer D (1997) Incidence and type of cervical spine injuries associated with mandibular fractures. Craniomaxillofac Trauma 3(2): 18–21
4. Bachulis BL, Long WB, Hynes GD, Johnson MC (1987) Clinical indications for cervical spine radiographs in the traumatized patient. Am J Surg 153(5):473–478
5. Barba CA, Taggert J, Morgan AS, Guerra J, Bernstein B, Lorenzo M, Gershon A, Epstein N (2001) A new cervical spine clearance protocol using computed tomography. J Trauma 51:652–657
6. Beirne JC, Butler PE, Brady FA (1995) Cervical spine injuries in patients with facial fractures: a 1-year prospective study. Int J Oral Maxillofac Surg 24(1 pt 1):26–29
7. Berne JD, Velmahos GC, El-Tawil Q, Demetriades D, Asensio JA, Murray JA, Cornwell EE, Belzberg H, Berne TV (1999) Value of complete cervical helical computed tomographic scanning in identifying cervical spine injury in the unevaluable blunt trauma patient with multiple injuries: a prospective study. J Trauma 47:896–902
8. Blahd WH, Iserson KV, Bjelland JC (1985) Efficacy of the post-traumatic cross table lateral view of the cervical spine. J Emerg Med 2:243–249
9. Bohlman HH (1979) Acute fractures and dislocations of the cervical spine. An analysis of three hundred hospitalized patients and review of the literature. J Bone Joint Surg 61A(8):1119–1142
10. Borock C, Gabram S, Jacobs L, Murphy M (1991) A prospective analysis of a two-year experience using computed tomography as an adjunct for cervical spine clearance. J Trauma 31:1001–1004
11. Brooks AR, Willett KM (2001) Evaluation of the Oxford protocol for total spinal clearance in the unconscious trauma patient. J Trauma 50:862–867
12. Brown CV, Antevil JL, Sise MJ, Sack DI (2005) Spiral computed tomography for the diagnosis of cervical, thoracic, and lumbar spine fractures: its time has come. J Trauma 58:890–895
13. Cadoux CG, White JD (1986) High-yield radiographic considerations for cervical spine injuries. Ann Emerg Med 15(3):236–239
14. Chiu WC, Haan JM, Cushing BM, Kramer ME, Scalea TM (2001) Ligamentous injuries of the cervical spine in unreliable blunt trauma patients: incidence, evaluation, and outcome. J Trauma 50:457–564
15. Cohn SM, Lyle WG, Linden CH, Lancey RA (1991) Exclusion of cervical spine injury: a prospective study. J Trauma 31:570–574
16. Como JJ, Thompson MA, Anderson JS, Shah RR, Claridge JA, Yowler CJ, Malangoni MA (2007) Is magnetic resonance imaging essential in clearing the cervical spine in obtunded patients with blunt trauma? J Trauma 63:544–549
17. Cox MW, McCarthy M, Lemmon G, Wenker J (2001) Cervical spine instability: clearance using dynamic fluoroscopy. Curr Surg 58:96–100
18. Daffner RH, Hackney DB (2007) ACR Appropriateness Criteria on suspected spine trauma. J Am Coll Radiol 4: 762–775
19. D'Alise MD, Benzel EC, Hart BL (1999) Magnetic resonance imaging evaluation of the cervical spine in the comatose or obtunded trauma patient. J Neurosurg 91(1 suppl):54–59
20. Davis JW, Kaups KL, Cunningham MA, Parks SN, Nowak TP, Bilello JF, Williams JL (2001) Routine evaluation of the cervical spine in head-injured patients with dynamic fluoroscopy: a reappraisal. J Trauma 50:1044–1047
21. Davis JW, Phreaner DL, Hoyt DB, Mackersie RC (1993) The etiology of missed cervical spine injuries. J Trauma 34:342–346
22. Diaz JJ, Aulino JM, Collier B, Roman C, May AK, Miller RS, Guillamondegui O, Morris JA (2005) The early work-up for isolated ligamentous injury of the cervical spine: does computed tomography scan have a role? J Trauma 59:897–903
23. Diliberti T, Lindsey RW (1992) Evaluation of the cervical spine in the emergency setting: who does not need an X-ray? Orthopedics 15:179–183
24. Domeier RM (1999) Indications for prehospital spinal immobilization. National Association of EMS Physicians Standards and Clinical Practice Committee. Prehosp Emerg Care 3(3):251–253
25. Doris PE, Wilson RA (1985) The next logical step in the emergency radiographic evaluation of cervical spine trauma: the five-view trauma series. J Emerg Med 3:371–385
26. Edwards M, Frankema S, Kruit MC, Bode PJ, Breslau PJ, van Vugt AB (2001) Routine cervical spine radiography for trauma victims: does everybody need it? J Trauma 50: 529–534
27. Fischer RP (1984) Cervical radiographic evaluation of alert patients following blunt trauma. Ann Emerg Med 13: 905–907
28. Freemyer B, Knopp R, Piche J, Wales L, Williams J (1989) Comparison of five-view and three-view cervical spine

series in the evaluation of patients with cervical trauma. Ann Emerg Med 18:818–821

29. Gale SC, Gracias VH, Reilly PM, Schwab CW (2005) The inefficiency of plain radiography to evaluate the cervical spine after blunt trauma. J Trauma 59:1121–1125

30. Gerrelts BD, Petersen EU, Mabry J, Petersen SR (1991) Delayed diagnosis of cervical spine injuries. J Trauma 31:1622–1626

31. Ghanta MK, Smith LM, Polin RS, Marr AB, Spires WV (2002) An analysis of Eastern Association for the Surgery of Trauma practice guidelines for cervical spine evaluation in a series of patients with multiple imaging techniques. Am Surg 68(6):563–567

32. Graber MA, Kathol M (1999) Cervical spine radiographs in the trauma patient. Am Fam Physician 59:331–342

33. Grogan EL, Morris JA, Dittus RS, Moore DE, Poulose BK, Diaz JJ, Speroff T (2005) Cervical spine evaluation in urban trauma centers: lowering institutional costs and complications through helical CT scan. J Am Coll Surg 200:160–165

34. Grossman MD, Reilly PM, Gillett T, Gillett D (1999) National survey of the incidence of cervical spine injury and approach to cervical spine clearance in US trauma centers. J Trauma 47(4):684–690

35. Hackl W, Hausberger K, Sailer R, Ulmer H, Gassner R (2001) Prevalence of cervical spine injuries in patients with facial trauma. Oral Surg Oral Med Oral Pathol Oral Radiol Endod 92(4):370–376

36. Hadley MN, Walters BC, Grabb PA, Oyesiku NM, Przybylski GJ, Resnick DK, Ryken TC, Mielke DH (2002) Guidelines for the management of acute cervical spine and spinal cord injuries. Clin Neurosurg 49:407–498

37. Harris JH (1986) Radiographic evaluation of spinal trauma. Ortho Clin North Am 17:75–86

38. Harris TJ, Blackmore CC, Mirza SK, Jurkovich GJ (2008) Clearing the cervical spine in obtunded patients. Spine 33:1547–1553

39. Harris MB, Kronlage SC, Carboni PA, Robert KQ, Menmuir B, Ricciardi JE, Chutkan NB (2000) Evaluation of the cervical spine in the polytrauma patient. Spine 25(22):2884–2891

40. Harris MB, Shilt JS (2003) The potentially unstable cervical spine: evaluation techniques. Tech Orthop 17:278–286

41. Haug RH, Wible RT, Likavec MJ, Conforti PJ (1991) Cervical spine fractures and maxillofacial trauma. J Oral Maxillofac Surg 49(7):725–729

42. Hoffman JR, Mower WR, Wolfson AB, Todd KH, Zucker MI (2000) Validity of a set of clinical criteria to rule out injury to the cervical spine in patients with blunt trauma. National Emergency X-Radiography Utilization Study Group. N Engl J Med 343(2):94–99

43. Hoffman JR, Schriger DL, Mower W, Luo JS, Zucker M (1992) Low-risk criteria for cervical-spine radiography in blunt trauma: a prospective study. Ann Emerg Med 21(12):1454–1460

44. Hoffman JR, Wolfson AB, Todd K, Mower WR (1998) Selective cervical spine radiography in blunt trauma: methodology of the National Emergency X-Radiography Utilization Study (NEXUS). Ann Emerg Med 32:461–469

45. Hogan GJ, Mirvis SE, Shanmuganathan K, Scalea TM (2005) Exclusion of unstable cervical spine injury in obtunded patients with blunt trauma: is MR imaging needed when multidetector row CT findings are normal? Radiology 237:106–113

46. Holmes JF, Akkinepalli R (2005) Computed tomography versus plain radiography to screen for cervical spine injury: a meta-analysis. J Trauma 58:902–905

47. Huelke D, O'Day J, Mandelsohn RA (1981) Cervical injuries suffered in automobile crashes. J Neurosurg 54:316–322

48. Isiklar ZU, Lindsey RW (1997) Low-velocity civilian gunshot wounds of the spine. Orthopedics 20(10):967–972

49. Jacobs LM, Schwartz R (1986) Prospective analysis of acute cervical spine injury: a methodology to predict injury. Ann Emerg Med 15:44–49

50. Jenkins MG, Curran P, Rocke LG (1999) Where do we go after the three standard cervical spine views in the conscious trauma patient? A survey. Eur J Emerg Med 6: 215–217

51. Kassel EE, Cooper PW, Rubinstein JD (1983) Radiology of spine trauma – practical experience in a trauma unit. Can Ass Radiol J 34:189–203

52. Kerr D, Bradshaw L, Kelly AM (2005) Implementation of the Canadian C-spine rule reduces cervical spine X-ray rate for alert patients with potential neck injury. J Emerg Med 28(2):127–131

53. Knopp R, Parker J, Tashjian J, Ganz W (2001) Defining radiographic criteria for flexion–extension studies of the cervical spine. Ann Emerg Med 38:31–35

54. Levi AD, Hurlbert RJ, Anderson P, Fehlings M, Rampersaud R, Massicotte EM, France JC, Le Huec JC, Hedlund R, Arnold P (2006) Neurologic deterioration secondary to unrecognized spinal instability following trauma – a multicenter study. Spine 31:451–458

55. Lewis LM, Docherty M, Ruoff BE et al (1991) Flexion–extension views in the evaluation of cervical-spine injuries. Ann Emerg Med 20:117–121

56. Lieberman IH, Webb JK (1994) Cervical spine injuries in the elderly. J Bone Joint Surg 76B(6):877–881

57. Lindsey RW, Diliberti TC, Doherty BJ, Watson AB (1993) Efficacy of radiographic evaluation of the cervical spine in emergency situations. South Med J 86:1253–1255

58. Lindsey RW, Gugala Z (1999) Spinal cord injury as a result of ballistic trauma. In: Chapman JR (ed) Spine: state of the art reviews. Spinal cord injuries, vol 13(3). Hanley & Belfus, Philadelphia, pp 529–547

59. Lindsey RW, Gugala Z (2005) Clearing of the cervical spine. In: Clark CR, Benzel EC, Currier BL, Dormans JP, Dvořák J, Eismont F, Garfin SR, Herkowitz HN, Ullrich CG, Vaccaro AR (eds) The cervical spine, 4th edn. The Cervical Spine Research Society Editorial Committee. Lippincott Williams & Wilkins, Philadelphia, pp 375–386

60. Lowery DW, Wald MM, Browne BJ, Tigges S, Hoffman JR (2001) Mower WR; NEXUS Group. Epidemiology of cervical spine injury victims. Ann Emerg Med 38(1):12–16

61. MacDonald RL, Schwartz ML, Mirich D, Sharkey PW, Nelson WR (1990) Diagnosis of cervical spine injury in motor vehicle crash victims: how many X-rays are enough? J Trauma 30:392–397

62. Mace SE (1985) Emergency evaluation of cervical spine injuries: CT versus plain radiographs. Ann Emerg Med 14:973–975

63. Marion DW, Domeier R, Dunham CM, Luchette FA, Haid R, Erwood SC (2000) EAST practice management guidelines for identifying cervical spine injuries following trauma. http://www.east.org/tpg/chap3.pdf. Accessed 18 August 2009

64. McCulloch PT, France J, Jones DL et al (2005) Helical computed tomography alone compared with plain radiographs with adjunct computed tomography to evaluate the cervical spine after high-energy trauma. J Bone Joint Surg 87A:2388–2394

65. McNamara RM, Heine E, Esposito B (1990) Cervical spine injury and radiography in alert, high-risk patients. J Emerg Med 8(2):177–182

66. Menaker J, Philp A, Boswell S, Scalea TM (2008) Computed tomography alone for cervical spine clearance in the unreliable patient – are we there yet? J Trauma 64:898–903

67. Mirvis SE (2001) Fluoroscopically guided passive flexion–extension views of the cervical spine in the obtunded blunt trauma patient: a commentary. J Trauma 50:868–870

68. Mower WR, Hoffman JR, Pollack CV, Zucker MI, Browne BJ, Wolfson AB; NEXUS Group. Use of plain radiography to screen for cervical spine injuries. Ann Emerg Med 2001;38:1-7.

69. Muchow RD, Resnick DK, Abdel MP, Munoz A, Anderson PA (2008) Magnetic resonance imaging (MRI) in the clearance of the cervical spine in blunt trauma: a meta-analysis. J Trauma 64:179–189

70. Orledge JD, Pepe PE (1998) Out-of-hospital spinal immobilization: is it really necessary? Acad Emerg Med 5(3):203–204

71. Pasquale M, Fabian TC (1998) Practice management guidelines for trauma from the Eastern Association for the Surgery of Trauma. J Trauma 44:941–957

72. Petri R, Gimbel R (1999) Evaluation of the patient with spinal trauma and back pain: an evidence based approach. Emerg Med Clin North Am 17(1):25–39

73. Platzer P, Hauswirth N, Jaindl M et al (2006) Delayed or missed diagnosis of cervical spine injuries. J Trauma 61:150–155

74. Pollack CV Jr, Hendey GW, Martin DR, Hoffman JR, Mower WR; NEXUS Group (2001) Use of flexion–extension radiographs of the cervical spine in blunt trauma. Ann Emerg Med 38:8–11

75. Ransohoff J, Fleischer A (1975) Head injuries. JAMA 234:861–864

76. Reid DC, Henderson R, Saboe L, Miller JD (1987) Etiology and clinical course of missed spine fractures. J Trauma 27:980–986

77. Roberge RJ, Samuels JR (1999) Cervical spine injury in low-impact blunt trauma. Am J Emerg Med 17:125–129

78. Roberge RJ, Wears RC (1992) Evaluation of neck discomfort, neck tenderness, and neurologic deficits as indicators for radiography in blunt trauma victims. J Emerg Med 10:539–544

79. Roberge RJ, Wears RC, Kelly M, Evans TC, Kenny MA, Daffner RD, Kremen R, Murray K, Cottington EC (1988) Selective application of cervical spine radiography in alert victims of blunt trauma: a prospective study. J Trauma 28(6):784–788

80. Ross SE, Schwab CW, David ET, Delong WG, Born CT (1987) Clearing the cervical spine: initial radiologic evaluation. J Trauma 27(9):1055–1060

81. Ryan MD, Henderson JJ (1992) The epidemiology of fractures and fracture-dislocations of the cervical spine. Injury 23(1):38–40

82. Schenarts PJ, Diaz J, Kaiser C, Carrillo Y, Eddy V, Morris JA (2001) Prospective comparison of admission computed tomographic scan and plain films of the upper cervical spine in trauma patients with altered mental status. J Trauma 51:663–668

83. Schuster R, Waxman K, Sanchez B, Becerra S, Chung R, Conner S, Jones T (2005) Magnetic resonance imaging is not needed to clear cervical spines in blunt trauma patients with normal computed tomographic results and no motor deficits. Arch Surg 140:762–766

84. Sees DW, Rodriguez-Cruz LR, Flaherty SF, Ciceri DP (1998) The use of bedside fluoroscopy to evaluate the cervical spine in obtunded trauma patients. J Trauma 45:768–777

85. Shaffer MA, Doris PE (1981) Limitation of the cross table lateral view in detecting cervical spine injuries: a retrospective analysis. Ann Emerg Med 10:508–513

86. Spain DA, Trooskin SZ, Flancbaum L, Boyarsky AH, Nosher JL (1990) The adequacy and cost effectiveness of routine resuscitation-area cervical-spine radiographs. Ann Emerg Med 19(3):276–278

87. Spivak JM, Weiss MA, Cotler JM, Call M (1994) Cervical spine injuries in patients 65 and older. Spine 19(20):2302–2306

88. Stäbler A, Eck J, Penning R, Milz SP, Bartl R, Resnick D, Reiser M (2001) Cervical spine: postmortem assessment of accident injuries-comparison of radiographic, MR imaging, anatomic, and pathologic findings. Radiology 221:340–346

89. Stassen NA, Williams VA, Gestring ML, Cheng JD, Bankey PE (2006) Magnetic resonance imaging in combination with helical computed tomography provides a safe and efficient method of cervical spine clearance in the obtunded trauma patient. J Trauma 60(1):171–177

90. Stelfox HT, Velmahos GC, Gettings E, Bigatello LM, Schmidt U (2007) Computed tomography for early and safe discontinuation of cervical spine immobilization in obtunded multiply injured patients. J Trauma 63:630–636

91. Stiell IG, Wells GA (1999) Methodologic standards for the development of clinical decision rules in emergency medicine. Ann Emerg Med 33:437–447

92. Stiell IG, Wells GA, Vandemheen KL, Clement CM, Lesiuk H, De Maio VJ, Laupacis A, Schull M, McKnight RD, Verbeek R, Brison R, Cass D, Dreyer J, Eisenhauer MA, Greenberg GH, MacPhail I, Morrison L, Reardon M, Worthington J (2001) The Canadian C-spine rule for radiography in alert and stable trauma patients. JAMA 286(15):1841–1848

93. Tomycz ND, Chew BG, Chang YF et al (2008) MRI is unnecessary to clear the cervical spine in obtunded/comatose trauma patients: the four-year experience of a level I trauma center. J Trauma 64:1258–1263

94. Turetsky DB, Vines FS, Clayman DA, Northup HM (1993) Technique and use of supine oblique views in acute cervical spine trauma. Ann Emerg Med 22:685–689

95. Vaccaro AR, Kreidl KO, Pan W et al (1998) Usefulness of MRI in isolated upper cervical spine fractures in adults. J Spinal Disord 11:289–293

96. Velmahos GC, Theodorou D, Tatevossian R, Belzberg H, Cornwell EE, Berne TV, Asensio JA, Demetriades D (1996) Radiographic cervical spine evaluation in the alert asymptomatic blunt trauma victim: much ado about nothing. J Trauma 40(5):768–774

97. Walter J, Doris PE, Shaffer MA (1984) Clinical presentation of patients with acute cervical spine injury. Ann Emerg Med 13:512–515

98. Widder S, Doig C, Burrowes P, Larsen G, Hurlbert RJ, Kortbeek JB (2004) Prospective evaluation of computed tomographic scanning for the spinal clearance of obtunded trauma patients: preliminary results. J Trauma 56(6):1179–1184

99. Williams CF, Bernstein TW, Jelenko C (1981) Essentiality of the lateral cervical spine radiograph. Ann Emerg Med 10:198–204

100. Woodring JH, Lee C (1993) Limitations of cervical radiography in the evaluation of acute cervical trauma. J Trauma 34:32–39

Imaging of Spinal Trauma

3

Brian Petersen

3.1 Introduction

Patients presenting with a suspicion of spine trauma remain a diagnostic challenge despite continued research and technological advances over the last decade. These patients confound physicians because they constitute a difficult subset of patients; significant trauma with distracting injuries and commonly obtunded, either chemically or from associated head trauma. Even when presenting coherently, the consequences of a missed or delayed diagnosis of spinal trauma are devastating, contributing to a general high level of anxiety en route to "clearing the spine" in this population of patients. The sheer volume of patients presenting to the Emergency Department already in a cervical collar has increased, fueled by a combination of more trauma and more litigation.

Plain radiography, with conventional tomography, was the primary modality of choice in the workup of spinal trauma prior to the widespread availability of CT and MRI. CT, once a slow modality, capable of imaging only in the axial plane, has become exceedingly fast, is available 24 h a day, and produces submillimeter volumetric acquisition, allowing reconstruction and evaluation of data in any orthogonal plane. CT can now be performed over large portions of the body in seconds and that data can be converted into discrete spinal imaging studies. It is common at level I trauma centers to routinely scan high mechanism trauma from head through pelvis, reconstructing the cervical, thoracic,

and lumbar spine studies from that initial data acquisition. This largely obviates the need for plain radiographs and can greatly speed the disposition of severely traumatized patients.

Similarly, MRI has become much more readily available and, although significantly more constrained in ease of acquisition compared to CT, has become extremely important in the imaging of spinal cord trauma and ligamentous injury.

The purpose of this chapter is to provide the reader with an overview of imaging of the spinal trauma. Although criteria for "clearing the spine" will be discussed relative to imaging, this subject is addressed elsewhere in this text in great detail. The role of advanced imaging will be explored, and its context within the radiographic and clinical workup of the spine trauma patient will be discussed in detail. Special consideration will be given to imaging of the pediatric, elderly, ankylotic, and athletic patient populations and the indications and appropriate workup for the evaluation of neurovascular injury.

Finally, a brief pictorial review of common spinal injuries and their radiographic findings will conclude the discussion.

3.2 To Image or Not To Image the Cervical Spine?

The evaluation of patients with cervical spinal trauma has been controversial for over 50 years. The consequences of a missed spine injury are devastating: a neurologically intact patient can progress to neurologic impairment with unrecognized unstable cervical spine injury. With older techniques, progression to neurologic compromise was up to 50% [70]. With the current

B. Petersen
University of Colorado, Denver,
PO BOX 6511, MS L954
Aurora, CO 80045, USA
e-mail: brian.petersen@ucdenver.edu.

V.V. Patel et al. (eds.), *Spine Trauma*,
DOI: 10.1007/978-3-642-03694-1_3, © Springer-Verlag Berlin Heidelberg 2010

emphasis on spinal stability with rigid cervical spine protection and backboard precautions for all trauma victims, the percentage is lower, but remains significant. Twenty years ago, 23% of 253 patients prospectively studied by Reid et al. had a delay in cervical spinal injury diagnosis. "Secondary deficits" occurred in 10% of this delayed diagnosis group compared to 1.4% of patients whose spinal injuries were identified at presentation [68]. Clearly, the clinical consequences of a delayed or missed diagnosis of spinal injury are significant.

Historically, cervical spine radiographs were obtained in great numbers with few positive findings. Only 1–3% of studies demonstrate visible fractures [44, 50, 80]. This widespread overutilization comes at a significant financial cost to high volume trauma centers. In a resource cost analysis of cervical spine radiographs from a level I trauma center, resource costs exceeded Medicare reimbursement for all risk strata [15].

Ideally, one would image only those patients at a high risk for cervical spine injury to increase pretest probability and control cost, but have a broad enough selection criteria so that neglecting spinal injury would be exceedingly rare. The imaging test performed should have high sensitivity to give adequate weight to a negative result in clinical decision making. So two questions arise: (1) Who should be imaged? (2) How should they be imaged?

3.2.1 Who Should Be Imaged?

According to the US Bone and Joint Decade website, a 2002 census reported 21 million ER trauma visits. Given the high volume of patients encountered by the United States trauma centers, there have been multiple iterations of attempted cost containment and efficient resource utilization through the last 20 years. Protocol-driven workup of cervical spine trauma, in which patients were uniformly imaged for cervical spine trauma regardless of symptoms or mechanism, was utilized for many years by trauma surgeons and emergency room physicians, but was clearly inefficient in identifying patients with cervical spine trauma. Mirvis et al. found a single C7 transverse process fracture in 138 asymptomatic patients who were imaged with CT following incomplete cervical spine radiographs at a cost of $59,202 [59], a significant amount of money for a single stable fracture.

Increasing efficiency and cost containment have helped focus attempts to identify patient populations that need spinal imaging. In response to protocol-driven imaging at Duke University, Vandemark, in collaboration with trauma physicians, developed clinical criteria to parse out those patients whose mechanism required spinal workup and those who could be clinically freed of the cervical collar [84]. Vandemark et al. emphasized the collaborative approach to "clearing the cervical spine," asking the clinicians to stratify patients into categories of risk, from Level 1 (no risk) to Level 4 (high risk). High-risk criteria, according to Vandemark, are listed in Table 3.1. Risk stratification dictated the radiographic series obtained: no films in Level 1, standing 3-view series in Level 2 (low risk), 3-view supine series followed by radiologist-approved upright obliques in Level 3 (moderate risk), and finally, 5-view radiographs in supine position in Level 4 (high-risk patients). Vandemark argued appropriately that risk stratification increased radiographic interpretation accuracy by allowing the radiologist to weigh the potential implications of subtle findings [84].

It has been proposed that a "well-positioned, optimally exposed complete radiographic series of the cervical spine," interpreted by an experienced radiologist, has a high sensitivity for significant injury [44, 54]. However, it is clear that the patients in whom obtaining a "well-positioned, optimally exposed, complete radiographic series of the cervical spine" is most challenging, are the patients who have sustained the most severe trauma, and are most likely to have a clinically significant cervical spine injury. A substantial number of clinically significant fractures are missed on routine trauma radiographs

Table 3.1 Vandemark's clinical and historical characteristics of the high-risk patient

High-velocity blunt trauma
Significant motor vehicle accident
Direct cervical region injury
Altered mental status at the time of trauma and/or during ER evaluation (includes alcohol, drugs, intoxication, loss of consciousness, and mental illness)
Falls/diving injuries
Significant head/facial injury
Abnormal neurologic examination
Prominent neck pain or tenderness
Thoracic or lumbar spine fracture
Rigid spine (ankylosing spondylitis, DISH etc.)

in patients who are severely traumatized or uncooperative [1, 88]. Primary CT screening of the cervical spine for trauma was reported by Nunez at the University of Miami for patients who "have sustained multisystem injury, have altered mental status, or are uncooperative" [62]. Hanson et al. at the University of Washington subsequently published a clinical decision rule based on criteria that would be immediately apparent to the treating trauma team upon presentation. This stratified patients into primary CT screening of the cervical and upper thoracic spine in combination with head CT. Those who did not satisfy the criteria underwent cervical spine radiographs [39]. They found, using the clinical decision rule summarized in Table 3.2, that true-positive detection rate for CT screening population was 10% (35/355), while those in the conventional radiography group yielded a true-positive rate of 0.2% (7/3684).

Although both Vandemark and Hanson succeeded in stratifying those patients who should be placed in the high-risk category, there was still a paucity of information regarding which group of patients should be placed in the "no-risk" category. The National Emergency X-Radiography Utilization Study Group (NEXUS Group) set out to perform a multicenter, prospective trial to validate simple clinical criteria that would place patients into a no-risk group that would not require imaging [44]. The NEXUS study prospectively looked at clinical criteria for imaging the cervical spine in 34,069 patients who had experienced blunt trauma. From those 34,069 patients, 818 patients had radiographically documented cervical spine injury. Of those 818, eight patients satisfied the criteria for "no-risk" stratification, and only two of eight had a "clinically significant" injury. The criteria were termed the NEXUS "No"s (Table 3.3) and had 99.8% negative predictive value, but only a 12.9% specificity.

Concomitantly with the NEXUS study, a multicenter Canadian study was undertaken to develop a clinical decision rule to obtain sensitivity and specificity in image acquisition of patients who were "alert and stable" [81]. Of 8,773 patients, 151 had a clinically important injury. No clinically important injuries were missed in the "no-risk" group. This yielded a sensitivity of 100% and a specificity of 42.5%. The Canadian C-Spine Rule applies initial high-risk criteria to force imaging; subsequent presence of low-risk criteria allows the patient to actively rotate his or her neck under physician supervision. If these criteria are met (absence of high-risk criteria → presence of low-risk criteria → ability to rotate neck 45° left and right), no imaging is indicated. Please see Table 3.4 for the summary of the Canadian C-Spine Rule.

The Canadian C-Spine Rule (CCR) and NEXUS criteria were prospectively compared by the same group that produced the CCR [80]. The results suggested that the CCR performed slightly better, but this

Table 3.3 NEXUS "No"s

NO posterior midline tenderness
NO focal neurologic deficit
*NOr*mal alertness
NO evidence of intoxication
NO painful distracting injury

Table 3.4 Canadian C-spine rule. Adapted from [81]

High-risk factors Age >65 years Dangerous mechanism Fall from >1 m/5 stairs Axial load to head (diving injury) High-speed MVA (>100 km/hr), rollover, ejection Motorized recreational vehicle injury Bicycle collision Paresthesias in extremities	If any high-risk factors are present proceed to radiography
Low-risk factors (if any low-risk factors are present and high-risk factors are absent proceed to ROM) Simple rear-end MVC or Sitting position in ED or Ambulatory at any time or Delayed onset neck pain or Absence of midline c-spine tenderness	If none of these are present proceed to radiography
Able to actively rotate neck 45° left or right?	If pain free no radiography necessary

Table 3.2 University of Washington Clinical Decision Rule to select patients to undergo helical CT C-spine

Injury mechanism High-speed (≥35 mph combined impact) MVA Crash with death at scene of MVA Fall from height of ≥10 ft
Clinical parameters based on primary patient survey Significant closed head injury (or intracranial hemorrhage seen on CT) Neurologic symptoms or signs referred to the cervical spine Pelvic or multiple extremity fractures
The presence of any one parameter places the patient at high risk

was controversial. Both had high sensitivity, but the CCR had higher specificity (45.2% vs. 36.8%) and resulted in lower rates of radiography (55.9% vs. 66.6%). This generated some controversy, however, as the CCR included in its study the fraction of patients on whom imaging was not performed based on clinical criteria (follow-up was confirmed by phone call) and NEXUS excluded these patients, resulting in lower specificity for the NEXUS criteria. Both of these clinical decision rules successfully identify patients with nearly zero risk of cervical spine trauma and succeed in decreasing the overall utilization of limited resources.

3.2.2 How Should We Image the Cervical Spine?

Regardless of the criteria used to select those patients who need imaging, the next point of decision is how best to image those patients. In suspected spinal trauma, the clearing of the cervical spine by imaging is a tricky proposition. Clinically, in a patient who does not fit neatly into the clinical decision rules, and whose

mechanism is not of significant severity to warrant CT of other body parts, high-quality radiographs are likely sufficient. In a study looking at CT and radiography in patients with "very low risk" or "low risk" of cervical spine injury, CT and radiography had the same sensitivities and specificities [60]; however, there were no injuries in these groups, so both modalities had a 100% sensitivity. AP, lateral, and open-mouth odontoid views of high quality and appropriate position may be able to effectively detect most clinically significant injuries in patients in the lower-risk strata. Using these three views, MacDonald et al. detected 99% of "significant injuries" in a retrospective review of 775 motor vehicle collision patients [54]. Variables such as the quality of the radiographs and the experience of the interpreter affect the sensitivity of radiography. For evaluation of unstable injuries, a technically adequate 3-view radiographic series of the cervical spine (Fig. 3.1) interpreted as "normal" in the NEXUS study had a 99.99% negative predictive value [44]. However, only 2/3 of the radiographs were technically adequate and of 1,496 cervical spine injuries, only 932 (62%) were identified on radiographs. In significantly traumatized patients, technically inadequate radiographs are common (Fig. 3.2).

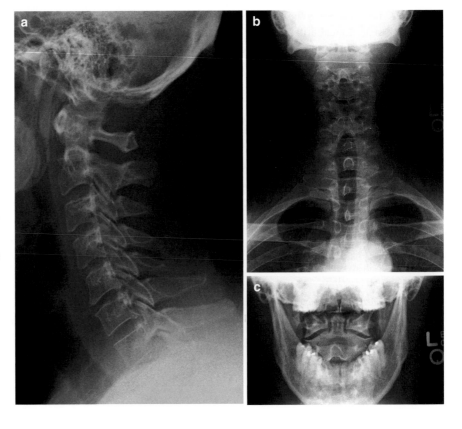

Fig. 3.1 Adequate 3-view of the cervical spine. The lateral radiograph (a) is adequately exposed to the C7/T1 disc space. The AP radiograph (b) is exposed to make the spinous processes and the lateral masses visible. The lung apices and superior ribs are included. Open-mouth odontoid view (c) shows the entirety of the dens, and the lateral masses are visualized without overlying structures. Occipital condyles are partially obscured

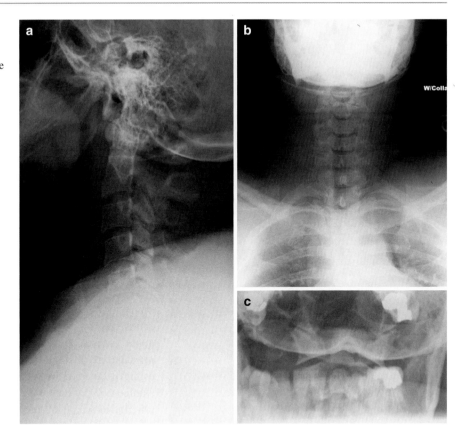

Fig. 3.2 Technically inadequate cervical radiograph series. Lateral radiograph (**a**) is a cross-table lateral which is adequately exposed only to the C4/C5 interspace. AP radiograph (**b**) is adequate, but is of the least utility in the evaluation of typical cervical spinal trauma. The occiput overlies much of the dens, and the margins of the C1/C2 articulation are obscured on the open-mouth odontoid view (**c**)

There are several studies touting a combination of radiography and focused cervical spine CT [6, 10]. This approach is based on evaluating areas not well seen on radiography. Historically, the combination of the two modalities was necessary given a subset of fractures that were not visualized on CT, but were readily apparent on radiography [1, 65] representing fractures that were oriented in-plane to the axial CT images. These studies, however, were conducted at a time when CT images were obtained axially, and the ability to reconstruct the data in coronal and sagittal planes was not feasible. With today's technology, helically acquired thin slices are able to be reconstructed in planes that make these axially oriented fractures obvious (Fig. 3.3).

The greatest number of fractures missed by radiography occur at the C1/C2 level [62]. The combination of CT and radiography to "clear" the cervical spine has been more recently advocated by combining routine cervical spine radiographs with CT imaging acquired at the same time as a head CT, extending the routine head CT imaging to the C3 vertebral body. This protocol has been adopted in several large volume trauma hospitals

and has been touted to be a time-saving and cost-effective way to evaluate the craniocervical junction and upper cervical spine; areas that are commonly injured and suboptimally evaluated by radiography. In a prospective study by Schenarts et al., 95/1,356 patients had injuries to the upper cervical spine. CT detected 96% of the injuries while radiography detected only 54% [73].

When weighing radiography alone against CT, most pertinent is the clear insensitivity of plain radiography in the severely traumatized patient. Those patients who are clinically unstable, intubated, and nonresponsive are commonly the ones whose complete radiographic evaluation is most challenging. Much time and energy has historically been spent attempting to obtain diagnostic radiographs on these patients who are unable to cooperate. In patients where the chance of spinal trauma is high, it is widely regarded as more efficient to study the spine by multidetector CT (MDCT), saving time and increasing sensitivity and specificity [23, 24]. This patient population commonly requires CT evaluation of the head, chest, abdomen, and pelvis due to associated injuries, and taking significant additional time to complete a radiographic spine series is inefficient. With the

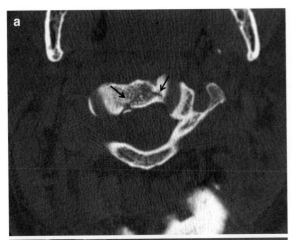

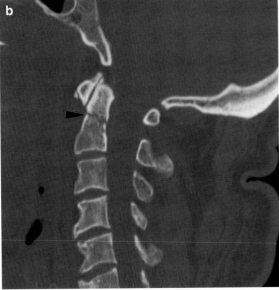

Fig. 3.3 The widespread use of multidetector CT (MDCT) allows thin acquisition and multiplanar reconstructions increasing the conspicuity of fractures that could have been missed with previous iterations of CT capable of only axial images. The type II dens fracture is less conspicuous on axial images (**a**, *arrows*) compared to sagittal reconstruction (**b**, *arrowheads*)

speed and volumetric acquisitions being possible with the current technologies, far less time is wasted by acquiring data through the cervical spine at the same time as the ubiquitous head CT. Coronal and sagittal reconstructions of the cervical spine are easily performed given the thin-section acquisition currently obtainable.

In a study of unconscious, intubated patients, Brohi et al. reported a 39.3% sensitivity for lateral radiographs (commonly acquired as part of the "Big 3" obtained portably upon ER arrival of the traumatized patient) for any fracture and 51.7% sensitivity for

unstable injuries [18]. The sensitivity of CT for fracture detection has been reported from 90–99% to specificities 72–89%, without caveat to the severity of injury. The sensitivity of the radiographs has been shown to be inversely related to the severity of the trauma [14, 16, 17, 37, 60, 73, 83, 87].

It is becoming clear that radiography's role for definitive evaluation of spinal fracture in the significantly traumatized patient may be nearing its end. Several recent studies have compared radiography and CT in the screening of the cervical spine in high mechanism trauma and have shown CT to significantly outperform even "adequate" radiographs. McCulloch et al. prospectively performed CT and 3-view radiography in 407 patients who had suffered priority I or II trauma. Of those patients, only 48% of the radiographs were deemed "adequate"; however, sensitivity for injury in the "adequate" subset was 52%, not significantly better than the sensitivity of 45% in the "inadequate" subset. Helical CT had a sensitivity of 98% missing only a single dens fracture, which was, interestingly, detected by radiography [57]. Mathen et al. studied 667 patients not clinically cleared by NEXUS criteria, in which 60 had c-spine injury. All of these injuries were detected by CT (four ligamentous injuries were detected by CT as well, subsequently confirmed on MRI) while 3-view radiography detected only 45% of injuries [56] (Fig. 3.4).

Some may suppose that increasing the number of radiographic views may increase the detection of fracture, but this does not appear to be the case. Comparing 5-view cervical spine radiography (AP, lateral, odontoid, and bilateral oblique views) with CT in blunt trauma patients with altered mental status, Diaz et al. showed CT to have a sensitivity of 97.4% and a specificity of 100% compared to 44 and 100% for radiography [30]. In a meta-analysis of seven studies that met inclusion criteria, the pooled sensitivity of MDCT was 98% compared with 52% for plain radiography [46].

In 2007, the Expert Panel on Musculoskeletal Imaging of the American College of Radiology updated the ACR appropriateness criteria for the imaging of suspected spine trauma. ACR appropriateness criteria utilize experts in the field to perform extensive literature review and make recommendations for the appropriateness of imaging modalities for multiple clinical scenarios. *The conclusion in the most recent recommendation was that "thin-section CT, and not radiography, is the primary screening study for suspected*

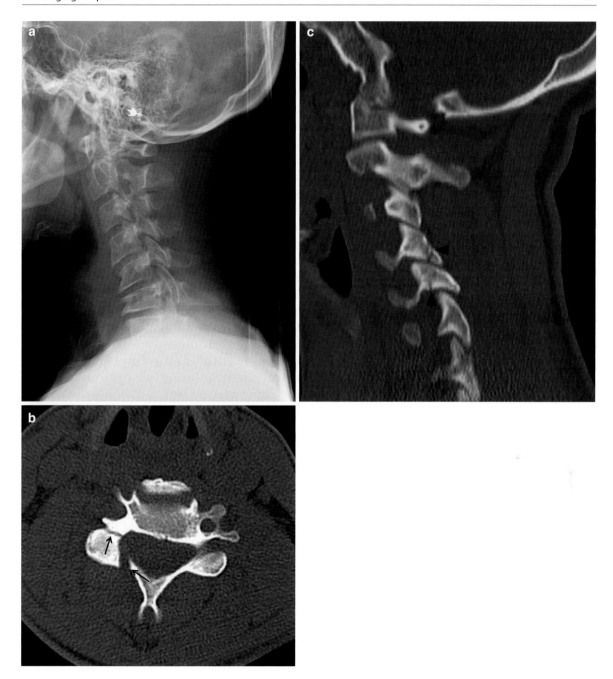

Fig. 3.4 Thirty-seven year old intoxicated male involved in a roll-over motor vehicle accident with radiographic series showing no fracture (**a**). C5 and C6 were degenerative on subsequent CT. Collar was removed based on the negative plain films, but patient complained of neck pain and CT was performed. CT found right C5 laminar and pedicle fractures (**b**, *arrows*) and right inferior articulating process fractures of C4 and C5 (**c**, *arrowheads*)

cervical spine injury. The 3-view radiographic study should be performed only when CT is not readily available and should not be considered a substitute for CT. Furthermore, the panel recommended that sagittal and coronal multiplanar reconstruction from the axial CT images be performed for all studies to improve identification and characterization of fractures and subluxations" [25].

3.2.3 Ligamentous/Soft Tissue Evaluation

Although osseous injury to the cervical spine demands most of the attention, the soft tissue stabilizers are equally important. The anterior longitudinal ligament (ALL), posterior longitudinal ligament (PLL), disk annulus, ligamentum flavum, facet joint capsules, uncovertebral joints, and interspinous ligaments all span the osseous structures of the cervical spine to confer stability. Soft tissue and ligamentous disruption can occur in the absence of osseous abnormality and, thus, be occult on both static radiographs and CT. In a somewhat expected display of radiographic insensitivity, an autopsy series of patients with fatal cranial trauma compared fine detail postmortem specimen radiographs with cryosections of the excised spinal column. These fine detail radiographs missed 198 facet, ligament, and disk lesions [47]. Even MRI detected only 11 of 28 soft tissue injuries in a similar study [78]. It is clear that most of the injuries missed in these postmortem exams are not of clinical significance. For clinically significant ligamentous injury, MRI has been shown to be accurate [9].

Flexion/extension radiographs can theoretically be diagnostic of ligamentous injury, but in an acute setting, muscle spasm commonly stabilizes an otherwise unstable spine, and can be falsely reassuring. Delayed radiographs after a period of time in a soft collar, allowing resolution of muscle spasm, has been shown to unmask otherwise occult ligamentous instability [41].

The practice of forced flexion/extension radiography or flexion/extension fluoroscopy in obtunded patients is no longer advocated. This has been shown to be insufficient to clear the cervical spine and is potentially dangerous. Anglen et al. showed forced flexion/extension radiographs to be of no value in the acute setting, finding only 4 suspicious cases out of 837 patients, with nearly 1/3 being technically inadequate [36]. In 123 patients studied by Freedman, forced flexion/extension identified only 3/7 significant ligamentous injuries [32]. More tragically, 1 patient developed quadriplegia as a result of forced flexion/extension fluoroscopy in a series of 301 patients submitted by Davis et al. [28]. Only two true positives were detected, both being stable injuries. A cervical traction protocol has been advocated by Bednar, where progressively greater cervical traction is applied to obtunded patients in the operating room with flexion/extension performed after the cervical lordosis has been "straightened." This is extreme, the lead author being the only one of eight spinal surgeons at his institution willing to perform it, and, clearly, cannot be advocated for general use [7]. The ACR Appropriateness Criteria suggests that dynamic flexion/extension radiography or fluoroscopy may retain utility in patients with equivocal MRI examinations, to scrutinize a particular level of suspected ligamentous sprain [25]. This would clearly exclude all the patients with markedly unstable spines, in which forced flexion/extension could lead to catastrophic consequences.

MRI should be performed in conjunction with CT and not in lieu of it, given the far superior ability of CT to identify fracture. The role of MRI in evaluating patients following a negative evaluation with MDCT is controversial. Three hundred and sixty six obtunded patients underwent MRI of the cervical spine after MDCT of the cervical spine was interpreted as normal, yielding four ligamentous injuries, all considered stable [45], *yielding a 100% negative predictive value for unstable ligamentous injury.* Conversely, Diaz et al. prospectively looked at 85 patients who had clinical or radiographic abnormalities without fracture and were studied with cervical MRI. CT was normal in 14/21 patients, and there were clinically significant injuries, including cord contusions and ligamentous injury requiring surgical stabilization. The analysis of Ghanta et al. also supports the use of MRI in patients with neurologic deficit and normal CT. Several pathologies – traumatic disc herniation, epidural hematoma, cord contusion, and nerve root avulsion – can be detected on MRI. Clinically unstable ligamentous injuries may be equally evaluated between the two if MDCT signs of disc space widening, facet uncovering, and interspinous distance widening are not overlooked (Fig. 3.5). However, Fig. 3.6 illustrates a case where radiographs and CT were interpreted as negative and presumably a ligamentous injury was missed. The patient returned 14 days later after a low mechanism fall with an unstable cervical spine ligamentous injury, demonstrating a bilateral facet dislocation (BFD). The high sensitivity of MRI for ligamentous injury can lead to false positive interpretations and need to be correlated to the patient's clinical presentation.

Fig. 3.5 Gapping of the anterior disc space of C4/C5 on CT (**a**, *arrow*) suggested ligamentous injury and prompted MRI. MRI demonstrated peeling of the anterior longitudinal ligament (ALL) (**b**, *white arrowhead*) and high signal within the anterior portion of the C4/C5 disc (*white arrowhead*). In addition, interspinous ligament injury was detected, with high signal in the posterior paraspinous musculature (*asterisk*)

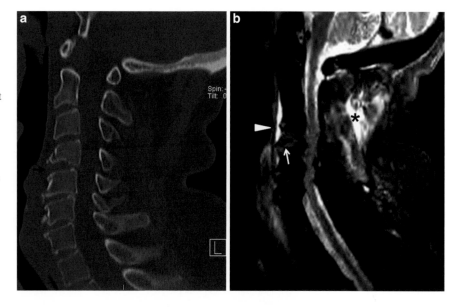

3.3 Special Considerations

3.3.1 Pediatric Patients

The risk of cervical spine injury in the pediatric population is low, shown to be <1% in several large series [4, 49, 85]. The NEXUS study included children; however, there were few cervical spine injuries in the 3,065 children in the study, and only 0.98% had a cervical spine injury by radiography. At 9 years of age, the anatomy of the spine approximates that of the adult and the NEXUS criteria can be applied to this patient population. Below this age, routine radiographic screening is advocated, with AP and lateral radiographs being suitable for children less than 5 years of age and the open-mouth odontoid view being added to those children between 5 and 8 years of age. 3-view radiography has a 94% sensitivity for fracture [89] in the pediatric population.

CT is not routinely advocated as a primary screening tool in patients less than 9 years of age. Hernandez et al. showed only four cervical spine fractures out of 606 patients under the age of 5. All the four injuries had abnormal radiographs as well [42]. In patients older than 9 years of age, with high mechanism of trauma and failing the NEXUS criteria, CT cervical spine screening may be advocated with low-dose protocol, given the radiosensitivity of the thyroid in young patients. A recent study attempting to gage the efficiency of obtaining diagnostic cervical spine radiographs vs cervical spine CT in pediatric patients with head injury requiring head CT concluded that cervical spine CT in this patient population decreased the need for repeat radiographs of the cervical spine [48]. It could be argued that CT would obviate the need for cervical spine radiographs in this patient population, rather than simply decreasing the number of additional views necessary.

There are a wide variety of protocols advocated for dealing with children presenting to the emergency room with the potential for cervical spine injury. These tend to be institution specific and few are published. Lee et al. published a protocol for cervical spine clearance in patients who were 8 years of age or younger [53], separating children who are conscious from those who are unconscious. Children who are conscious are evaluated using clinical information very similar to the NEXUS criteria, with AP, lateral, and odontoid radiographs obtained in those patients failing to fulfill these criteria. In patients undergoing head CT, imaging is extended inferiorly to include C1 and C2 and the odontoid radiograph is excluded. All the patients who are unconscious receive AP and lateral radiographs and cervical spine CT to the T1 vertebral body. MRI is performed if patients have neurologic deficit without radiographic abnormality or have findings on radiography or CT that suggest spinal cord or

Fig. 3.6 CT and radiographs were interpreted as normal at presentation (**a, b**) and patient was discharged from the Emergency Department. Fourteen days later with low mechanism fall, the patient returned to the Emergency Department with neurologic deficit and radiography, CT, and MRI (**c, d, e**) showing focal C5/C6 kyphosis (**c**, *white arrow*) associated with bilateral facet dislocation (BFD), interspinous ligament disruption (**e**, *asterisk*), and spinal cord injury (**e**, *arrow*). (Images courtesy of Dr. David Symonds, Denver Health Medical Center, Denver, CO)

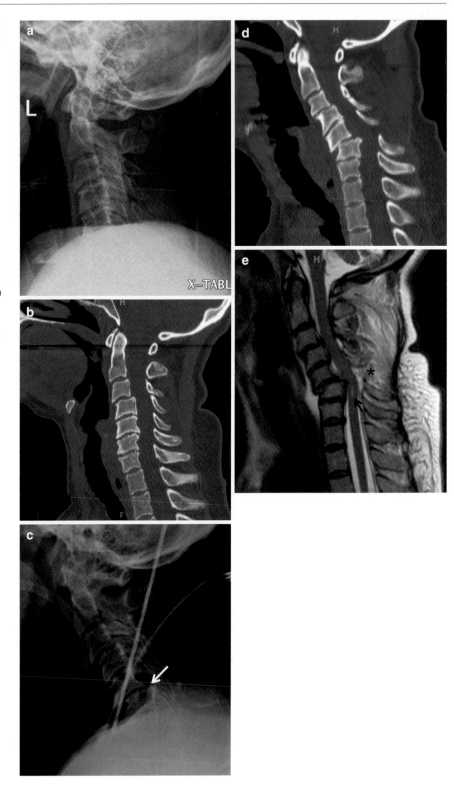

ligamentous injury. Within the institution of this protocol, they noted a statistically significant decrease in the time to c-spine clearance in conscious patients and a trend toward statistical significance in unconscious patients.

Anderson et al. prospectively studied a protocol in which all the children who present to the emergency room in a cervical collar are evaluated with C-spine radiographs (3-view in children older than 5 years of age and limited to AP and lateral in children 5 years of age or less). If radiographs are normal, then the NEXUS clinical criteria is employed on communicative children who are 3 years of age or older. If NEXUS criteria are met, the cervical spine is clear. All the children who are less than 3 years of age are cleared by a Neurosurgery consult. If NEXUS clinical criteria are not met, the child undergoes flexion/extension radiographs and cleared if those are normal. The study was divided into two study periods. Phase I, prior to protocol implementation showed 9% of patients undergoing CT and 3% undergoing MR yielding 2–3% injury rate and only eight fractures (0.9%). Phase II, after the protocol was instituted, saw an increase in CT and MR utilization (24 and 7% respectively) without significant increase in the number of injuries detected (2.8%). It would seem that the protocol increases radiation dose and the utilization of advanced imaging without real benefit; however, the authors pointed out that CT of the cervical spine is not part of the protocol and the majority of the increased utilization occurred in community hospitals prior to referral to the primary children's hospital.

Pediatric patients suffer a different injury pattern compared to adults. The majority of injuries in patients less than 10 years of age occurs at the craniocervical junction and upper cervical spine [43]. In addition, the ligamentous laxity and horizontally oriented facets in the young patient, although decreasing the number of fractures seen, increase the likelihood of spinal cord injury without radiographic abnormality (SCIWORA). This term, first coined by Pang and Wilberger [64], described children with clinical neurologic deficits without radiographic abnormality. It is clear that many of these injuries are now visible on MRI with the prognosis of recovery largely dependent on the severity of the MRI findings [63].

3.3.2 Elderly Patients

Evaluation of the cervical spine in the elderly population can be challenging. Clinically, a clear history is commonly absent, and low mechanism trauma, usually not sufficient to cause injury in the general population, can cause cervical spine injury due to osteopenia and lack of ligamentous flexibility. The elderly are more at risk for fracture for all clinical scenarios according to the clinical prediction rule developed by Bub et al. [19] showing risk of fracture ranging from 24.2% in patients with focal neurologic deficit to 0.4% in patients with low-energy trauma (fall from standing).

In the elderly population, fractures have been reported as more common in the upper cervical spine (dens fractures) compared to the general population, an area that can be difficult to assess on radiographs [27, 77]. Daffner's 10-year review of cervical spine injuries in patients who were 65 years of age or older demonstrated over 2/3 (69%) of injuries occurring at C1 or C2. In addition, the mechanisms leading to cervical spine injury differ greatly from the general population, with 170/231 sustained due to fall (73.5%). This is in comparison to those who are younger than 65 in whom motor vehicle accidents dominate, causing 629 of 741 (85%) cervical spine fractures.

Although plain radiography is of great importance in this population, the accuracy and sensitivity of radiographs is less, due to associated degenerative change. It is difficult to accurately detect post-traumatic spondylolisthesis, given the common degenerative listheses that commonly coexist in the elderly spine. There seems to be an association between degenerative changes of the spine and increased risk of fracture as 90% of patients over the age of 40 with cervical spine fracture had moderate to severe spondylosis in a series conducted by Regenbogen [67]. The sensitivity of radiography in detecting fractures in the elderly appears to be comparable to the severely traumatized patient population, and suspicion of cervical spine injury should prompt CT evaluation despite absence of fracture on radiographs.

3.3.3 The Ankylotic Spine

Patients who suffer from spine anklyosis, either from diffuse idiopathic skeletal hyperostosis (DISH) or ankylosing spondylitis, are at significantly greater risk for cervical spine fracture compared to the general population [20, 38]. This is due to the marked decrease in the compliance of the spine at crucial pivot points. Hyperextension, hyperflexion, and rotational forces are poorly tolerated by cervical spines afflicted with ankylosis. Although typical clinical assessment of these patients should still be performed, the threshold for radiographic and CT evaluation should be low. The injuries sustained by this patient population are commonly severe, with fractures extending through all three spinal columns (Fig. 3.7).

3.3.4 The Athlete

Athletic cervical spine injury accounts for approximately 9–10% of the 11,000 cervical spine injuries per year [33, 55]. These are managed like other cervical spine traumatic mechanisms and the NEXUS criteria and CCR can be applied to this patient population with accuracy. Neurologic deficits in this group can be transient, spanning the spectrum from transient quadraparesis of hyperextension to the common "stinger," from either traction or compressive forces on the nerve roots of the brachial plexus. These commonly improve over a short period of time, but may prompt imaging. The risk of hyperextension ligamentous injury in this patient population is high and MRI may be necessary for accurate diagnosis. Flexion/extension radiographs have been advocated in the past to evaluate for these

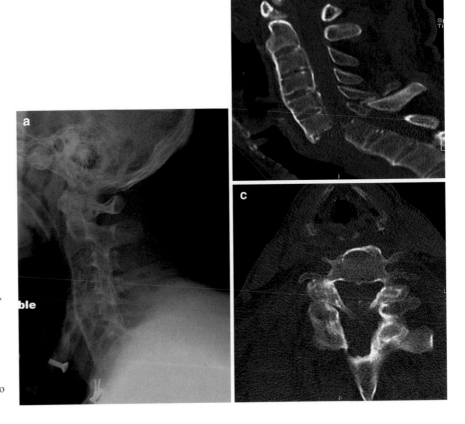

Fig. 3.7 Patient with ankylosing spondylitis suffering a hyperextension fracture dislocation at C6/C7, inferior to the area of coverage on suboptimal lateral radiograph (**a**), but clearly confirmed on CT (**b**) with marked canal compromise due to anterior displacement of C6 relative to C7 (**b** and **c**)

ligamentous instabilities, but transient muscle spasm associated with the acute injury can mask instability in the acute setting. Soft collar application and follow-up flexion/extension radiographs after resolution of muscle spasm has been shown to unmask previously unsuspected ligamentous instability [41].

3.3.5 Neurovascular Injury

The incidence of vascular injury related to blunt trauma is low, with overall incidence of 0.86% in the ground-breaking work done by Biffl et al [12]. The Denver Health group advocated 4-vessel cerebral angiography for patients satisfying clinical and imaging criteria (Table 3.5). Of those screened, 18% had vascular injury, the majority of those being asymptomatic. Initially, CT angiography (CTA) was not advocated as it was shown to be inaccurate and insensitive and 4-vessel digital angiography was performed. Subsequent advances in CT technology have largely allowed replacement of conventional 4-vessel angiography with CTA. *CTA has been shown to be accurate and sensitive to clinically significant arterial injuries* [11].

Carotid artery injury can occur due to extreme hyperextension of the carotid vessels across the articular processes of C1–C3 (Fig. 3.8) or from the extension of the line of force through the carotid canal in the setting of skull base fracture. For our purposes, secondary signs of vertebral artery injury will be addressed, with cervical spine lateral mass fractures extending into the foramen transversarium, where the vertebral artery is fixed and is

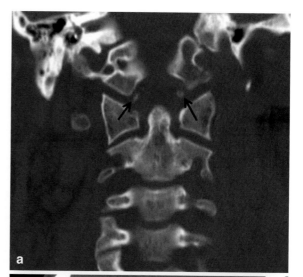
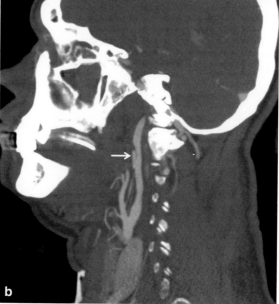

Fig. 3.8 Patient with hyperextension injury resulting in bilateral alar ligament avulsion from the occipital condyles (**a**, *black arrows*). The hyperextension mechanism resulted in traction force on the carotid artery resulting in grade III carotid injury (**b**, *white arrow*). (Images courtesy of Dr. David Symonds, Denver Health Medical Center, Denver, CO)

Table 3.5 Denver criteria for blunt neurovascular injury screening [12]

Signs/symptoms
Arterial hemorrhage or expanding hematoma
Cervical bruit
Focal neurological deficit
Neurological exam inconsistent with head CT findings
Stroke on follow-up head CT

Risk factors
LeForte II or III fracture pattern
Cervical spine fracture
Basilar skull fracture with the involvement of the carotid canal
Diffuse axonal injury with GCS <6
Near hanging with anoxic brain injury

most susceptible to injury (Fig. 3.9). Extension of fracture through the foramen transversarium should prompt CTA to evaluate for vertebral artery injury [22]. Notably, in the series of Cothren et al., only 69/92 patients with vertebral artery injuries had cervical spine fractures, and of those, only 26% had an extension of fracture through

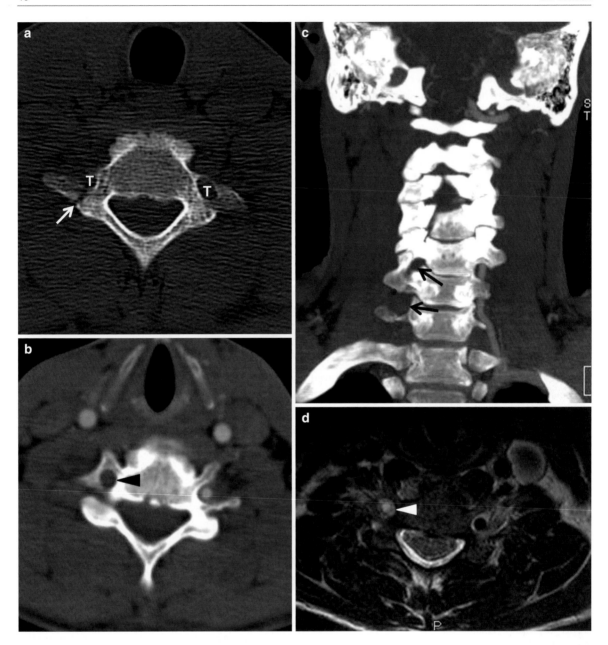

Fig. 3.9 Fracture of the right C7 transverse process (*white arrow*) extends to the right foramen transversarium (T) of C7. CT angiogram confirms right vertebral artery occlusion both on axial source images (**b**, *arrowhead*) and coronal maximum intensity projection (**c**, *black arrows*). Axial T2 weighted MRI shows high signal thrombus within the right vertebral artery (**d**, *white arrowhead*)

the foramen transversarium, 55% had fractures associated with the subluxation of vertebral bodies, and the remaining 18% of fractures involved the upper cervical spine. So, although the extension of fracture through the foramen transversarium should incite arterial interrogation, cervical spinal fractures of all types can be associated with vertebral artery injury. Vertebral artery injuries are commonly treated with anticoagulation, but failure to treat can lead to subsequent stroke in 20% of patients [13]. Also when considering surgical treatment, if a vertebral artery is injured, every precaution should be taken to avoid injury to the contralateral side.

3.4 Cervical Spine Injury

3.4.1 Normal Cervical Spine Radiographs

Despite the relative insensitivity of radiographs for cervical spine injury, they are still commonly performed in Emergency Departments across the country. A single lateral view of the cervical spine is included in the "Big 3" upon arrival to the Emergency Department on nearly every significantly traumatized patient. The need to accurately interpret traumatic cervical spine radiographs remains high.

Radiographic evaluation of the cervical spine can be performed with many views. The standard 3-view of AP, lateral, and open-mouth odontoid have been shown to be the most efficient way to gain a relatively high sensitivity for cervical spine injury. The routine addition of bilateral obliques or flexion/extension views in the acute setting, have not been shown to be of high yield [30].

The properly positioned lateral view yields the most information in a traumatized spine. In evaluating the lateral cervical spine, there should be smooth cervical arcs connecting the ventral margins of the cervical vertebral bodies, the dorsal margin of the vertebral bodies, and the spinolaminar line (Fig. 3.10). The laminar space (Fig. 3.11) is uniform in a properly positioned film and acute variation in this space can indicate a rotational injury [90]. The ubiquitous presence of the cervical collar can straighten the normal cervical lordosis (Fig. 3.12). Muscle spasm can also contribute to straightening the cervical spine and even cause some smooth reversal of the normal cervical lordosis. The facets should be properly positioned and uniformly covered, resembling

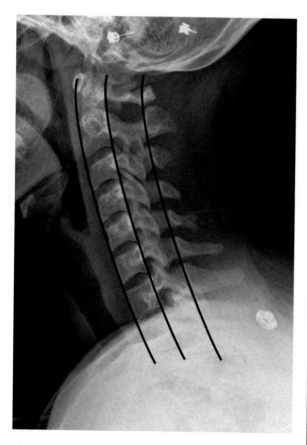

Fig. 3.10 Normal lateral radiograph demonstrating the normal cervical arcs. The eye should be drawn along the ventral and dorsal margins of the vertebral bodies and along the spinolaminar line. Discontinuity of these typically smooth arcs can be due to degenerative change, but may prompt cross-sectional evaluation of the cervical spine with an adequate clinical history

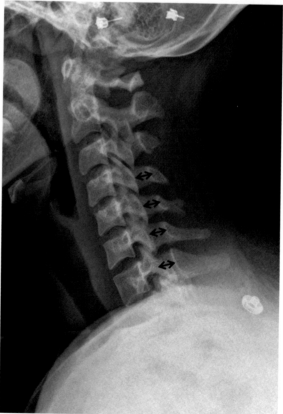

Fig. 3.11 Laminar space (*double arrows*) should be uniform in a properly positioned lateral radiograph. Acute changes in the laminar space can indicate a rotational injury

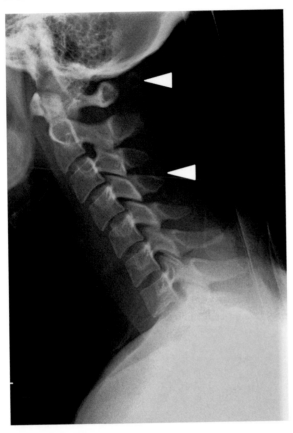

Fig. 3.12 Smooth reversal of the normal cervical lordosis associated with muscle spasm and the presence of a cervical collar. The cervical collar snaps are visible radiographically (*arrowheads*). This patient had no cervical spine injury

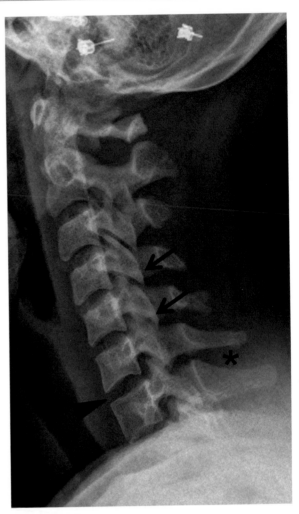

Fig. 3.13 The inferior articulating processes of the facets should appropriately cover the lateral masses of the vertebral body below (*arrows*). The intervertebral disc spaces should be uniform from anterior to posterior (*arrowhead*). The interspinous distances should be relatively uniform (*asterisk*)

shingles on a roof (Fig. 3.13). The interspinous and intervertebral distances should be uniform (Fig. 3.13). The atlantodental interval should be assessed and not be greater than 3 mm in adults and 5 mm in children (Fig. 3.14). The prevertebral soft tissues have a predictable contour and should not exceed 7 mm anterior to C3 and 20 mm anterior to C6/C7 where the esophagus typically originates (Fig. 3.15). A normal bulge of the prevertebral soft tissues is seen anterior to the arch of C1 with a reliable indentation just caudal and cranial to the anterior C1 tubercle (Fig. 3.15). Normal prevertebral soft tissue contours are reassuring and abnormal contours should raise suspicion, although abnormal contours can be caused by swallowing during image acquisition or presence of adenoidal tissue in the superior pharynx.

Evaluation of the craniocervical junction on the lateral radiograph is difficult given the overlapping shadows of the cranium, mandible, and overlying soft tissues. Radiography is insensitive to craniocervical injuries, but there are clues to injury in this area. Occipital condyle

fractures without the displacement of fracture fragments are almost universally occult on radiography. The prevertebral soft tissue distension commonly associated with these injuries may be the only clue (Fig. 3.16). The normal relationship between the cranium and the atlas can be measured on the lateral radiograph in several different ways. The Powers ratio and Lee's X-line require the visualization of the opisthion (the occipital contribution to the foramen magnum) which is inconsistently seen on trauma lateral radiographs [51, 66]. Wackenheim's line relies on the slant of the clivus which is also variable [86]. More reliable and based on the visualization of structures on the traumatic lateral radiograph is the method proposed by Harris [40]. This set of

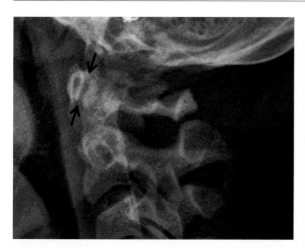

Fig. 3.14 Normal atlantodental interval (*arrows* mark the superior and inferior aspects of the interval). The atlantodental interval should not exceed 3 mm in adults and 5 mm in children, measured from the ventral cortex of the dens to the dorsal cortex of the anterior C1 arch

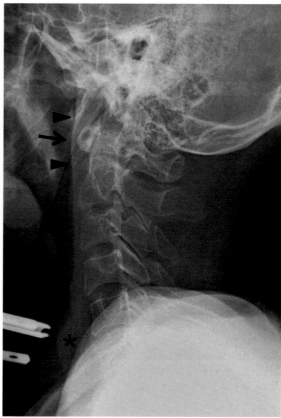

Fig. 3.15 Normal prevertebral soft tissue (PVST) contours. There is a normal bulge at the level of C1 (*arrow*) with slight concavity on either side off the anterior arch of C1 (*arrowheads*). Esophagus at the level of C5/C6 accounts for the normal PVST bulge typically seen in this area (*asterisk*)

measurements places the basion (tip of the clivus) within 12 mm anterior of a line drawn cephalad from the posterior cortex of C2 (the basion-axial interval – BAI) and within 12 mm of the tip of the dens (basion-dental interval – BDI) (Fig. 3.17), with distances greater than these suggesting crianiocervical instability or frank craniocervical dissociation (Fig. 3.18).

Adequate open-mouth odontoid view should include the entire dens, both lateral mass articulations of C1/C2 and, ideally, the occipital condyles. The lateral atlantoaxial interval should be symmetric and the lateral masses of the C1 should align with C2 (Fig. 3.19). Subtle alignment abnormalities can be caused by rotation of the head (Fig. 3.20). The AP radiograph should be scrutinized for proper midline alignment of the spinous processes to exclude a rotational injury.

CT has the advantage of tomographically depicting the cervical spine in any plane, and even small fractures can be demonstrated with accuracy. Fractures can be easily missed when they travel in the plane of the tomographic acquisition and axially oriented fractures are commonly occult on axial images. Now, with the widespread use of MDCT, multiplanar reformats have largely solved this problem with previously occult fractures now conspicuous (Fig. 3.3b). It should be understood that reconstructions in the sagittal and coronal plane are useful only when reconstructed from thin data sets. As illustrated in Fig. 3.21, the reconstruction from 3 mm axial images and that from 1 mm axial images differ greatly in their resolution and diagnostic

value. Moreover, motion on the original axial acquisitions is transmitted through all the reconstructions and makes evaluation of these areas impossible (Fig. 3.22). The sensitivity of CT is high, but specificity can suffer in inexperienced hands, with commonly encountered vascular channels simulating fractures (Fig. 3.23). Similar to radiographs, sagittal and coronal reconstructions can be evaluated, with the assessment of the normal cervical arcs, prevertebral soft tissues, and alignment of the craniocervical junction.

3.4.2 Mechanisms of Injury

The common cervical spine injuries will be broken down into the common predominant mechanisms of injury. These include axial load, hyperflexion, hyperflexion and rotation, and hyperextension.

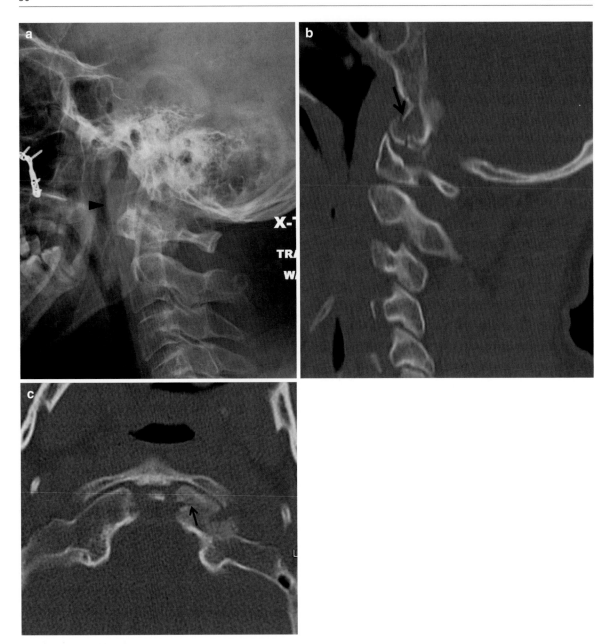

Fig. 3.16 (**a**) Lateral radiograph demonstrating focal PVST swelling above the anterior C1 arch (*arrowhead*). (**b, c**) Axial and sagittal CT reconstruction shows left sided occipital condyle fracture (*arrow*)

3.4.2.1 Axial Load: Occipital Condyle Fractures

When Anderson and Montesano published their series of occipital condyle fractures in 1998, they called them "rare" with only "20 cases reported in the literature" [3]. With the recent widespread use of MDCT, occipital condyle fractures are clearly more prevalent than once thought. They are very difficult to see radiographically and, commonly, the only clue to their presence is loss of the normal prevertebral soft tissue contour above the anterior C1 arch (Fig. 3.16). They may be directly visible on the open-mouth odontoid view, but the presence of overlapping bones and teeth often make this diagnosis difficult to confirm. Most commonly, they are diagnosed on MDCT where they are readily visible (Fig. 3.16).

Anderson and Montesano divided occipital condyle fractures into 3 types:

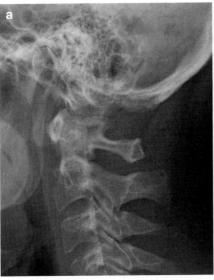
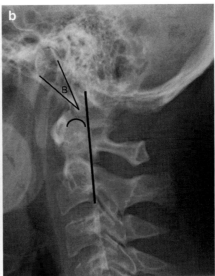

Fig. 3.17 Measurements for the assessment of appropriate craniocervical alignment on lateral radiograph (**a**, *unmarked* and **b**, *annotated*). The black line represents the posterior axial line drawn along the posterior aspect of the C2 vertebral body and dens. The tip of the clivus (basion, B) is outlined in black. The distance from the basion to the posterior axial line is the basion-axial interval (BAI) and should not exceed 12 mm. The distance from the basion to the tip of the dens (outlined with *curved black line*) is the basion-dental interval (BDI) and should not exceed 12 mm. Increased distances indicate craniocervical instability

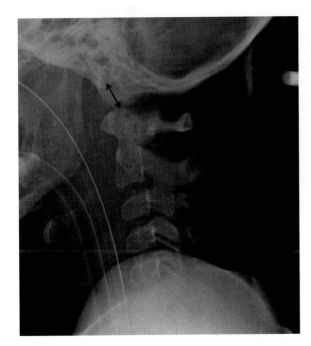

Fig. 3.18 Seven-year old with craniocervical dissociation. Note the significant distance between the clivus and the tip of the dens (double arrow), and the frank dislocation of the occipital condyles from their normal articulation with the lateral masses of C1. (Images courtesy of Dr. David Symonds, Denver Health Medical Center, Denver, CO)

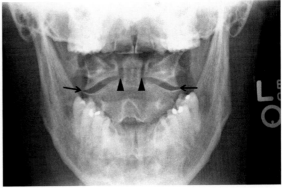

Fig. 3.19 The lateral masses of C1 should be scrutinized for symmetric articulation with C2 (*arrows*) and the distance between the dens and the lateral masses of C1 should be symmetric (*arrowheads*). Asymmetry of the C1/C2 articular distance can be caused by rotation. The occipital condyles are suboptimally evaluated due to overlying incisors

Type I: axial load mechanism, without instability, treated with bracing

Type II: skull base fracture that propagates into the condyles, usually stable and treated with bracing

Type III: avulsion fracture by alar ligament, unstable, and require rigid fixation (Fig. 3.8)

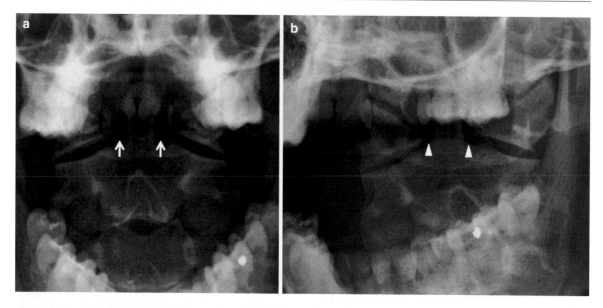

Fig. 3.20 Open-mouth odontoid view in neutral position (**a**) shows symmetric distance between the lateral masses of C1 and the C2 dens (*arrows*). Open-mouth odontoid view with head turned to the right produces slight asymmetry (**b**, *arrowheads*)

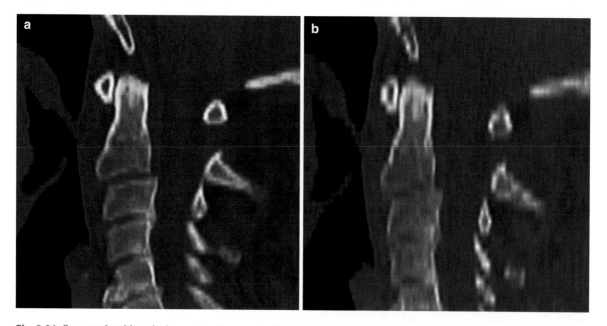

Fig. 3.21 Same study with sagittal reconstructions made with (**a**) 1 mm slices and (**b**) 3 mm slices. It is imperative that reconstructions are made from thin source images

3.4.2.2 Axial Load: Jefferson Burst Fracture

Jefferson burst fracture (JBF) is a result of a direct axial load on the atlas, causing a bursting of the C1 ring. The C1 ring cannot fracture in a single location – like trying to break only one point in a pretzel – the ring must fracture in at least two places. The classic JBF has two fracture points anteriorly and two fracture points posteriorly,

at the margins of the lateral masses with the C1 body. However, this pattern is less common and fractures can occur in diverse patterns, with the end result being radial displacement of the lateral masses.

This injury is an important plain film diagnosis, and has findings on both the lateral and open-mouth odontoid views. On the lateral view, there are common clues to aid in the diagnosis to include: (1) prevertebral soft

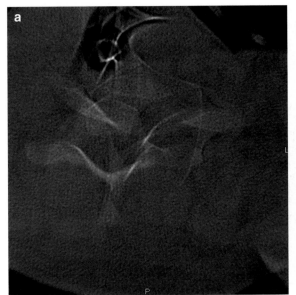

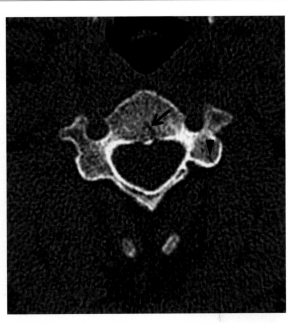

Fig. 3.23 Vascular channel in a typical location at the point of coalescence of the vertebral body venous plexus (*arrow*) and within the left lateral mass (*arrowhead*). Vascular channels can occur anywhere and can be mistaken for fractures if care is not taken

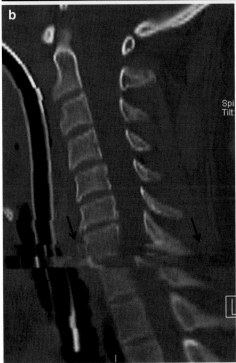

Fig. 3.22 (a) Axial CT image showing excessive motion artifact. (b) Any motion artifact on source images is propagated through all reconstructed images (*arrows*)

tissue swelling (Fig. 3.24a) (2) posterior displacement of the C1 portion of the spinolaminar line (Fig. 3.24a) and (3) direct visualization of the posterior fracture line. On open-mouth odontoid view, the lateral masses are directly visualized displacing radially from the C2 peg . The lateral mass articulations are offset and the

distance between the C1 lateral mass and the C2 peg is increased (Fig. 3.24b).

The majority of JBF injuries are stable and are treated with halo or brace fixation. There is evidence to suggest that the degree of displacement of the lateral masses has implications regarding the stability of the fracture. The "Rule of Spence" states that a combined overhang of C1 lateral masses on C2 of 7 mm suggests transverse ligament disruption, a potentially unstable situation, perhaps requiring surgical rigid fixation. Acutely traumatic anterior atlantodental interval (AADI) >3 mm has also been shown to be a secondary sign of transverse ligament disruption.

3.4.2.3 Axial Load: Cervical Burst Fracture

Cervical burst fractures are rare, but compared to their thoracolumbar counterparts, are more commonly associated with neurologic deficits (Fig. 3.25). In a series of 169 burst fractures, 15 were located in the cervical spine and all involved C5, C6, or C7 (JBFs excluded). Interestingly, 26% of all the burst fractures associated with sporting injury were cervical and sporting injury mechanism accounted for 40% of the cervical spine burst fractures [8].

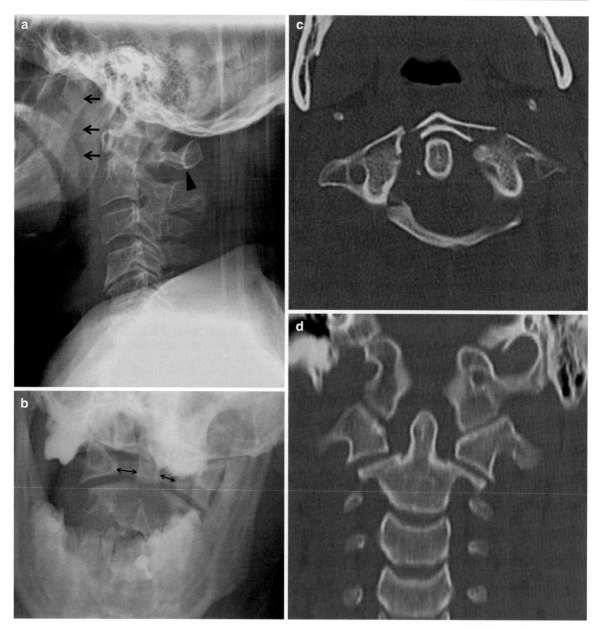

Fig. 3.24 C1 burst fracture (Jefferson burst fracture) on lateral radiograph (**a**) showing anterior PVST swelling (*arrows*) and slight posterior displacement of the C1 contribution to the spinolaminar line (*arrowhead*). Open-mouth odontoid view (**b**) shows radial displacement of the articular pillars of C1 (*double headed arrows*). These findings are confirmed on axial CT (**c**) and coronal reconstruction (**d**)

3.4.2.4 Hyperflexion: Hyperflexion Sprain

Hyperflexion sprain results in injury to the extensive ligamentous complex of the posterior and middle columns of the cervical spine. These structures include the posterior interspinous ligament, the ligamentum flavum, facet joint capsule, PLL, and variable involvement of the dorsal disc annulus and disc. The radiographic findings can be subtle but should not be overlooked. This ligamentous injury can produce cord injury acutely, or subsequently result in chronic instability predisposing to neuropathy from repetitive cord damage.

Radiographic findings (Fig. 3.26) include: (1) focal widening of the interspinous distance at the level of

Fig. 3.25 Lateral cervical radiograph (**a**) component of the "Big 3" upon arrival at the Emergency Department shows height loss of the C5 and C6 vertebral bodies. The bursting type C5 fracture was confirmed with CT as demonstrated on coronal and sagittal reconstructions (**b, c**) with radial displacement of C5 fracture fragments. Lateral displacement is best demonstrated on coronal reconstructions, with posterior displacement seen on sagittal reconstruction (*arrowhead*)

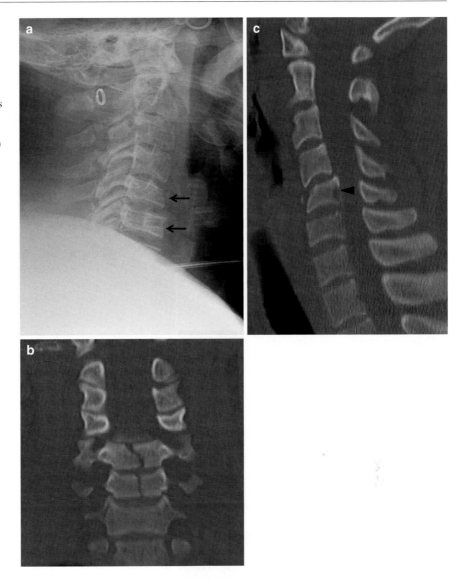

injury (2) acute kyphosis with the narrowing of the anterior disc space and widening of the posterior disc space (3) uncovering of the facets (4) and variable degrees of anterior subluxation. Anterior subluxation is usually less than 3 mm if present. This injury can be radiographically occult in neutral position and is the basis of including flexion/extension radiographs in the traumatized patient. It has been suggested, however, that muscle spasm associated with acute injury can brace the spine sufficiently to hide signs of ligamentous instability. As a result, bracing of a patient with persistent neck pain, without visible fracture, with flexion and extension radiographs obtained 7–10 days

later, after the muscle spasm has resolved, has been advocated to "uncover" occult ligamentous hyperflexion sprain injuries. The acute kyphosis of hyperflexion sprain is usually discernable from the smooth kyphotic curvature related to the presence of the ubiquitous cervical collar (Fig. 3.12).

Similar to radiographs, CT can show the sequelae of hyperflexion sprain. CT lacks sufficient soft tissue contrast to confidently assess ligamentous disruption directly (Fig. 3.26b). MRI can provide direct visualization of the injured structures, with edema present within the broad interspinous ligament and discontinuity of the ligamentum flavum and PLL (Fig. 3.26c).

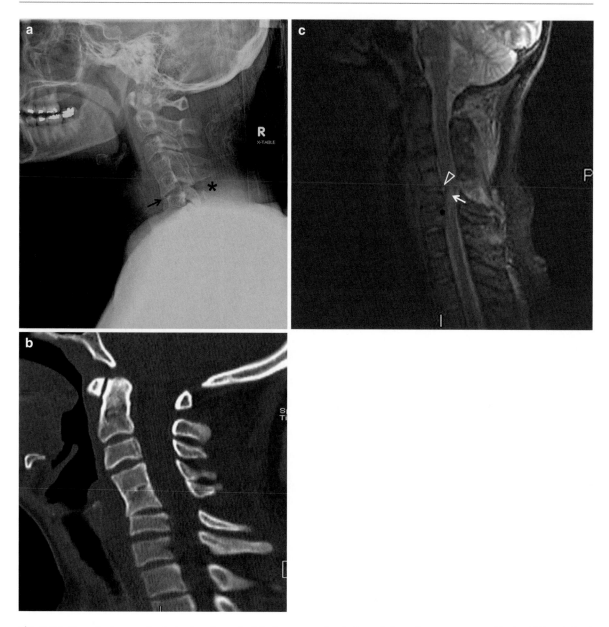

Fig. 3.26 Hyperflexion sprain. Lateral radiograph (**a**) shows focal kyphosis (*arrow*) and splaying of the spinous processes (*asterisk*) at C5/C6 below the level of previous cervical fusion at C4/C5. Subsequent CT with sagittal reconstruction (**b**) confirmed kyphosis, widening of the posterior C5/C6 disc space, and splaying of the spinous processes. Sagittal T2 weighted MRI (**c**) demonstrates severe hyperflexion injury with disruption of the interspinous ligament, ligamentum flavum, and posterior longitudinal ligament (PLL) (*white arrowhead*) with cord injury (*white arrow*)

3.4.2.5 Hyperflexion: Bilateral Facet Dislocation

Bilateral facet dislocation (BFD) is a more severe form of hyperflexion sprain, with greater hyperflexion injury resulting in bilateral facet capsule disruption, facet dislocation, and anterior subluxation of the more cephalic vertebral body by approximately 50% the vertebral body width (Fig. 3.27). The inferior articulating facets of the more cephalic vertebral body come to rest either anterior to the superior articulating processes of the caudal vertebral body or are perched on top of them. When the facets become "perched," acute kyphotic angle is commonly present. Complete dislocation and anterior translation results in greater anterolisthesis and less kyphosis. Small chip fractures are commonly present on CT, but these are usually radiographically occult and clinically insignificant compared to the ligamentous, capsular, and spinal cord injury.

This injury is usually conspicuous on initial trauma lateral imaging (if the level is visible) but the necessity of further imaging is controversial. There is a relatively high incidence of acute traumatic disk herniation accompanying BFD, and closed reduction in these patients can exacerbate or instigate neurologic compromise. Some have advocated MRI of these patients prior to reduction to exclude the presence of a large disk herniation. Others attempt closed reduction on alert patients, with MRI to follow, and obtain MRI on obtunded patients prior to reduction. The choice of MRI imaging in these patients may be related to the emergent availability of MRI, as the closed reduction of these injuries is going to be beneficial in the majority of patients and risk of unreduced unstable injury may outweigh the risk of reduction in cases where MRI is not readily obtainable.

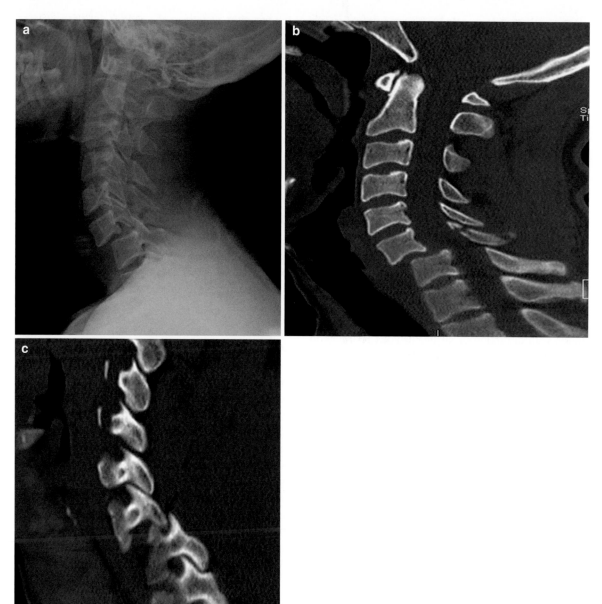

Fig. 3.27 Bilateral facet dislocation (BFD). Lateral radiograph showing bilateral jumped facets at C6/C7 with anterior translation of C6 by approximately 50%. Sagittal reconstructions of the CT cervical spine confirm the diagnosis demonstrating subluxation (**b**) and bilateral perched facets (**c, d** *black arrows*). Axial CT source image (**e**) also demonstrates the jumped inferior articulating processes of C6 (*white arrows*) anterior to the superior articulating processes of C7 (*white arrowheads*)

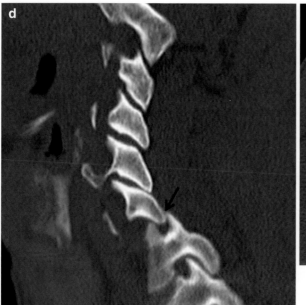

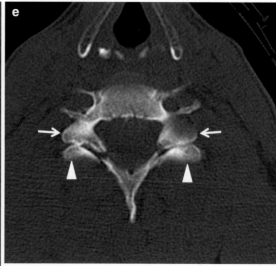

Fig. 3.27 (continued)

3.4.2.6 Hyperflexion: Hyperflexion Teardrop

This catastrophic injury is the result of severe hyperflexion and comminuted fracture of the cervical vertebral body. It is, by definition, associated with acute anterior cervical cord syndrome with complete quadriplegia with intact posterior cord sensations. This is a three column injury, with disruption of all ligamentous restraints to the cervical spine. The two segments of the disrupted cervical spine then move independently of each other, resulting in severe cord injury. Radiographic findings (Fig. 3.28) include: (1) triangular facture fragment donated by the anteroinferior aspect of the affected vertebral body in line with the more inferior cervical spine, (2) retropulsion of the affected vertebral body into the spinal canal, maintaining alignment with the more superior cervical spine, (3) focal and acute kyphosis, and (4) fanning of the spinous processes at the affected level.

3.4.2.7 Hyperflexion: Wedge Compression Fracture

This injury usually presents with mild impaction to the superior endplate of the affected vertebral body and can be stable, if the PLL is intact. When it accompanies signs of hyperflexion sprain, the risk of delayed instability with interspinous and PLL involvement may require MRI confirmation and surgical stabilization of the ligamentous injury. Radiographic findings consist of anterior superior endplate compression with less than 25% loss of vertebral body height. Small ventral cortical buckle fracture is commonly seen along with prevertebral soft tissue swelling.

3.4.2.8 Hyperflexion: Clay Shoveler's Fracture

The clay shoveler's fracture is an avulsion of the spinous process of a low cervical vertebral body. T1 is commonly involved as well. This results from hyperflexion and subsequent tensioning of the interspinous ligament. The name comes from Australian clay shovelers who would dig their shovel into dense clay which would become stuck, forcing the necks of the workers into acute hyperflexion with downward traction on the shoulder girdle. The clay shoveler's fracture has an oblique horizontal orientation (Fig. 3.29). Common anatomic variations including unfused apophysis and ossification of ligamentum nuchae (Fig. 3.29b) can be commonly confused with this injury.

3.4.2.9 Hyperflexion with Rotation: Unilateral Facet Dislocation

Unilateral facet dislocation (UFD) requires hyperflexion as well as rotation. This results in the disruption of

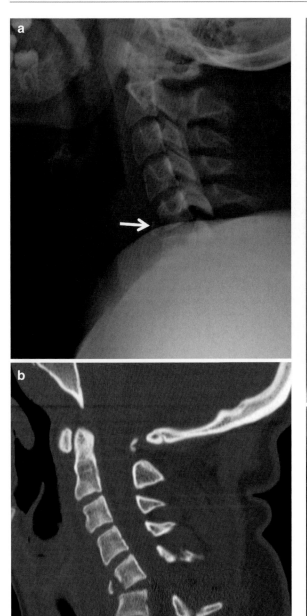

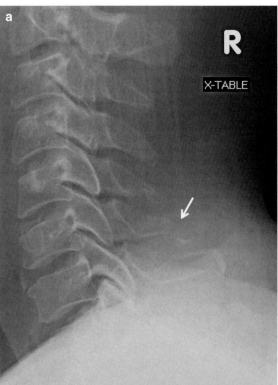

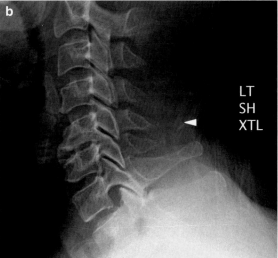

Fig. 3.29 Clay shoveler's fracture of C6 (**a**, *white arrow*). This hyperflexion injury can be mimicked by unfused spinous process apophysis (not pictured) and ligamentum nuchae ossification (**b**, *arrowhead*)

Fig. 3.28 C5 flexion teardrop fracture on lateral radiograph (**a**) and sagittal reconstruction (**b**). The anterior inferior fracture fragment (*white arrow*) of the C5 vertebral body has retained relatively normal orientation with the subjacent vertebral body. Posterior subluxation of C5 and acute kyphosis indicates complete disruption of all supporting ligamentous structures and results in acute cord syndrome. This patient presented with acute quadraparesis. (Images courtesy of Dr. David Symonds, Denver Health Medical Center, Denver, CO)

the interspinous ligament, unilateral facet capsule disruption, ligamentum flavum injury and PLL injury. The inferiorly articulating facet of the affected side (contralateral to the direction of rotational force) is displaced, coming to rest anterior to the superior articulating facet of the caudal vertebral body. This causes

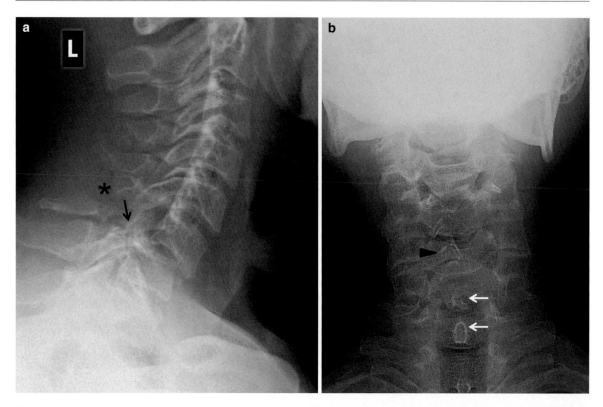

Fig. 3.30 Unilateral facet dislocation (UFD). Lateral radiograph demonstrating approximately 25% anterolisthesis of C6 on C7 associated with right sided UFD. The inferior articulating facet of C6 (*arrow*) is projecting anterior to the superior articulating facet of C7. On AP radiograph (**b**), there is commonly a rotational component with lateral rotation of the affected level spinous process relative to the level below. In this patient, the rotational component is less conspicuous as there is a C6 spinous process fracture (**a**, *asterisk*), with C6 spinous process remaining in anatomic location with regard to C7 (*white arrows*). The C5 spinous process (*black arrowhead*) is slightly rotated compared to the position of C6 and C7 spinous processes

narrowing of the ipsilateral neural foramen and may cause radicular symptoms. Spinal cord injury is rare [75]. The position of the facets results in a stable position, invoking the moniker "locked facets".

Radiographic findings in UFD (Fig. 3.30) include: (1) focal kyphosis at the affected level (2) widening of the interspinous distance (3) anterolisthesis of 25–50% of the vertebral body width (4) superimposition of the facets causing a "bowtie" appearance (5) focal narrowing of the laminar space on lateral view and offset of the spinous processes on the AP view. CT may be useful to evaluate for adjacent level fracture. MRI is indicated if patient is exhibiting neurologic symptoms.

3.4.2.10 Hyperextension: Dens Fractures

Dens fractures occur from diverse mechanisms with hyperextension being one of them. For the sake of simplicity, these fractures are included in the hyperextension group, but hyperextension is clearly not a necessity to cause dens fractures. Anderson and D'Alonso [2] described three types of dens fractures. Type I involves the superior tip of the dens and is thought to be an alar ligament avulsion. This implies craniocervical instability with disruption of the "check" ligament and should be treated as an unstable fracture. This fracture may be visible in the open-mouth odontoid view, but CT is commonly required to separate this injury from an accessory ossification center (Fig. 3.31).

Type II fracture is a transverse fracture of the base of the dens, without significant extension into the C2 vertebral body. This is the most common of the dens fractures (Fig. 3.32). The degree of displacement has been submitted as predictive of the rate of nonunion with the greatest rates of nonunion occurring with the displacement of the fractured C2 peg greater than 6 mm [35]. The type II dens fracture is commonly visualized on open-mouth odontoid, but overlying mach lines from the occiput or the teeth can simulate a fracture (Fig. 3.33). Prevertebral

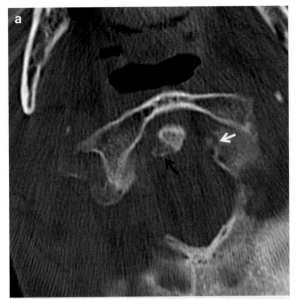

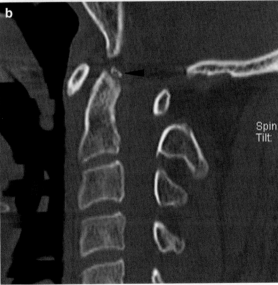

Fig. 3.31 Type I dens fracture. Axial CT image is degraded by streak artifact from dental hardware, but a small avulsion fracture is demonstrated off the right aspect of the dens tip (a, *arrow*). Left alar ligament avulsion fracture is demonstrated from the occipital condyle (*white arrow*). Sagittal CT reconstruction (b) shows the small dens tip avulsion (*arrowhead*)

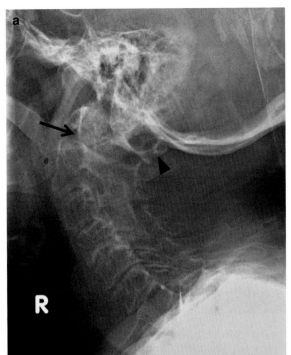

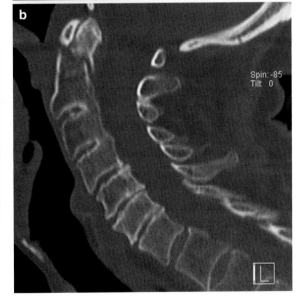

Fig. 3.32 Type II dens fracture. Lateral trauma radiograph (a) demonstrates fracture line at the base of the dens (*arrow*) with posterior displacement of the C1/C2 dens complex causing posterior displacement of the C1 posterior elements and discontinuity of the spinolaminar line (*arrowhead*). (b)Sagittal CT reconstruction confirms the diagnosis

soft tissues are usually abnormal in the setting of an acute C2 fracture. The axial orientation of this fracture was the source of missed injuries on initial experience with CT for cervical spine injury, and prompted the recommendation that all CT cervical spines be accompanied by a radiographic cervical spine series. With the more widespread use of MDCT with excellent sagittal and coronal reconstructions, the risk of missing this fracture is no

longer real and, in the presence of a good quality CT of the cervical spine, the need for radiographs is obviated.

Type III fracture (Fig. 3.34) involves the base of the dens with extension into the vertebral body. These

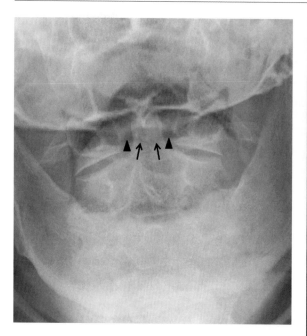

Fig. 3.33 Mach line form the superimposed occiput, traversing the dens can simulate fracture to the untrained eye (*arrows*). Note the extension of the linear lucency outside the osseous confines of the dens (*arrowheads*)

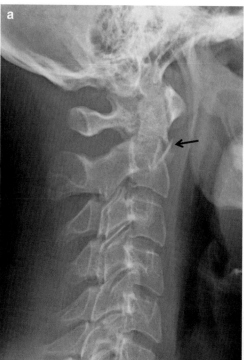

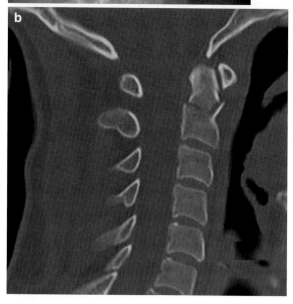

Fig. 3.34 Type III dens fracture. Lateral radiograph shows fracture of the ventral cortex of C2 (**a**, *arrow*) with prevertebral soft tissue swelling. Anterolisthesis of C2 dens is mild with associated discontinuity of the spinolaminar line. Sagittal CT reconstruction confirms extension of fracture into the body of C2

have variable conspicuity on radiographs, but prevertebral soft tissues are usually distended. Open-mouth odontoid views are very useful, but mach lines from occiput or teeth, or residual physis, can cause false positive results. The "fat C2" sign [76] can be a useful tool in occult fractures (Fig. 3.35a), but is nonspecific, and can be present with any type of C2 body fracture. CT is confirmatory. Type III injuries are commonly treated nonoperatively as the rate of nonunion is much lower compared to type II fractures.

3.4.2.11 Hyperextension: Hangman's Fracture

Traumatic spondylolysis of C2 is the second most common fracture to involve the C2 vertebral body. The mechanism involves traumatic forceful head extension and axial loading, overloading the posterior elements of C2 and resulting in vertical bilateral C2 pars interarticularis fractures. This was described as the mechanism of injury for death related to hanging [74], thus acquiring the exciting moniker of Hangman's fracture. More accurately, it would be termed the Hangedman's fracture, but in reality, death by judicial hanging probably occurs from a variety of mechanisms.

Radiographic visualization of this injury is usually in the lateral projection, with the orientation of the fracture line making the injury occult on the open-mouth odontoid or AP view of the cervical spine. The fat C2 sign is

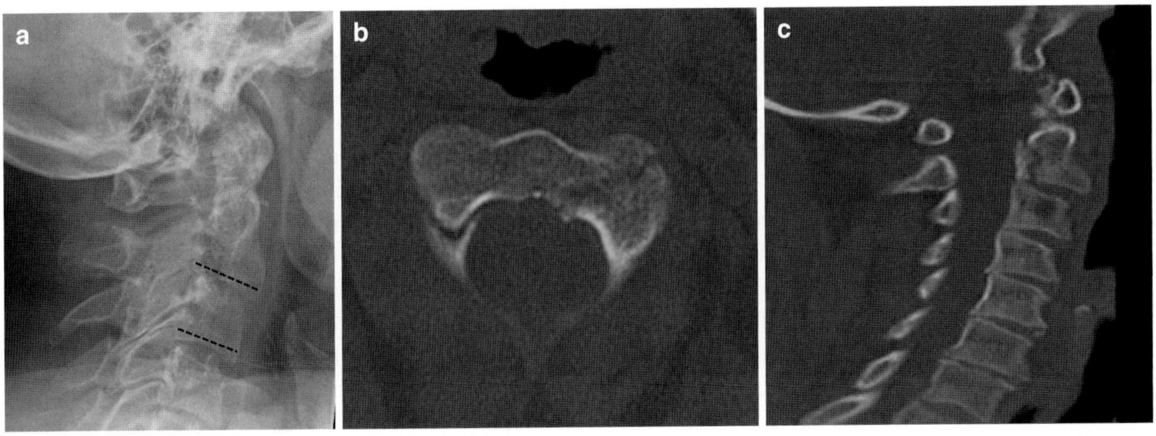

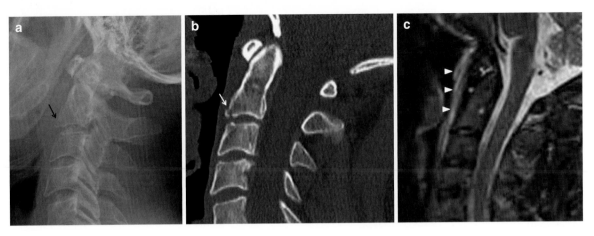

Fig. 3.35 Fat C2 sign associated with traumatic spondylolysis of C2 (Hangedman's fracture). Lateral radiograph (**a**) shows the AP diameter of the C2 vertebral body to be greater than that of C3 (*dashed lines*). C2 pars and body fractures confirmed on axial CT (**b**) and sagittal CT reconstruction (**c**)

useful (Fig. 3.35). On the lateral view, there is commonly posterior displacement of the posterior elements of C2, resulting in spinolaminar line discontinuity at the C2 level. The vertical fracture line can be difficult to appreciate depending on the degree of displacement.

In a retrospective review of 142 patients with C2 ring fractures, Effendi et al. proposed a classification that has implications regarding the treatment of these injuries. Type I injuries were nondisplaced fractures, treated with splinting. Type II fractures demonstrated displacement of fracture fragments >3 mm, and extension or flexion tilt to the C2 vertebral body indicating disruption of the C2/C3 disc. These injuries were treated with halo stabilization with the majority healing without surgical intervention. Type III injuries were displaced fractures with a jumped C2 facet. These injuries are generally treated surgically.

Acute neurologic deficit in type I and II injuries are rare due to the autodecompression of the spinal canal. Type III injuries can be neurologically impaired due to spinal cord injury.

3.4.2.12 Hyperextension: Hyperextension Teardrop

Hyperextension teardrop is an avulsion fracture of the ALL resulting from excessive hyperextensive traction mechanism. This most commonly occurs at the anterior inferior margin of C2 in osteoporotic elderly patients and is not commonly associated with neurologic dysfunction in this patient population (Fig. 3.36).

Fig. 3.36 Hyperextension teardrop fracture of C2. Lateral radiograph (**a**) shows the small avulsion fracture fragment from the anterior inferior vertebral body of C2 (*arrow*). Sagittal CT reconstruction (**b**) confirms the small fracture fragment and subsequent sagittal STIR MR sequence (**c**) suggests anterior ligamentous injury with edema of the prevertebral soft tissues (*arrowhead*)

In the younger patient, with normal osseous integrity, the forces required to cause this injury are much greater. The injury, typically occurring in the lower cervical spine, is accompanied by significant prevertebral soft tissue swelling, and central cord syndrome in 80% [52].

The fracture is well seen on the lateral radiograph, and has a characteristic morphology, with the vertical height of the fracture fragment equal to, or greater, than the horizontal component of the fracture. Flexion teardrop fracture fragments are generally larger and associated with focal kyphosis.

3.4.2.13 Hyperextension: Hyperextension Avulsion of Anterior Arch of C1

The ALL attaches on the anterior tubercle of the C1. Hyperextension results in a horizontally oriented fracture isolated to the anterior arch of C1. On radiographs, this injury is typically associated with prevertebral soft tissue swelling and is apparent on the lateral view. The injury is commonly occult on AP or open-mouth odontoid views.

3.4.2.14 Hyperextension: Hyperextension Sprain/Fracture Dislocation

Hyperextension mechanism can result in variable soft tissue and osseous injury depending on the magnitude of force. Hyperextension sprain is isolated injury to the ALL without avulsion fracture. Radiographically, this can manifest as subtle widening of the anterior disc space, with the diagnosis easily made by direct visualization of the disrupted ALL on MRI (Fig. 3.37).

If the magnitude of hyperextensive force is sufficient, ligamentous injury can extend through all the vertebral stabilizing structures with disruption of the ALL, disc at the level of injury, tear of the PLL, and disruption of the ligamentum flavum. The interspinous ligament is compressed and usually not torn due to the hyperextension mechanism of injury. Osseous components to include teardrop avulsion fracture of the anterior inferior vertebral body and posterior element fractures associated with posterior element compressive force may be demonstrated on radiographs or CT. The severity of this injury is commonly underestimated on radiography. In the setting of neurologic deficit, MRI should be used to accurately characterize the degree of ligamentous disruption as well as the presence of spinal cord injury.

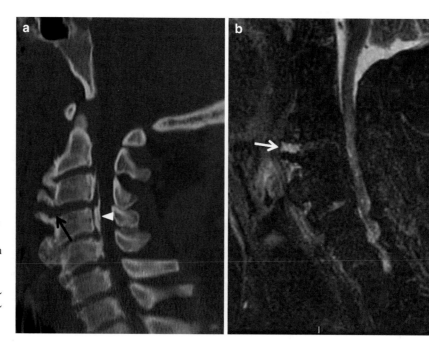

Fig. 3.37 Hyperextension sprain injury. Sagittal CT reconstruction (**a**) shows slight anterior widening of the C3/C4 disc space (*arrow*) with prevertebral soft tissue (PVST) swelling. Ossification of the PLL is also noted (*white arrowhead*). Sagittal STIR sequence confirms ALL injury with edema of the ALL at the C3/C4 level (*arrowhead*)

Hyperextension fracture dislocation is much more common in the noncompliant ankylotic spine in patients with ankylosing spondylitis and DISH (Fig. 3.7).

3.5 Injury to the Thoracic and Lumbar Spine

3.5.1 Indications for Imaging

Fractures of the thoracic and lumbar spines are exceedingly common, predominantly occurring in the elderly patient population as pathologic wedge compression deformities of osteoporotic vertebral bodies. Osteoporotic wedge compression fractures rarely require more than a radiograph for initial evaluation. Subsequent workup may include MRI or bone scan to assess for continued micromotion in workup prior to percutaneous treatment with fractureplasty, but rarely is advanced imaging necessary in the acute setting.

In trauma patients, thoracic and lumbar spinal fractures commonly accompany trauma to the thorax, abdomen, and pelvis. The indications for dedicated thoracolumbar spinal imaging in the acutely traumatized patients have not been studied as extensively as those for cervical spine imaging. It is clear that the prevalence of thoracolumbar spinal fractures in patients with high mechanism trauma is significant, and this has prompted the advocacy of liberal imaging of the thoracolumbar spine. The mechanism is largely the one of acute deceleration with the majority of thoracolumbar spinal fractures being attributed to either falls or motor vehicle collisions [31, 58, 69, 71, 72, 79, 82].

In a retrospective review of their trauma database, as well as a review of the literature, Hsu et al. arrived at the following recommendations for imaging the thoracolumbar spine: (1) back pain or midline tenderness (2) local signs of thoracolumbar injury (3) abnormal neurological signs (4) cervical spine fracture (5) GCS <15 (6) major distracting injury and (7) alcohol or drug intoxication.

The utility of radiographic screening of the thoracolumbar spine is high in the pediatric population but drops in the adult population. With the widespread use of MDCT, reformatted spine images are easily acquired from CT studies of the chest, abdomen, and pelvis. The indications for thoracolumbar spinal imaging overlap with those for imaging of the chest, abdomen, and pelvis for routine trauma evaluations, so attention to the spine should be high in these patients, and sagittal and coronal reconstructions should be included in the routine postprocessing of trauma patients.

The need for whole spine screening in patients with confirmed spinal fracture has been advocated given the high incidence of noncontiguous level involvement. MRI may be necessary in patients with neurological symptoms. Isolated ligamentous injury in the thoracolumbar spine in the absence of fracture is extremely uncommon.

3.5.2 Concept of Thoracic and Lumbar Fracture Stability

The three column concept of thoracolumbar spinal stability put forth by Francis Denis, is a simple and effective model for classifying potentially unstable fractures. Denis submitted a three column model and proposed that two column involvement is necessary for instability (Fig. 3.38). The anterior column consists of the anterior half of the vertebral body, the ALL, and the anterior half of the annulus fibrosis. The middle column consists of

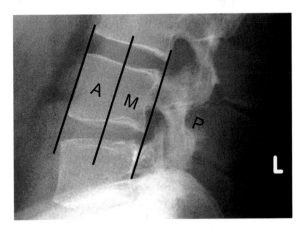

Fig. 3.38 Columns of Denis. The anterior column (A) consists of the ALL and the anterior half of the annulus fibrosis. The middle column (M) consists of the posterior half of the annulus fibrosis and the PLL. The posterior column (P) consists of the posterior osseous neural arch, the ligamentum flavum, facet joint capsule, and the interspinous ligament

the posterior margin of the vertebral body, the PLL, and the posterior half of the annulus fibrosis. The posterior column consists of the posterior neural osseous arch and the posterior ligamentous complex to include the ligamentum flavum, the facet capsule, and the interspinous ligament [29].

For additional discussion on spine stability, please refer to chapters 5, 18, and 22.

3.5.3 Wedge Compression Fracture

Wedge compression fracture results from hyperflexion force overcoming the integrity of the anterior half of the vertebral body. Depending on the degree of force applied, the middle and posterior column can be involved. Radiographic hallmarks for instability have been proposed by Daffner et al. They include: (1) displacement/translation of >2 mm (2) widening of the interspinous space, facet joints, or interpediculate distance (3) disruption of the posterior vertebral body line (4) widened vertebral canal (5) vertebral body height loss >50% and (6) kyphosis >20°.

Simple wedge compression fracture results in less than 50% loss of anterior vertebral body height and is considered a stable fracture if the middle column is not involved (Fig. 3.39). However, the ability of radiography to accurately exclude second column involvement has been shown to be poor [5, 21]. The involvement of the middle column has prognostic and treatment implications and CT has thus been advocated to make this important distinction.

Severe wedge compression fracture with >50% anterior vertebral body height loss implies middle column involvement [26]. CT of wedge compression fractures is necessary to accurately characterize the extent and assess stability.

3.5.4 Burst Fracture

Burst fracture is due to an axially compressive force overcoming the integrity of the vertebral body. This results in first and second column involvement. However, the instability of the two column burst fracture is controversial, but the involvement of the posterior column significantly affects the clinical treatment and outcome.

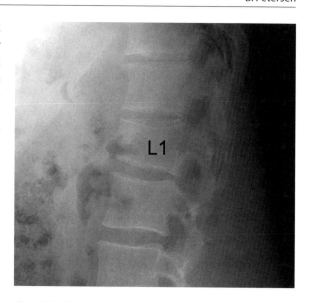

Fig. 3.39 Simple wedge compression fracture of L1. Lateral radiograph shows mild anterior wedging of the L1 vertebral body with approximately 20% vertebral body height loss. This is likely a stable compression deformity, but radiographic sensitivity for middle column involvement is low

Neurologic deficits result from retropulsion of osseous fragments and CT is necessary to accurately quantify central spinal canal narrowing resulting from retropulsed fragments.

Radiographic signs of burst fracture include: (1) significant loss of vertebral body height loss on both the lateral and AP projections (2) widening of the interpediculate distance on the AP radiograph and (3) indistinctness of the posterior vertebral body cortex on lateral view (Fig. 3.40).

CT of burst fractures is useful to evaluate the degree of spinal canal compromise. The AP diameter of the spinal canal above and below the level of fracture is used to obtain an average. The AP diameter of the spinal canal at the injured level is then divided into this denominator to arrive at a percentage canal narrowing. CT is also important for the assessment of the posterior elements as the degree of instability of burst fractures increases with third column involvement. The presence of a sagittally oriented laminar fracture is an important finding as it has been associated with the presence of a dural tear. Burst fractures in the presence of a dural tear have a high incidence of neurologic deficits and require a posterior approach and repair of the dura prior to surgical reduction and fixation (Fig. 3.41).

Fig. 3.40 T12 burst fracture. Lateral radiograph (**a**) demonstrates significant anterior wedging of the T12 vertebral body (*arrow*) with anterior height loss of approximately 70%. Dorsal margin of the vertebral body is indistinct and displaced posteriorly (*black arrowheads*). Frontal radiograph (**b**) confirms burst fracture with widening of the interpediculate distance (*double headed arrow*). Axial CT (**c**) more accurately assesses the degree of spinal canal narrowing by posterior displaced burst fracture fragment (*white arrowheads*), with 50% canal compromise

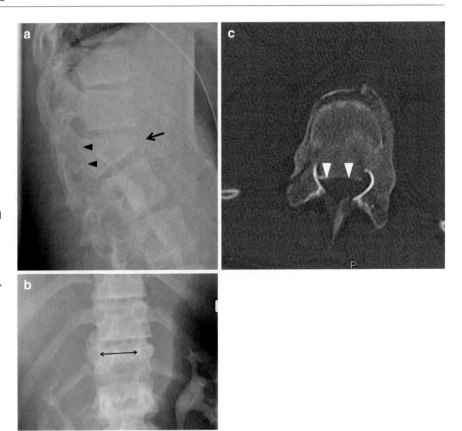

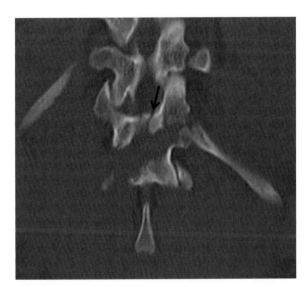

Fig. 3.41 Coronal CT reconstruction shows a vertically oriented laminar fracture. Vertical laminar fracture associated with T12 burst fracture has a high incidence of dural tear (*arrow*)

3.5.5 Chance Fracture

The thoracolumbar junction (T12–L2) is an area that is particular vulnerable to injury. Approximately, two-thirds of all spine injuries occur in this region [61]. This segment represents a transition from the relatively stiff thoracic spine to the more mobile lumbar segment. The Chance fracture occurs exclusively at the thoracolumbar junction and is a unique spinal injury deserving special consideration.

Chance fracture (Fig. 3.42) is due to hyperflexion at the thoracolumbar junction and is characterized by a distraction of the posterior and middle columns with compression fracture of the anterior column. This was prevalent in motor vehicle collisions with victims wearing only a lap belt, where the anterior abdominal wall served as the fulcrum, but the incidence has decreased with the advent and widespread use of the shoulder harness component of seatbelts.

Radiographically, the classic Chance fracture includes a distracted fracture of the pedicles, transverse processes, and spinous process with horizontal fracture through the

Fig. 3.42 L1 Chance fracture with extension of injury through all three columns. Lateral radiograph (**a**) demonstrates the focal kyphosis with fracture of L1 (*arrow*). Axial (**b**) and sagittal (**c**) CT confirms the line of force extending through the posterior elements and the marked spinal canal compromise. Sagittal T2 weighted MRI (**d**) shows complete disruption of the PLL (*white arrow*), and edema in the interspinous space and dorsal soft tissue hematoma (*asterisk*)

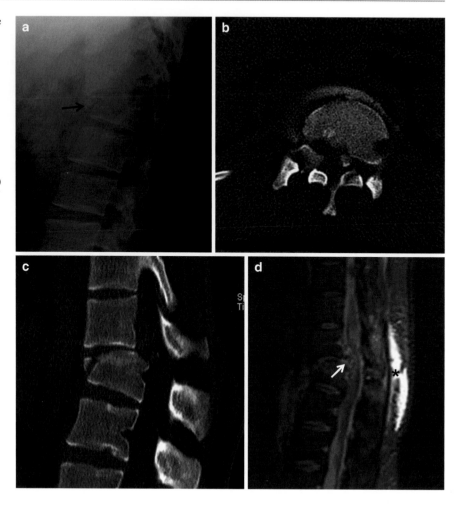

vertebral body. The middle column may be spared as the center of spinal hyperflexion rotation. On radiographs, the anterior compression injury to the vertebral body is visible on the lateral view as is the distraction of the posterior elements. Depending on the degree of fragment displacement, pedicle fractures and spinous process fractures can be demonstrated on the lateral view as well. On the AP view, transverse fracture through the pedicles and transverse processes are commonly demonstrated. Soft tissue Chance injuries can occur without osseous abnormality, with the line of force directed through the disc space and the ligamentous supports of the posterior column.

Attention must be paid to the high association of intra-abdominal injuries in the setting of osseous or soft tissue Chance injury. The incidence of injury to the mesentery, duodenum, or pancreas has been reported to be as high as 50% [34]. Patients with Chance-type injuries should be imaged with CT, to evaluate both the spinal and intra-abdominal sequelae.

3.6 Conclusion

Imaging of spinal trauma has evolved significantly over the past decades, from radiography and conventional tomography, to MRI and MDCT capable of submillimeter resolution and rapid multiplanar reconstructions. Despite significant technological advancement and extensive research, imaging of the traumatic spine continues to be a difficult problem, with the high incidence of suspected spine trauma and the grave consequences of a missed or delayed diagnosis contributing to the high level of anxiety in dealing with these patients. However, a clear shift in emphasis has occurred over the last 5–10 years. In traumatized adult patients, the high rate of technically inadequate radiographs has emphasized the need for early CT imaging of the spine, saving time and increasing accuracy. Pediatric and elderly patient populations, as well as those patients with noncompliant and ankylotic spines, deserve special consideration. Despite the shift toward cross-sectional imaging, accurate evaluation of radiographs and intimate familiarity of the common injuries and their radiographic manifestations is crucial. A combination of good physical exam, history, and clinical judgement, appropriate and technically excellent imaging, and expert image interpretation continue to be the combination necessary to appropriately manage this challenging patient population.

References

1. Acheson MB, Livingston RR, Richardson ML, Stimac GK (1987) High-resolution CT scanning in the evaluation of cervical spine fractures: comparison with plain film examinations. AJR Am J Roentgenol 148(6):1179–1185
2. Anderson LD, D'Alonzo RT (1974) Fractures of the odontoid process of the axis. J Bone Joint Surg Am 56(8): 1663–1674
3. Anderson PA, Montesano PX (1988) Morphology and treatment of occipital condyle fractures. Spine 13(7):731–736
4. Anderson RC, Kan P, Hansen KW, Brockmeyer DL (2006) Cervical spine clearance after trauma in children. Neurosurg Focus 20(2):E3
5. Ballock RT, Mackersie R, Abitbol JJ, Cervilla V, Resnick D, Garfin SR (1992) Can burst fractures be predicted from plain radiographs? J Bone Joint Surg Br 74(1):147–150
6. Barba CA, Taggert J, Morgan AS et al (2001) A new cervical spine clearance protocol using computed tomography. J Trauma 51(4):652–656, discussion 656–657
7. Bednar DA, Toorani B, Denkers M, Abdelbary H (2004) Assessment of stability of the cervical spine in blunt trauma patients: review of the literature, with presentation and preliminary results of a modified traction test protocol. Can J Surg 47(5):338–342
8. Bensch FV, Koivikko MP, Kiuru MJ, Koskinen SK (2006) The incidence and distribution of burst fractures. Emerg Radiol 12(3):124–129
9. Benzel EC, Hart BL, Ball PA, Baldwin NG, Orrison WW, Espinosa MC (1996) Magnetic resonance imaging for the evaluation of patients with occult cervical spine injury. J Neurosurg 85(5):824–829
10. Berne JD, Velmahos GC, El-Tawil Q et al (1999) Value of complete cervical helical computed tomographic scanning in identifying cervical spine injury in the unevaluable blunt trauma patient with multiple injuries: a prospective study. J Trauma 47(5):896–902, discussion 902–893
11. Biffl WL, Egglin T, Benedetto B, Gibbs F, Cioffi WG (2006) Sixteen-slice computed tomographic angiography is a reliable noninvasive screening test for clinically significant blunt cerebrovascular injuries. J Trauma 60(4):745–751, discussion 751–742
12. Biffl WL, Moore EE, Ryu RK et al (1998) The unrecognized epidemic of blunt carotid arterial injuries: early diagnosis improves neurologic outcome. Ann Surg 228(4):462–470
13. Biffl WL, Moore EE, Elliott JP et al (2000) The devastating potential of blunt vertebral arterial injuries. Ann Surg 231(5):672–681
14. Blackmore CC, Mann FA, Wilson AJ (2000) Helical CT in the primary trauma evaluation of the cervical spine: an evidence-based approach. Skeletal Radiol 29(11):632–639
15. Blackmore CC, Zelman WN, Glick ND (2001) Resource cost analysis of cervical spine trauma radiography. Radiology 220(3):581–587
16. Blackmore CC, Ramsey SD, Mann FA, Deyo RA (1999) Cervical spine screening with CT in trauma patients: a cost-effectiveness analysis. Radiology 212(1):117–125
17. Brandt MM, Wahl WL, Yeom K, Kazerooni E, Wang SC (2004) Computed tomographic scanning reduces cost and time of complete spine evaluation. J Trauma 56(5):1022–1026, discussion 1026–1028
18. Brohi K, Healy M, Fotheringham T et al (2005) Helical computed tomographic scanning for the evaluation of the cervical spine in the unconscious, intubated trauma patient. J Trauma 58(5):897–901
19. Bub LD, Blackmore CC, Mann FA, Lomoschitz FM (2005) Cervical spine fractures in patients 65 years and older: a clinical prediction rule for blunt trauma. Radiology 234(1):143–149
20. Callahan EP, Aguillera H (1993) Complications following minor trauma in a patient with diffuse idiopathic skeletal hyperostosis. Ann Emerg Med 22(6):1067–1070
21. Campbell SE, Phillips CD, Dubovsky E, Cail WS, Omary RA (1995) The value of CT in determining potential instability of simple wedge-compression fractures of the lumbar spine. AJNR Am J Neuroradiol 16(7):1385–1392
22. Cothren CC, Moore EE, Biffl WL et al (2003) Cervical spine fracture patterns predictive of blunt vertebral artery injury. J Trauma 55(5):811–813
23. Daffner RH (2000) Cervical radiography for trauma patients: a time-effective technique? AJR Am J Roentgenol 175(5):1309–1311
24. Daffner RH (2001) Helical CT of the cervical spine for trauma patients: a time study. AJR Am J Roentgenol 177(3):677–679
25. Daffner RH, Hackney DB (2007) ACR Appropriateness Criteria on suspected spine trauma. J Am Coll Radiol 4(11): 762–775
26. Daffner RH, Deeb ZL, Goldberg AL, Kandabarow A, Rothfus WE (1990) The radiologic assessment of post-traumatic vertebral stability. Skeletal Radiol 19(2):103–108
27. Daffner RH, Goldberg A, Evans TC, Hanlon DP, Levy DB (1998) Cervical vertebral injuries in the elderly: a 10-year study. Emerg Radiol 5(1):38–42
28. Davis JW, Kaups KL, Cunningham MA et al (2001) Routine evaluation of the cervical spine in head-injured patients with dynamic fluoroscopy: a reappraisal. J Trauma 50(6):1044–1047
29. Denis F (1983) The three column spine and its significance in the classification of acute thoracolumbar spinal injuries. Spine 8(8):817–831
30. Diaz JJ Jr, Gillman C, Morris JA Jr, May AK, Carrillo YM, Guy J (2003) Are five-view plain films of the cervical spine unreliable? A prospective evaluation in blunt trauma patients with altered mental status. J Trauma 55(4):658–663, discussion 663–654
31. Frankel HL, Rozycki GS, Ochsner MG, Harviel JD, Champion HR (1994) Indications for obtaining surveillance thoracic and lumbar spine radiographs. J Trauma 37(4):673–676

32. Freedman I, van Gelderen D, Cooper DJ et al (2005) Cervical spine assessment in the unconscious trauma patient: a major trauma service's experience with passive flexion-extension radiography. J Trauma 58(6):1183–1188

33. Ghiselli G, Schaadt G, McAllister DR (2003) On-the-field evaluation of an athlete with a head or neck injury. Clin Sports Med 22(3):445–465

34. Green DA, Green NE, Spengler DM, Devito DP (1991) Flexion-distraction injuries to the lumbar spine associated with abdominal injuries. J Spinal Disord 4(3):312–318

35. Greene KA, Dickman CA, Marciano FF, Drabier JB, Hadley MN, Sonntag VK (1997) Acute axis fractures. Analysis of management and outcome in 340 consecutive cases. Spine 22(16):1843–1852

36. Griffiths HJ, Wagner J, Anglen J, Bunn P, Metzler M (2002) The use of forced flexion/extension views in the obtunded trauma patient. Skeletal Radiol 31(10):587–591

37. Grogan EL, Morris JA Jr, Dittus RS et al (2005) Cervical spine evaluation in urban trauma centers: lowering institutional costs and complications through helical CT scan. J Am Coll Surg 200(2):160–165

38. Hanson JA, Mirza S (2000) Predisposition for spinal fracture in ankylosing spondylitis. AJR Am J Roentgenol 174(1):150

39. Hanson JA, Blackmore CC, Mann FA, Wilson AJ (2000) Cervical spine injury: a clinical decision rule to identify high-risk patients for helical CT screening. AJR Am J Roentgenol 174(3):713–717

40. Harris JH Jr, Carson GC, Wagner LK (1994) Radiologic diagnosis of traumatic occipitovertebral dissociation: 1. Normal occipitovertebral relationships on lateral radiographs of supine subjects. AJR Am J Roentgenol 162(4):881–886

41. Herkowitz HN, Rothman RH (1984) Subacute instability of the cervical spine. Spine 9(4):348–357

42. Hernandez JA, Chupik C, Swischuk LE (2004) Cervical spine trauma in children under 5 years: productivity of CT. Emerg Radiol 10(4):176–178

43. Hill SA, Miller CA, Kosnik EJ, Hunt WE (1984) Pediatric neck injuries. A clinical study. J Neurosurg 60(4):700–706

44. Hoffman JR, Mower WR, Wolfson AB, Todd KH, Zucker MI (2000) Validity of a set of clinical criteria to rule out injury to the cervical spine in patients with blunt trauma. National Emergency X-Radiography Utilization Study Group. N Engl J Med 343(2):94–99

45. Hogan GJ, Mirvis SE, Shanmuganathan K, Scalea TM (2005) Exclusion of unstable cervical spine injury in obtunded patients with blunt trauma: is MR imaging needed when multi-detector row CT findings are normal? Radiology 237(1):106–113

46. Holmes JF, Akkinepalli R (2005) Computed tomography versus plain radiography to screen for cervical spine injury: a meta-analysis. J Trauma 58(5):902–905

47. Jonsson H Jr, Bring G, Rauschning W, Sahlstedt B (1991) Hidden cervical spine injuries in traffic accident victims with skull fractures. J Spinal Disord 4(3):251–263

48. Keenan HT, Hollingshead MC, Chung CJ, Ziglar MK (2001) Using CT of the cervical spine for early evaluation of pediatric patients with head trauma. AJR Am J Roentgenol 177(6):1405–1409

49. Kokoska ER, Keller MS, Rallo MC, Weber TR (2001) Characteristics of pediatric cervical spine injuries. J Pediatr Surg 36(1):100–105

50. Kreipke DL, Gillespie KR, McCarthy MC, Mail JT, Lappas JC, Broadie TA (1989) Reliability of indications for cervical spine films in trauma patients. J Trauma 29(10):1438–1439

51. Lee C, Woodring JH, Goldstein SJ, Daniel TL, Young AB, Tibbs PA (1987) Evaluation of traumatic atlantooccipital dislocations. AJNR Am J Neuroradiol 8(1):19–26

52. Lee JS, Harris JH, Mueller CF (1997) The significance of prevertebral soft tissue swelling in extension teardrop fracture of the cervical spine. Emerg Radiol 4(3):132–139

53. Lee SL, Sena M, Greenholz SK, Fledderman M (2003) A multidisciplinary approach to the development of a cervical spine clearance protocol: process, rationale, and initial results. J Pediatr Surg 38(3):358–362, discussion 358–362

54. MacDonald RL, Schwartz ML, Mirich D, Sharkey PW, Nelson WR (1990) Diagnosis of cervical spine injury in motor vehicle crash victims: how many X-rays are enough? J Trauma 30(4):392–397

55. Maroon JC, Bailes JE (1996) Athletes with cervical spine injury. Spine 21(19):2294–2299

56. Mathen R, Inaba K, Munera F et al (2007) Prospective evaluation of multislice computed tomography versus plain radiographic cervical spine clearance in trauma patients. J Trauma 62(6):1427–1431

57. McCulloch PT, France J, Jones DL et al (2005) Helical computed tomography alone compared with plain radiographs with adjunct computed tomography to evaluate the cervical spine after high-energy trauma. J Bone Joint Surg Am 87(11):2388–2394

58. Meldon SW, Moettus LN (1995) Thoracolumbar spine fractures: clinical presentation and the effect of altered sensorium and major injury. J Trauma 39(6):1110–1114

59. Mirvis SE, Diaconis JN, Chirico PA, Reiner BI, Joslyn JN, Militello P (1989) Protocol-driven radiologic evaluation of suspected cervical spine injury: efficacy study. Radiology 170(3 Pt 1):831–834

60. Nguyen GK, Clark R (2005) Adequacy of plain radiography in the diagnosis of cervical spine injuries. Emerg Radiol 11(3):158–161

61. Nicoll EA (1949) Fractures of the dorso-lumbar spine. J Bone Joint Surg Am 31B(3):376–394

62. Nunez DB Jr, Zuluaga A, Fuentes-Bernardo DA, Rivas LA, Becerra JL (1996) Cervical spine trauma: how much more do we learn by routinely using helical CT? Radiographics 16((6):1307–1318, discussion 1318–1321

63. Pang D (2004) Spinal cord injury without radiographic abnormality in children, 2 decades later. Neurosurgery 55(6):1325–1342, discussion 1342–1323

64. Pang D, Wilberger JE Jr (1982) Spinal cord injury without radiographic abnormalities in children. J Neurosurg 57(1):114–129

65. Pech P, Kilgore DP, Pojunas KW, Haughton VM (1985) Cervical spinal fractures: CT detection. Radiology 157(1):117–120

66. Powers B, Miller MD, Kramer RS, Martinez S, Gehweiler JA Jr (1979) Traumatic anterior atlanto-occipital dislocation. Neurosurgery 4(1):12–17

67. Regenbogen VS, Rogers LF, Atlas SW, Kim KS (1986) Cervical spinal cord injuries in patients with cervical spondylosis. AJR Am J Roentgenol 146(2):277–284

68. Reid DC, Henderson R, Saboe L, Miller JD (1987) Etiology and clinical course of missed spine fractures. J Trauma 27(9):980–986

69. Richter D, Hahn MP, Ostermann PA, Ekkernkamp A, Muhr G (1996) Vertical deceleration injuries: a comparative study of the injury patterns of 101 patients after accidental and intentional high falls. Injury 27(9):655–659

70. Rogers WA (1957) Fractures and dislocations of the cervical spine; an end-result study. J Bone Joint Surg Am 39-A(2): 341–376

71. Saboe LA, Reid DC, Davis LA, Warren SA, Grace MG (1991) Spine trauma and associated injuries. J Trauma 31(1):43–48

72. Samuels LE, Kerstein MD (1993) 'Routine' radiologic evaluation of the thoracolumbar spine in blunt trauma patients: a reappraisal. J Trauma 34(1):85–89

73. Schenarts PJ, Diaz J, Kaiser C, Carrillo Y, Eddy V, Morris JA Jr (2001) Prospective comparison of admission computed tomographic scan and plain films of the upper cervical spine in trauma patients with altered mental status. J Trauma 51(4):663–668, discussion 668–669

74. Schneider RC, Livingston KE, Cave AJ, Hamilton G (1965) "Hangman's Fracture" Of The Cervical Spine. J Neurosurg 22:141–154

75. Shapiro S, Snyder W, Kaufman K, Abel T (1999) Outcome of 51 cases of unilateral locked cervical facets: interspinous braided cable for lateral mass plate fusion compared with interspinous wire and facet wiring with iliac crest. J Neurosurg 91(1 Suppl):19–24

76. Smoker WR, Dolan KD (1987) The "fat" C2: a sign of fracture. AJR Am J Roentgenol 148(3):609–614

77. Spivak JM, Weiss MA, Cotler JM, Call M (1994) Cervical spine injuries in patients 65 and older. Spine 19(20): 2302–2306

78. Stabler A, Eck J, Penning R et al (2001) Cervical spine: postmortem assessment of accident injuries–comparison of radiographic, MR imaging, anatomic, and pathologic findings. Radiology 221(2):340–346

79. Stanislas MJ, Latham JM, Porter KM, Alpar EK, Stirling AJ (1998) A high risk group for thoracolumbar fractures. Injury 29(1):15–18

80. Stiell IG, Clement CM, McKnight RD et al (2003) The Canadian C-spine rule versus the NEXUS low-risk criteria in patients with trauma. N Engl J Med 349(26):2510–2518

81. Stiell IG, Wells GA, Vandemheen KL et al (2001) The Canadian C-spine rule for radiography in alert and stable trauma patients. Jama 286(15):1841–1848

82. Terregino CA, Ross SE, Lipinski MF, Foreman J, Hughes R (1995) Selective indications for thoracic and lumbar radiography in blunt trauma. Ann Emerg Med 26(2):126–129

83. Tins BJ, Cassar-Pullicino VN (2004) Imaging of acute cervical spine injuries: review and outlook. Clin Radiol 59(10): 865–880

84. Vandemark RM (1990) Radiology of the cervical spine in trauma patients: practice pitfalls and recommendations for improving efficiency and communication. AJR Am J Roentgenol 155(3):465–472

85. Viccellio P, Simon H, Pressman BD, Shah MN, Mower WR, Hoffman JR (2001) A prospective multicenter study of cervical spine injury in children. Pediatrics 108(2):E20

86. Wackenheim A (1985) Cervico-occipital joint: exercises in radiological diagnosis. Springer-Verlag, New York

87. Widder S, Doig C, Burrowes P, Larsen G, Hurlbert RJ, Kortbeek JB (2004) Prospective evaluation of computed tomographic scanning for the spinal clearance of obtunded trauma patients: preliminary results. J Trauma 56(6):1179–1184

88. Woodring JH, Lee C (1993) Limitations of cervical radiography in the evaluation of acute cervical trauma. J Trauma 34(1):32–39

89. Yngve DA, Harris WP, Herndon WA, Sullivan JA, Gross RH (1988) Spinal cord injury without osseous spine fracture. J Pediatr Orthop 8(2):153–159

90. Young JW, Resnik CS, DeCandido P, Mirvis SE (1989) The laminar space in the diagnosis of rotational flexion injuries of the cervical spine. AJR Am J Roentgenol 152(1):103–107

4.1 Pathophysiology of Spinal Cord Injury (SCI)

4.1.1 Primary SCI

The primary injury to the spinal cord is a result of mechanical forces applied to the bony elements and/or the spinal cord at the time of trauma impact. These forces can lead to translocation of fracture fragments or disk material into the spinal canal, leading to an acute compromise of the spinal canal and potential compression of the spinal cord. Mechanical damage to axons will consecutively alter the physiological flow of electrical signals to target organs, resulting in motor and sensory deficits below the level of injury [28]. However, the posttraumatic axonal and myelin damage is not exclusively related to the severity of the primary SCI. The primary traumatic impact initiates a secondary inflammatory cascade, with potentially detrimental effects on the injured spinal cord.

4.1.2 Secondary SCI

While primary lesions are directly caused by the mechanical impact, secondary SCI is initiated by a delayed host-mediated inflammatory response [28, 41] (Fig. 4.1). Resident spinal cord cells are rapidly activated by the primary injury and initiate an exquisitely orchestrated proinflammatory response, involving numerous inflammatory mediators [28]. The resulting

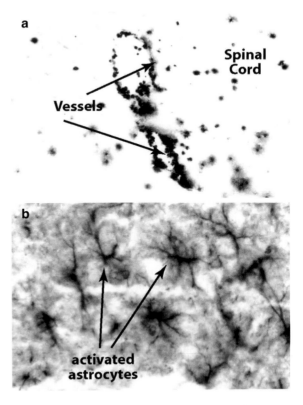

Fig. 4.1 Immunohistochemical staining of perivascular neutrophil infiltration (**a**) and reactive astrocytosis (**b**) in the spinal cord in a rodent model of experimental spinal cord injury

P.F. Stahel (✉) M.A. Flierl A. Dwyer
Department of Orthopaedic Surgery, Denver Health Medical Center, University of Colorado School of Medicine, 777 Bannock Street, Denver, CO 80204, USA
e-mail: philip.stahel@dhha.org

K.M. Beauchamp
Department of Surgery, Division of Neurosurgery, Denver Health Medical Center, University of Colorado School of Medicine, 777 Bannock Street, Denver, CO 80204, USA

V.V. Patel et al. (eds.), *Spine Trauma*,
DOI: 10.1007/978-3-642-03694-1_4, © Springer-Verlag Berlin Heidelberg 2010

chemoattraction induces transmigration of hematogenous inflammatory cells, such as neutrophils, macrophages, and lymphocytes. In conjunction with activated resident cells of the spinal cord, leukocytes subsequently release copious amounts of neurotoxic oxygen species, nitrogen species, proteases, cytokines, chemokines, and complement activation products [59, 60]. These events ultimately lead to the breakdown of the blood-spinal cord barrier (BSCB). Once the BSCB is profoundly compromised, multiple systemic molecules and further inflammatory cells leak into the spinal cord, resulting in additional neuronal damage and progressive expansion of the lesion. This inflammatory vicious cycle culminates in spinal edema with subsequent delayed neuropathology. The underlying, highly complex pathophysiological events of this inflammatory downward spiral are briefly illustrated in the following section.

4.2 Posttraumatic Immunological Response

4.2.1 Disruption of the Blood-Spinal Cord Barrier

Under physiological conditions, the BSCB tightly regulates the microenvironment of the spinal and controls fluids and molecules that enter the spinal tissue. The primary traumatic impact itself leads to vascular injury, bleeding, ischemia, and functional disruption of this physical barrier between systemic circulation and spinal parenchyma [41, 47, 70]. These events result in increased permeability of the BSCB and enable previously blocked, large hematogenous molecules, exudates, and inflammatory cells to leak into the spinal tissue and induce spinal edema [51]. Simultaneously, resident cells of the central nervous system (CNS) are activated by the trauma. In parallel, cascade systems like the complement system and the coagulation system become locally activated and generate a proinflammatory environment. The cytokines and chemokines released by resident spinal cord cells induce nearby endothelial cells to upregulate their cellular adhesion molecules, such as intracellular adhesion molecule (ICAM)-1, P-selectin, or E-selectin, which in turn facilitate intraspinal

leukocyte recruitment (Fig. 4.1a). Attracted by the chemotactic gradient, hematogenous neutrophils and monocytes attach to these "cell anchors" and transmigrate to the site of injury, where they unleash proinflammatory mediators, cytotoxic proteases, and reactive oxygen and nitrogen species. This further exacerbates the deterioration of the BSCB, increases spinal edema, and leads to an excessive inflammatory response. As a consequence, this secondary cascade, rather than the initial trauma, is responsible in large part for the protracted cranio-caudal expansion of the SCI-induced lesion [42].

4.2.2 Cellular and Molecular Neuroinflammatory Reactions

Shortly after the initial insult, injured neurons and glial cells undergo necrotic or apoptotic cell death, with subsequent recruitment and activation of microglia and transmigrating neutrophils and monocytes/macrophages (Fig. 4.1a) [14]. In response to the primary trauma, microglia, the resident phagocytes in the CNS, alter their morphology, phenotype, and profile of secreted inflammatory mediators [37, 49]. Following transformation into phagocytes, microglia then migrate to the site of injury, where they activate complement proteins and secrete various neurotoxic factors, such as proinflammatory cytokines, reactive oxygen species, and proteases [24, 38]. This chain of events has been termed *reactive microgliosis*. Microglial production of proinflammatory cytokines has been found to contribute to pathophysiological changes seen in neuroinflammation as well as neurodegeneration [2, 21, 33]. By secreting various cytokines and chemokines, activated microglia stimulate the proliferation and hypertrophy of astrocytes, a process referred to as *reactive astrogliosis* (Fig. 4.1b). Within a few days after trauma, reactive astrocytes then form a dense border around the site of injury, most likely to "wall-off" damaged tissue and prevent further spread of injurious molecules and inflammatory cells into adjacent healthy tissue [19, 43]. This inflammatory process greatly complicates the subsequent neuronal repair [55, 68].

Microvascular neutrophil margination in the spinal cord is evident within few hours after injury [44]. After neutrophils localize to regions of hemorrhagic

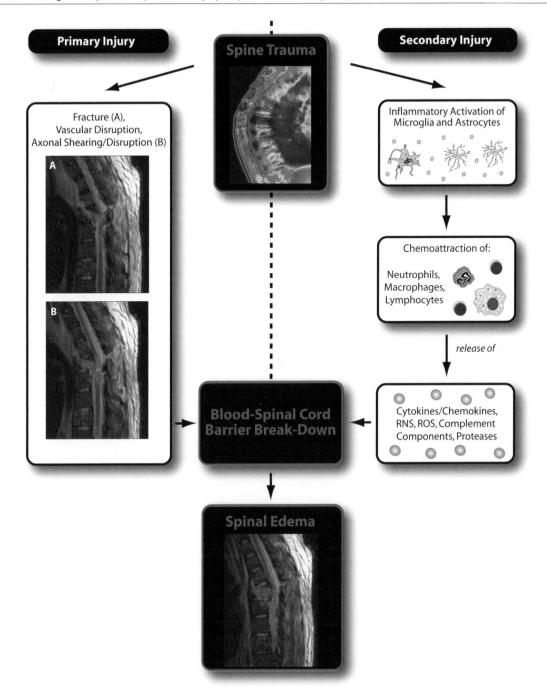

Fig. 4.2 Pathophysiology of primary and secondary spinal cord injury. Further downstream, both injury types converge in the disruption of the blood-spinal cord barrier with subsequent development of spinal edema. *RNS*, reactive nitrogen species *ROS*, reactive oxygen species

necrosis and neuronal damage, they release an inflammatory weaponry. However, by doing so, neutrophils not only degrade injured tissue and invading pathogens, but also harm intact CNS cells, which, for the most part, have poor regenerative capacity. The resulting damage to viable CNS cells might exceed their threshold of repair and further increase the size of the lesion [29, 69].

Activation of resident microglia precedes the onset of hematogenous monocyte entry into the site of injury, which starts within 2–3 days postinjury [50, 54]. Transmigrated monocytes rapidly differentiate into tissue macrophages. Like neutrophils, resident microglia and recruited monocytes/macrophages produce and secrete multiple neurotoxic mediators and generate a sophisticated proinflammatory microenvironment [18, 71]. The released neurotoxic factors have been shown to contribute to the demyelination of neurons following SCI [3–5]. This acute hyperinflammatory state is mainly driven by overshooting activity of the innate immune response, which is referred to as the "systemic inflammatory response syndrome" (SIRS) (Fig. 4.3).

Between 2 and 4 weeks posttrauma, there is a decline in the expression of proinflammatory activation markers as well as neutrophil and macrophage counts [54]. This marks the immunological shift from acute hyperinflammation to an increasingly anti-inflammation state that is predominantly driven by the adaptive immune system. T-lymphocytes start to invade the injured tissue during the first week after trauma [64]. The exact impact of lymphocytes on secondary injury following SCI remains controversial [52]. However, there is evidence that CNS antigens might drive T-cell attraction and activation. While not as numerous as transmigrated neutrophils and macrophages, T cells seem to be vital for the orchestration of the downstream inflammatory response [40]. Through close interaction between T cells and microglia, and intercommunication via mediator release, an important bridge between innate and adaptive immunity is formed. By releasing various cytokines and neurotrophic factors, activated T cells are able to cause microvascular injury [46], impair axonal conduction [35, 73], induce

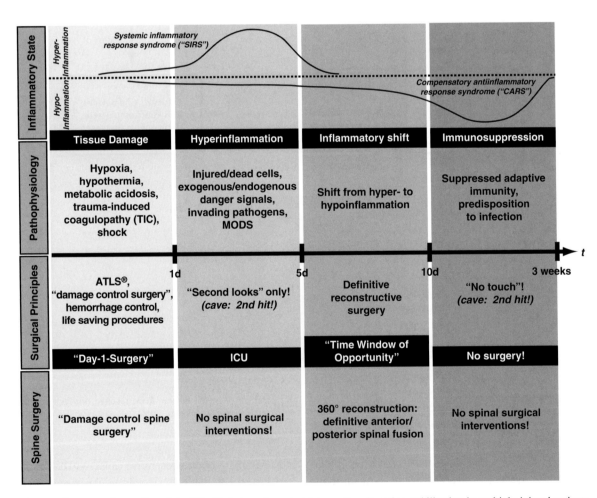

Fig. 4.3 Current understanding of the "ideal" timing of surgical intervention for spine stabilization in multiply injured patients, depending on the immunological state and susceptibility to "2nd hit" injuries. Modified from [17, 65]

neuronal cytotoxicity [20], or promote neuronal survival [61]. This "dual" function renders T cells a "double-edged sword" in the inflammatory pathophysiology of SCI. T cells further facilitate antibody production by B lymphocytes, and therefore initiate the shift from the rapid but undirected innate immune response to the more targeted adaptive immune response. Over time, the adaptive immune response then diverts from an initial proinflammatory T-cell response to an anti-inflammatory T-cell response, which can result in profound immunosuppression. The resulting critical state, which predisposes patients to serious infection, is also known as "compensatory anti-inflammatory response syndrome" (CARS) (Fig. 4.3).

4.2.3 "No-Go" – The Future Way to Go?

Multiple therapeutic approaches have attempted to ameliorate the severe inflammatory detrimental improve of secondary SCI. Unfortunately, most trials targeting secondary injury failed or showed only very modest improvement of SCI [6, 34]. This may be due to the fact that the inflammatory neuroimmune response is not only involved in destructive events, but also plays a critical role in neuronal repair and reorganization following injury [13, 53]. One of the currently most promising therapeutic approaches involves the protein Nogo-A, which is expressed in the mammalian CNS mainly by oligodentrocytes [27, 72]. Nogo has a crucial role in restricting axonal regeneration and compensatory fiber growth following SCI [58]. Recent in vivo studies using anti-Nogo-A neutralizing antibodies have been shown to induce long-distance axonal regeneration with impressive enhancement of functional recovery [9, 23, 45, 57]. These findings were confirmed by the use of Nogo "knock-out" mice [32, 62], blockade of the Nogo receptor (NgR) [12, 39], or inhibition of intracellular signaling after Nogo-A-NgR-interaction [1, 15, 48]. Most importantly, even when application was delayed for as long as 7 days, NgR-blockade enhanced sprouting of the corticospinal tract [39]. Encouragingly, these results were translatable into nonhuman primates [16], prompting a multicenter trial for humanized Nogo-A antibodies in acute SCI, which is currently under way [22]. The results will be of great interest and will hopefully advance pharmacological treatment strategies following SCI in the future.

4.3 Impact on the Timing of Surgery

4.3.1 Timing of Surgery – Is It Important?

While concepts of fracture fixation for isolated spinal fractures, with or without neurological compromise, are well defined in the pertinent literature, the question about the "ideal" time-point of spine fracture fixation in severely injured patients remains an ongoing topic of debate. Secondary to the lack of scientific evidence from prospective randomized trials, a consensus has not yet been reached. Advocates of early spine fixation cite multiple advantages dictated by "common sense" when managing severely injured patients with unstable spine fractures. As such, the prolonged bed rest and the inability of adequate positioning and mobilization of polytrauma patients have been associated with severe posttraumatic complications. These include the development of pressure sores and thromboembolic events. Furthermore, prolonged bed rest may induce and exacerbate pulmonary complications related to ventilatory restrictions, leading to atelectasis, pneumonia, and ultimately to pulmonary organ failure (acute respiratory distress syndrome ARDS). Patients with multiple injuries are at increased risk of sustaining such adverse events, due to a profound immunological dysfunction, characterized by an early state of hyperinflammation, followed by a phase of immunosuppression with increased susceptibility to infection and multiple organ failure (Fig. 4.3) [30, 65, 67]. Polytrauma patients require unrestricted options of mobilization and positioning in the intensive care unit (ICU), including the upright seated position for the treatment of head injuries and prone positioning for respiratory therapy of acute lung injury (ALI) or ARDS [7, 17]. Finally, spine fractures that are not stabilized may contribute to the "antigenic load" of trauma by increasing stress and pain, which may contribute to the secondary deterioration of critically injured patients [30, 65]. This rationale provides a strong argument for the early clearance of bed rest and log-roll precautions in multiply injured patients [25, 26, 36]. In contrast, the opponents of early fracture stabilization cite different disadvantages, such as the risk of an iatrogenic insult related to prolonged surgery, as well as the inconvenience of surgical scheduling on a 24/7 basis.

Recently, opponents of early spine fixation provided evidence that surgical spine fixation within 48 h after trauma increased mortality significantly, from 2.5% to

7.6% [31]. However, a drawback of the study by Kerwin et al. which was based on a retrospective analysis of a prospective database on 361 trauma patients with operative spine injuries, is that the authors did not stratify by modality of spine fixation [31]. Provocatively speaking, those patients who died during the "early" time-window of spine fixation within 48 h may have undergone prolonged surgical procedures for anterior spinal fusion and decompression, which is associated with increased intraoperative blood loss and may have contributed to the increased mortality rate by aggravating the vicious cycle of postinjury coagulopathy [8, 63, 66]. It remains a matter of speculation as to whether these patients may have had a decreased mortality rate by applying a staged concept of initial posterior fixation and delayed anterior fusion during the physiological safer time-window, after the endpoints of resuscitation have been accomplished [26, 30, 65]. Beyond a doubt, a defined subset of critically injured patients may not be candidates to undergo a spine surgical procedure on day 1, related to an unjustifiable risk of postoperative morbidity and mortality. This includes polytrauma patients *"in extremis,"* related to a state of severe traumatic-hemorrhagic shock, and patients with traumatic coagulopathy who are at increased risk of increased intraperioperative bleeding with the potential for a secondary injury to the spinal cord [66].

Currently, there is an ongoing controversy about the use of steroids in SCI. The 8th revised ATLS course manual states that, at present, there is insufficient evidence to support the use of steroids in SCI. Based on the results of the National Acute Spinal Cord Injury Study (NASCIS)-trials, administration of methylprednisolone for SCI may only be beneficial for patients with nonpenetrating injury and when administered within 8 h after trauma. However, there is a lively debate about the scientific value and interpretability of the NASCIS trials due to their statistical weaknesses. As a result, administration of methylprednisolone for spinal cord injuries is currently neither considered a standard of care nor indicated in many spine trauma centers until more conclusive and evidence-based data emerge.

4.3.2 The Concept of "Spine Damage Control"

Despite the ongoing debate in the field, the pertinent literature has unequivocally shown that the early surgical spine fixation and the early mobilization of patients with unstable thoracolumbar fractures have been associated with a decreased incidence of posttraumatic complications and a shorter hospital and ICU stay. In a landmark article, Croce et al. performed a retrospective analysis of a prospective database on 291 consecutive patients with unstable spine fractures requiring surgical fixation [11]. Patients were matched for injury severity and stratified by the level of spine injury into two distinct cohorts, depending on the timing of fracture fixation: "early" fixation ($\leq$3 days, $n=142$) vs. "late" fixation (>3 days, $n=149$). The authors found that the "early" fixation of thoracic spine fractures resulted in a lower incidence of pneumonia, fewer ventilator-dependent days, a shorter ICU stay, and reduced hospital charges [11]. Similarly, Cengiz et al. recently reported data from a randomized prospective pilot study on 27 patients who underwent surgical stabilization of an unstable fracture in the thoracolumbar region (T8–L2) [10]. Patients were randomized depending on the timing of surgery within 8 h ($n=12$) or more than 3 days ($n=15$). The authors found that those patients who underwent spine fixation within 8 h had a significantly decreased incidence of pulmonary complications, such as pneumonia, and shorter length of ICU and hospital stay, compared to the group with delayed spine fixation [10]. Even though this study has some significant shortcomings and limitations, such as the small patient population and the flawed randomization procedure (surgeon's convenience based on their operative schedule), these preliminary findings make a strong point that early fracture fixation is feasible and safe, and potentially beneficial for the patients [10]. This notion was confirmed by a recent systematic review of the pertinent peer-reviewed literature in the field [56]. The authors reviewed all published articles in Medline and Embase databases, which provided a comparison between different time-points of surgical stabilization of thoracic or lumbar spine fractures. Ten papers encompassing 1,427 patients met the inclusion criteria. Based on their systematic review, the authors concluded that the early intervention for fracture stabilization in the thoraco-lumbar spine is safe, advantageous, and associated with a significantly decreased incidence of postoperative complications [56]. An example of successful "spine damage control" is shown in Figs. 4.4–4.6.

4.4 Conclusion

The trauma-induced inflammatory response renders patients with spine injuries vulnerable to "2nd hit" injury, either related to inadequate timing or procedure

Fig. 4.4 Clinical example of "damage control" spine surgery (1). A 33-year-old female was involved in a high-speed, unrestrained motor vehicle accident. She sustained an unstable T11/T12 fracture-dislocation with translational and rotational instability (AO/OTA type 52-C2.3). The patient was taken to the OR on the same day for posterior reduction and instrumentation from T10–L2

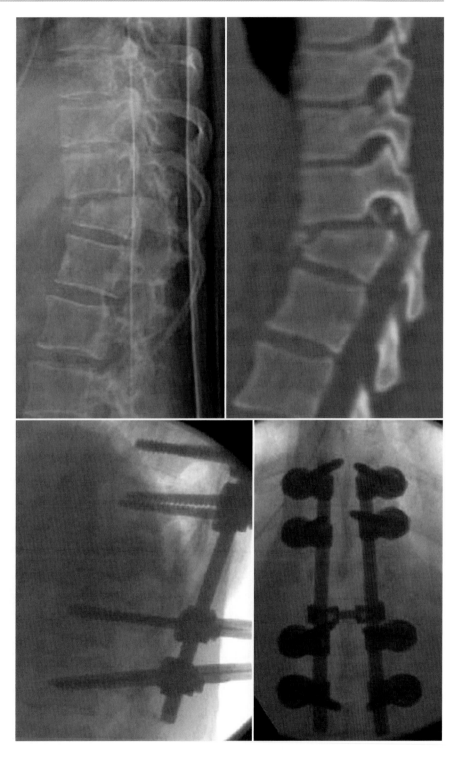

of spine fixation (Fig. 4.3) [30, 65]. Until present, there is no consensus on the "ideal" timing and modality of spine fracture fixation in multiply injured patients. Furthermore, no pharmacological "golden bullet" has yet been identified that may prevent or delay the onset of secondary SCI. The identification of *Nogo* as a therapeutic target represents a promising "bench-to-bedside" strategy, which, however, is still far from a standardized

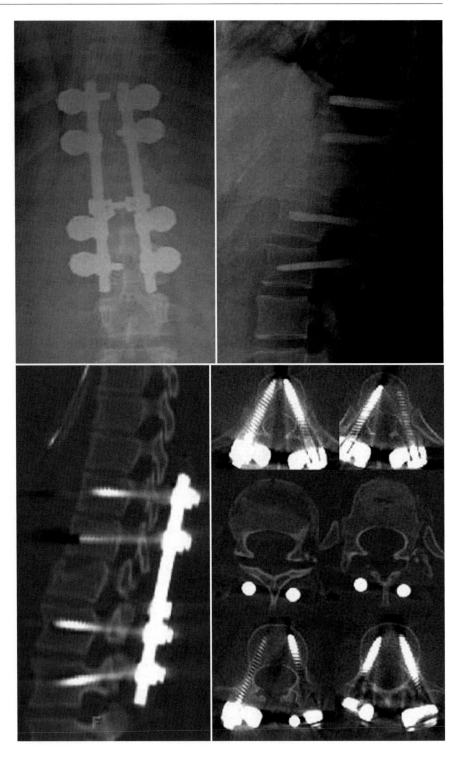

Fig. 4.5 Clinical example of "damage control" spine surgery (2). Postoperative X-rays and CT scan of the same patient depicted in Fig. 4.4. At this point, the fracture was considered stable for unrestricted patient positioning in the intensive care unit, for therapies related to associated injuries, e.g., pulmonary contusions and traumatic brain injury

implementation into clinical practice [22]. Thus, until present, we continue to rely on optimized surgical strategies for the management of unstable spine injuries in polytrauma patients. Delaying surgical fixation of unstable spine fractures has been associated with an increased risk of severe complications attributed to

Fig. 4.6 Clinical example of "damage control" spine surgery (3). The patient shown in Figs. 4.4 and 4.5 was taken back to the OR for an anterior completion corpectomy and fusion during the physiological "time-window of opportunity" on day 8 after trauma. She recovered well and was mobilized with physical and occupational therapy as early as day 1 after the initial "damage control" posterior fixation

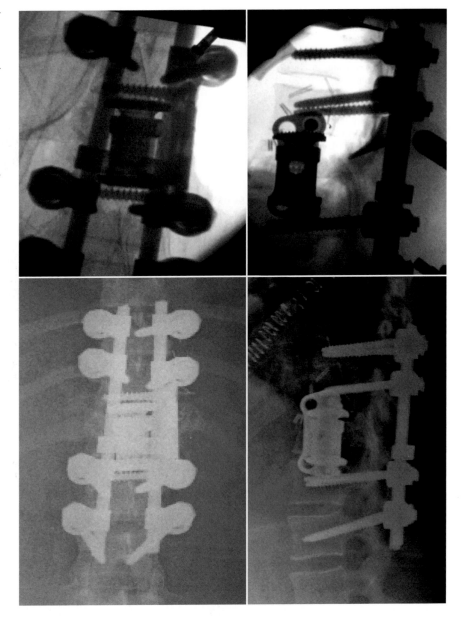

restrictions in mobilization of severely injured patients. On the other hand, early spine fixation through anterior approaches for acute anterior decompression and corpectomy with anterior fusion within the first 48 h after trauma has been associated with increased mortality [31], possibly due to extensive bleeding in hypothermic and coagulopathic trauma patients [8, 63, 66]. Based on these insights, the new concept of "spine damage control" has been advocated as a safe staged procedure of early posterior reduction and instrumentation,

followed by a scheduled anterior completion during a physiological "window of opportunity". Although this concept appears to be supported by metaanalyses of the pertinent literature on the timing of spine fixation [56], until present, "spine damage control" has only been advocated in anecdotal reviews and case reports, and a scientific proof of concept is still lacking. The safety and feasibility of the "spine damage control" strategy will have to be validated in well-designed, prospective studies on large cohorts of multiply injured patients.

References

1. Bandtlow CE, Schmidt MF, Hassinger TD et al (1993) Role of intracellular calcium in NI-35-evoked collapse of neuronal growth cones. Science 259:80–83

2. Bartholdi D, Schwab ME (1997) Expression of pro-inflammatory cytokine and chemokine mRNA upon experimental spinal cord injury in mouse: an in situ hybridization study. Eur J NeuroSci 9:1422–1438

3. Blight AR (1985) Delayed demyelination and macrophage invasion: a candidate for secondary cell damage in spinal cord injury. Cent Nerv Syst Trauma 2:299–315

4. Blight AR, Cohen TI, Saito K, Heyes MP (1995) Quinolinic acid accumulation and functional deficits following experimental spinal cord injury. Brain 118(Pt 3):735–752

5. Boutin H, LeFeuvre RA, Horai R et al (2001) Role of IL-1alpha and IL-1beta in ischemic brain damage. J Neurosci 21:5528–5534

6. Bracken MB, Shepard MJ, Collins WF et al (1990) A randomized, controlled trial of methylprednisolone or naloxone in the treatment of acute spinal-cord injury. Results of the Second National Acute Spinal Cord Injury Study N Engl J Med 322:1405–1411

7. Bream-Rouwenhorst HR, Beltz EA, Ross MB, Moores KG (2008) Recent developments in the management of acute respiratory distress syndrome in adults. Am J Health Syst Pharm 65:29–36

8. Brohi K, Singh J, Heron M, Coats T (2003) Acute traumatic coagulopathy. J Trauma 54:1127–1130

9. Brosamle C, Huber AB, Fiedler M et al (2000) Regeneration of lesioned corticospinal tract fibers in the adult rat induced by a recombinant, humanized IN-1 antibody fragment. J Neurosci 20:8061–8068

10. Cengiz SL, Kalkan E, Bayir A et al (2008) Timing of thoracolumbar spine stabilization in trauma patients - impact on neurological outcome and clinical course: a real prospective randomized controlled study. Arch Orthop Trauma Surg 128:959–966

11. Croce MA, Bee TK, Pritchard E et al (2001) Does optimal timing for spine fracture fixation exist? Ann Surg 233:851–858

12. David S, Fry EJ, Lopez-Vales R (2008) Novel roles for Nogo receptor in inflammation and disease. Trends Neurosci 31:221–226

13. Donnelly DJ, Popovich PG (2008) Inflammation and its role in neuroprotection, axonal regeneration and functional recovery after spinal cord injury. Exp Neurol 209:378–388

14. Dusart I, Schwab ME (1994) Secondary cell death and the inflammatory reaction after dorsal hemisection of the rat spinal cord. Eur J NeuroSci 6:712–724

15. Fournier AE, Takizawa BT, Strittmatter SM (2003) Rho kinase inhibition enhances axonal regeneration in the injured CNS. J Neurosci 23:1416–1423

16. Freund P, Schmidlin E, Wannier T et al (2006) Nogo-A-specific antibody treatment enhances sprouting and functional recovery after cervical lesion in adult primates. Nat Med 12:790–792

17. Gebhard F, Huber-Lang M (2008) Polytrauma-pathophysiology and management principles. Langenbecks Arch Surg 393:825–831

18. Giulian D, Corpuz M, Chapman S et al (1993) Reactive mononuclear phagocytes release neurotoxins after ischemic and traumatic injury to the central nervous system. J Neurosci Res 36:681–693

19. Giulian D, Lachman LB (1985) Interleukin-1 stimulation of astroglial proliferation after brain injury. Science 228:497–499

20. Giuliani F, Goodyer CG, Antel JP, Yong VW (2003) Vulnerability of human neurons to T cell-mediated cytotoxicity. J Immunol 171:368–379

21. Gonzalez-Scarano F, Baltuch G (1999) Microglia as mediators of inflammatory and degenerative diseases. Annu Rev Neurosci 22:219–240

22. Gonzenbach RR, Schwab ME (2008) Disinhibition of neurite growth to repair the injured adult CNS: focusing on Nogo. Cell Mol Life Sci 65:161–176

23. GrandPre T, Li S, Strittmatter SM (2002) Nogo-66 receptor antagonist peptide promotes axonal regeneration. Nature 417:547–551

24. Hanisch UK (2002) Microglia as a source and target of cytokines. Glia 40:140–155

25. Haschtmann D, Stahel PF, Heyde CE (2009) Management of a multiple trauma patient with extensive instability of the lumbar spine as a result of a bilateral facet dislocation and multiple complete vertebral burst fractures. J Trauma 66:922–930

26. Heyde CE, Ertel W, Kayser R (2005) Management of spine injuries in polytraumatized patients. Orthopade 34:889–905

27. Huber AB, Weinmann O, Brosamle C et al (2002) Patterns of Nogo mRNA and protein expression in the developing and adult rat and after CNS lesions. J Neurosci 22:3553–3567

28. Jones TB, McDaniel EE, Popovich PG (2005) Inflammatory-mediated injury and repair in the traumatically injured spinal cord. Curr Pharm Des 11:1223–1236

29. Katoh S, Ikata T, Tsubo M et al (1997) Possible implication of leukocytes in secondary pathological changes after spinal cord injury. Injury 28:215–217

30. Keel M, Trentz O (2005) Pathophysiology of polytrauma. Injury 36:691–709

31. Kerwin AJ, Frykberg ER, Schinco MA et al (2007) The effect of early surgical treatment of traumatic spine injuries on patient mortality. J Trauma 63:1308–1313

32. Kim JE, Li S, GrandPre T et al (2003) Axon regeneration in young adult mice lacking Nogo-A/B. Neuron 38:187–199

33. Klusman I, Schwab ME (1997) Effects of pro-inflammatory cytokines in experimental spinal cord injury. Brain Res 762:173–184

34. Knoller N, Auerbach G, Fulga V et al (2005) Clinical experience using incubated autologous macrophages as a treatment for complete spinal cord injury: phase I study results. J Neurosurg Spine 3:173–181

35. Koller H, Siebler M, Hartung HP (1997) Immunologically induced electrophysiological dysfunction: implications for inflammatory diseases of the CNS and PNS. Prog Neurobiol 52:1–26

36. Kossmann T, Trease L, Freedman I, Malham G (2004) Damage control surgery for spine trauma. Injury 35:661–670

37. Kreutzberg GW (1996) Microglia: a sensor for pathological events in the CNS. Trends Neurosci 19:312–318

38. Lee YB, Nagai A, Kim SU (2002) Cytokines, chemokines, and cytokine receptors in human microglia. J Neurosci Res 69:94–103

39. Li S, Strittmatter SM (2003) Delayed systemic Nogo-66 receptor antagonist promotes recovery from spinal cord injury. J Neurosci 23:4219–4227
40. Lodge PA, Sriram S (1996) Regulation of microglial activation by TGF-beta, IL-10, and CSF-1. J Leukoc Biol 60:502–508
41. Maikos JT, Shreiber DI (2007) Immediate damage to the blood-spinal cord barrier due to mechanical trauma. J Neurotrauma 24:492–507
42. Mautes AE, Weinzierl MR, Donovan F, Noble LJ (2000) Vascular events after spinal cord injury: contribution to secondary pathogenesis. Phys Ther 80:673–687
43. McGraw J, Hiebert GW, Steeves JD (2001) Modulating astrogliosis after neurotrauma. J Neurosci Res 63:109–115
44. Means ED, Anderson DK (1983) Neuronophagia by leukocytes in experimental spinal cord injury. J Neuropathol Exp Neurol 42:707–719
45. Merkler D, Metz GA, Raineteau O et al (2001) Locomotor recovery in spinal cord-injured rats treated with an antibody neutralizing the myelin-associated neurite growth inhibitor Nogo-A. J Neurosci 21:3665–3673
46. Naparstek Y, Cohen IR, Fuks Z, Vlodavsky I (1984) Activated T lymphocytes produce a matrix-degrading heparan sulphate endoglycosidase. Nature 310:241–244
47. Nelson E, Gertz SD, Rennels ML et al (1977) Spinal cord injury. The role of vascular damage in the pathogenesis of central hemorrhagic necrosis Archives of neurology 34:332–333
48. Niederost B, Oertle T, Fritsche J et al (2002) Nogo-A and myelin-associated glycoprotein mediate neurite growth inhibition by antagonistic regulation of RhoA and Rac1. J Neurosci 22:10368–10376
49. Popovich PG (2000) Immunological regulation of neuronal degeneration and regeneration in the injured spinal cord. Prog Brain Res 128:43–58
50. Popovich PG, Hickey WF (2001) Bone marrow chimeric rats reveal the unique distribution of resident and recruited macrophages in the contused rat spinal cord. J Neuropathol Exp Neurol 60:676–685
51. Popovich PG, Horner PJ, Mullin BB, Stokes BT (1996) A quantitative spatial analysis of the blood-spinal cord barrier. I. Permeability changes after experimental spinal contusion injury. Exp Neurol 142:258–275
52. Popovich PG, Jones TB (2003) Manipulating neuroinflammatory reactions in the injured spinal cord: back to basics. Trends Pharmacol Sci 24:13–17
53. Popovich PG, Longbrake EE (2008) Can the immune system be harnessed to repair the CNS? Nat Rev Neurosci 9:481–493
54. Popovich PG, Wei P, Stokes BT (1997) Cellular inflammatory response after spinal cord injury in Sprague-Dawley and Lewis rats. J Comp Neurol 377:443–464
55. Ridet JL, Malhotra SK, Privat A, Gage FH (1997) Reactive astrocytes: cellular and molecular cues to biological function. Trends Neurosci 20:570–577
56. Rutges JP, Oner FC, Leenen LP (2007) Timing of thoracic and lumbar fracture fixation in spinal injuries: a systematic review of neurological and clinical outcome. Eur Spine J 16:579–587
57. Schnell L, Schwab ME (1990) Axonal regeneration in the rat spinal cord produced by an antibody against myelin-associated neurite growth inhibitors. Nature 343:269–272
58. Schwab ME (2004) Nogo and axon regeneration. Curr Opin Neurobiol 14:118–124
59. Schwartz M, Yoles E (2006) Immune-based therapy for spinal cord repair: autologous macrophages and beyond. J Neurotrauma 23:360–370
60. Segal JL (2005) Immunoactivation and altered intercellular communication mediate the pathophysiology of spinal cord injury. Pharmacotherapy 25:145–156
61. Serpe CJ, Kohm AP, Huppenbauer CB et al (1999) Exacerbation of facial motoneuron loss after facial nerve transection in severe combined immunodeficient (scid) mice. J Neurosci 19:RC7
62. Simonen M, Pedersen V, Weinmann O et al (2003) Systemic deletion of the myelin-associated outgrowth inhibitor Nogo-A improves regenerative and plastic responses after spinal cord injury. Neuron 38:201–211
63. Spahn DR, Cerny V, Coats TJ et al (2007) Management of bleeding following major trauma: a European guideline. Crit Care 11:R17
64. Sroga JM, Jones TB, Kigerl KA et al (2003) Rats and mice exhibit distinct inflammatory reactions after spinal cord injury. J Comp Neurol 462:223–240
65. Stahel PF, Heyde CE, Ertel W (2005) Current concepts of polytrauma management. Eur J Trauma 31:200–211
66. Stahel PF, Moore EE, Schreier SL et al (2009) Transfusion strategies in postinjury coagulopathy. Curr Opin Anaesthesiol 22:289–298
67. Stahel PF, Smith WR, Moore EE (2007) Role of biological modifiers regulating the immune response after trauma. Injury 38:1409–1422
68. Steeves JD, Tetzlaff W (1998) Engines, accelerators, and brakes on functional spinal cord repair. Ann N Y Acad Sci 860:412–424
69. Taoka Y, Naruo M, Koyanagi E et al (1995) Superoxide radicals play important roles in the pathogenesis of spinal cord injury. Paraplegia 33:450–453
70. Tator CH, Fehlings MG (1991) Review of the secondary injury theory of acute spinal cord trauma with emphasis on vascular mechanisms. J Neurosurg 75:15–26
71. van der Laan LJ, Ruuls SR, Weber KS et al (1996) Macrophage phagocytosis of myelin in vitro determined by flow cytometry: phagocytosis is mediated by CR3 and induces production of tumor necrosis factor-alpha and nitric oxide. J Neuroimmunol 70:145–152
72. Wang X, Chun SJ, Treloar H et al (2002) Localization of Nogo-A and Nogo-66 receptor proteins at sites of axon-myelin and synaptic contact. J Neurosci 22:5505–5515
73. Yarom Y, Naparstek Y, Lev-Ram V et al (1983) Immunospecific inhibition of nerve conduction by T lymphocytes reactive to basic protein of myelin. Nature 303:246–247

The Role of Orthosis in Spinal Injury

David F. Apple, Courtney W. Brown, and Lesley M. Hudson

5.1 Introduction

The management of spinal column fractures, especially when associated with spinal cord injury, was largely ignored until World War II when a spinal injury program at Stoke-Mandeville, England, was started under the direction of Sir Ludwig Guttman. Soldiers and civilians with fractured spines and most with paralysis were treated in an organized fashion commencing with postural reduction. The reduction was maintained by traction in the case of cervical injuries while the patient remained on a turning frame or padded bed until fracture stability or healing was achieved. Thoracic and lumbar fractures were reduced posturally, and the same type frame or bed was utilized until stabilization or healing was obtained (Figs. 5.1 and 5.2). In complex fractures, occasionally cervical-pelvic or cervical-femoral traction was required to achieve reduction (Table 5.1).

Over time, the use of cervical and thoraco-lumbar orthoses was introduced to shorten the time spent in bed, and thus evolved the concept of earlier mobilization of the patient to decrease secondary complications (Figs. 5.3 and 5.4)

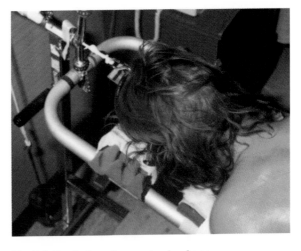

Fig. 5.1 Cervical traction on a turning frame

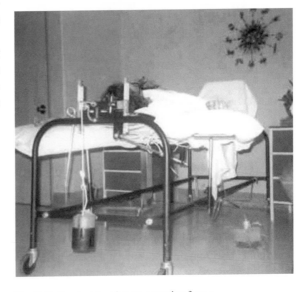

Fig. 5.2 Cervical traction on a turning frame

D.F. Apple (✉) and L.M. Hudson
Shepherd Center, 2020 Peachtree Rd NW, Atlanta,
GA 30309, USA
e-mail: david_apple@shepherd.org

C.W. Brown
Panorama Orthopaedics and Spine Center, 2660 Golden Ridge
Road, Golden, CO 80401-9522, USA

V.V. Patel et al. (eds.), *Spine Trauma*,
DOI: 10.1007/978-3-642-03694-1_5, © Springer-Verlag Berlin Heidelberg 2010

Table 5.1 Cervical traction weight

Cervical traction weight	
8–10#	Anchoring effect
10–20#	Physiology alignment
20–60#	Correct deformity
10#	Forehead
5#	For each cervical level

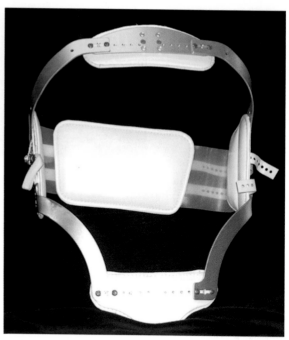

Fig. 5.4 Thoracic orthosis – Jewett Brace

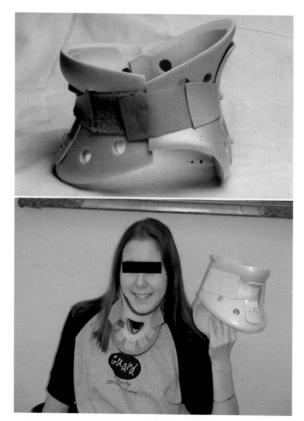

Fig. 5.3 Cervical orthosis – Philadelphia collar

5.2 Principles of Spinal Orthotic Immobilization

A properly applied orthotic, whether for the cervical spine or thoracolumbar spine, should provide stabilization in anatomic or near anatomic alignment. The orthosis should allow muscle relaxation and thus a reduction in pain. It must prevent deformity by limiting motion. An effective orthosis will provide partial unloading of the spine, especially necessary in the cervical spine, because of the weight of the head. The ideal orthosis

should also provide adequate distribution of pressure to avoid ischemic sores. In cervical orthosis, the problem areas that develop are on the chin and at the posterior base of the skull. In the case of the thoracic-lumbar orthosis, the most common problem occurs when the orthosis is fitted in the lying position; the orthosis should always be fitted in the sitting position or in the case of the neurologically intact patient in the standing position. A simple design is best as the orthosis should be easy to put on and take of. The orthotic material should be durable with allowances made for moisture and temperature control. Finally, an orthosis should be as comfortable as possible to increase compliance [17].

5.3 Motion Control

The most important issue for choosing an orthosis for the cervical spine or the thoracolumbar spine is how effectively it controls motion. This is more critical in the cervical spine because of the weight of the head, the smaller size of the supporting muscles, and the capacity of motion when compared to the thoracolumbar spine. Ferlic [9] in 1962 calculated the normal range of motion of all age groups to be flexion extension 127°, right and left lateral motion 73°, and right and left rotation 142°. Johnson et al. [10] in 1977 evaluated five cervical orthoses for motion restriction. Table 5.2 summarizes the percentage of restriction for flexion extension, rotation, and lateral bending.

Studies on the immobilizing effect of orthoses on the thoracolumbar spine have been multiple, but the results have been variable. In the thoracic spine, there is a decreased need for bracing because of the stabilizing effect of the rib cage and the limited motion of the thoracic vertebrae. Below T_{12}–L_1, flexion extension, lateral bending, and torsion become more of an issue. Numerous investigators starting with Norton and Brown [16] have tried to assess the use of orthoses in reducing motion in the lumbosacral spine. Although many braces were investigated, the emphasis was on the Jewett brace, the Williams brace, and plaster of Paris jackets with the end

result being the development of a new brace. The effects of motion restriction were different at each vertebral level, by each brace tested, and by the position of the patient. The conclusion was that no one brace will work in all cases and that a team approach be used to prescribe a well-fitted brace that accomplishes the restriction of motion desired at the correct lumbar level. The discussion suggested using a simple brace, then placing a thumbtack at the location where motion is not wanted, which would serve as a reminder to the patient of the undesirable motion. Cholewick et al. [7] looked at motion restriction and trunk stiffness provided by three thoracolumbosacral orthoses: Aspen TLSO, Boston body jacket, and CAMP TSLO. The results showed no statistical differences in the three in flexion/extension, anterior/posterior, pelvic tilt, and trunk lateral binding. The braces decreased full ROM by 39–45%, but allowed 55–61% of motion to be unrestricted. Thus, the authors suggested that comfort should be the determining issue to increase compliance.

Miller et al. [14] studied the three most commonly used thoracolumbar orthoses, the lumbosacral corset, the Jewett brace, and the plastic thoracolumbar orthosis (TLSO), by roentgenograms. The lumbosacral corset provided virtually no immobilization at L_{3-4}, L_{4-5}, L_5–S_1, whereas the Jewett and the TLSO did provide moderate decreased motion at L_{3-4}, and L_{4-5}

Table 5.2 Percent of normal motion

	F/E	Rotation	Lateral bend
Soft	74	83	92
Philadelphia	29	44	66
Some	28	34	66
HCTO	13	18	51
Halo	4	4	4

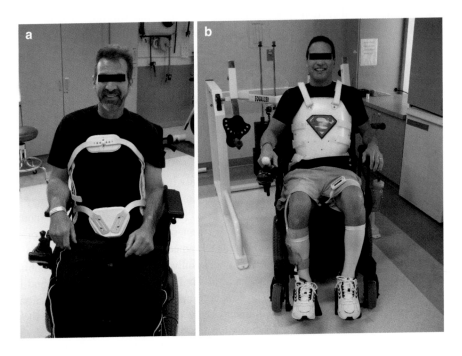

Fig. 5.5 (**a**, **b**) The two most commonly used thorcolumber orthoses

(Fig. 5.5a, b) but like the corset little immobilization at L_5–S_1. Lantz and Schultz [13], and Buchalter et al.'s [5] assessment of four orthoses was similar. Some have advocated adding hip extension to the lumbosacral orthoses to provide additional spine immobilization, especially at L_5–S_1. However, Axelsson et al. [3] studied roentgenograms of ten patients first with no orthosis and then an orthosis with hip extensions added and found no effect on sagittal, vertical, or transverse intervertebral translations in the lumbar spine. The study of four lumbosacral orthoses by Fidler and Plasmans [17], one being a hip extension orthosis, showed significant restriction of motion at the L_{4-5} segment. Vander Kooi et al. [20], utilizing fluoroscopy to study motion loss with respect to TLSO, concluded that the TLSO reduced total horizontal motion at L_{3-5}, from 20 to 50°, with a thigh extender reducing the motion to 10°.

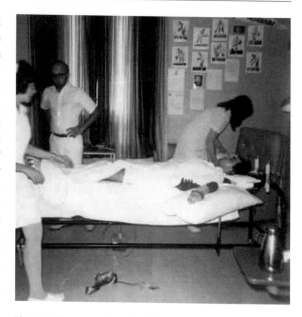

Fig. 5.6 Treatment of cervical fracture on a turning frame until healing occurs

5.4 Orthoses as a Treatment for Spine Fracture

In a world where operative management of spine fractures has improved due to better internal fixation implants and better operative techniques, it must not be forgotten that most, injuries can be managed safely nonoperatively. The original nonoperative treatment of cervical spine fracture was cervical traction in bed for the entire healing time (Fig. 5.6). This method has two disadvantages: the cost of hospitalization and the morbidity of inactivity. The introduction of cervical collars, first soft then rigid, began to reduce these disadvantages. Introduction of the halo vest in the 1960s [15] provided a more reliable immobilization of especially the upper cervical spine and allowed earlier mobilization of the patient (Fig. 5.7a, b).

Seljeskog [19] in 1978 wrote about the use of the halo vest that had been introduced by Nickel et al. [15] in 1960. Seljeskog recommended this method for use in Hangman's fractures, fractures of the atlas, odontoid fractures, and Jefferson fractures. Koivikko et al. [12] compared operative vs. nonoperative management of cervical burst fractures in patients with paralysis and no paralysis. Although the operative and nonoperative groups were not exactly similar, the healing was similar, with the operative group healing with less deformity. Complications were similar. The groupings were not large enough to be statistically significant. The conclusion was that it was safe to treat a cervical "burst" fracture nonoperatively.

Razak et al. [18] reviewed 53 patients treated with a halo vest for upper and lower cervical spine injures resulting in a 96% healing rate. The average time in the halo vest was 10.4 weeks. Vieweg and Schultheib [21] in a literature review of 35 studies involving 682 patients who were immobilized in a halo vest found the healing rate was 86%. The review recommended the use of the halo vest for isolated Jefferson's fractures, stable Hangman's fractures, and type II and III well-aligned odontoid fractures. The halo vest was not a suitable treatment for ligament injuries without associated fractures, i.e., bilateral facet dislocations or unilateral facet dislocations with or without associated fractures.

Nonoperative treatment of the cervical or thoracolumbar spine is a viable option even in these days of improving implant fixation. The initial treatment is anatomic body alignment in bed with or without traction (Fig. 5.8). Traction may be applied utilizing femoral traction alone or may require combination with cervical traction. If anatomic or near anatomic alignment is achieved, a thoracolumbar spinal orthosis can be applied so that early patient mobilization can be started. This is usually best done around 10–14 days postinjury. If postural attempts at reduction are not successful and there is X-ray evidence that the pedicles are intact, reduction can be attempted by hyperextension of the spine by

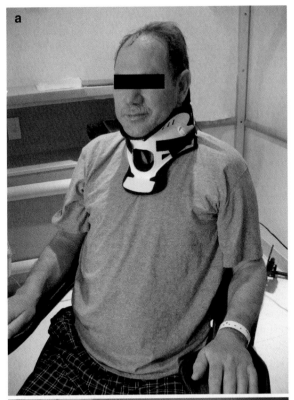

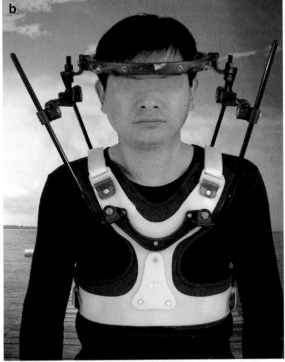

Fig. 5.7 (a, b) A cervical collar and a halo vest for the treatment of cervical spine fractures, both allowing early mobilization

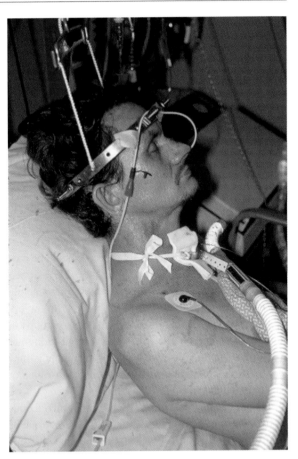

Fig 5.8 Fracture of the cervical spine in a patient with Marie-Strampells arthritis being maintained in "anatomic" position by traction

suspension of the patient between two gurneys, one supporting the pelvis and other the shoulders with the patient prone. From a historical standpoint, there are probably not many Goldthwaithe frames available, but previously this frame was an option for applying a body jacket with the spine in a hyperextended position. Jones et al. [11] in 1987 conducted a prospective study of 33 thoracic and lumbar fractures utilizing a TLSO after 6–8 weeks of bed rest. The levels ranged from T_3 to L_3. This treatment was not without problems, i.e., none improved neurologically, but none worsened; several ultimately required surgery. The conclusion was that nonoperative treatment was an alternative.

Davies et al. [8] compared the results of 34 patients treated nonoperatively with a group of 95 patients treated nonoperatively and operatively reviewed by Dickson et al. and concluded the results were similar regarding neurological improvement, loss of deformity, and main-tenance of deformity at follow-up. However, the authors felt surgical intervention was required if there was an unsuccessful nonoperative reduction of either a fracture or a dislocation, an uncooperative patient, or suspicion of soft tissue interposition. More recently, Butler et al. [6] reviewed 31 patients with L_1 burst fractures, 26 of whom were available for a mean of 43 months follow-up, 11 treated surgically, and 15 nonsurgically. The non-operative group had a shortened hospitalization, less pain at follow-up, and a higher rate of follow-up. The operative group had better correction of the kyphotic deformity, which gradually was lost in follow-up. The authors admitted the groups had different fracture char-acteristics, but felt indications for surgery should be nar-rowed. Yil et al. [22] surveyed 53 patients with assigned randomly to operative and nonoperative groups stable thoracolumbar fractures with a 44-month follow-up. There was no statistical difference in the two groups in functional outcome. The cost and complication rate were higher in the operative group. The authors admit-ted the sample size was small and the clinical use cannot be supported on the basis of this trial.

In conclusion, it is difficult to do a randomized con-trolled study of operative vs. nonoperative treatment, so it will be difficult to get level-one evidence to sup-port an opinion either way. But at least there is the implication that nonoperative treatment, if used prop-erly, is a safe alternative. Most authors will agree that an operative approach is indicated in soft tissue inju-ries alone, i.e., bilateral facet dislocations or unreduced unilateral facet dislocations, or when disk material can be proven to be causing cord compression.

5.5 Postsurgical Orthoses

The standard for postsurgical immobilization of the spine, whether cervical or thoracic, or lumbar, has been the use of an orthosis for 3 months. This recommenda-tion was based on the biological time taken for a fusion to mature or a fracture to heal enough to be unsup-ported. There has been no level-one evidence, new or old, to demonstrate how much each type of orthosis actually immobilizes the spinal area. The choice of the orthosis was divided into hard or rigid, or soft.

In volume one of *Campbell's Operative Orthopaedics* [1] the postoperative treatment for cervical fracture was continued cervical traction until the wound was healed followed by a chin-occiput brace for 4–6 months. For a thoracic fracture, the postoperative regi-men was continued bed rest until the sutures were removed followed by application of a plaster jacket using a Goldthwaite frame for fitting. The patient was continued on bed rest for 10 weeks.

Much has changed in the past 35 years with much less bed rest, less rigid mobilization, and shorter times utilizing external support being suggested [4]. In that time span, internal fixation implants have been engi-neered to provide more rigid fixation to allow fracture healing and graft incorporation to take place in a favor-able environment for healing. Additionally, braces have been developed that, although costly, can be easily fabricated and applied. Surgeons, not because of any controlled research studies, have been gradually decreasing the time and amount of postoperative brac-ing. Generally, it is recommended that a cervical collar be worn for 2–4 weeks of immobilization followed by resumption of near normal activity. In specific cases there may be reasons for longer immobilizations as determined by the surgeon. For thoracic and lumbar fracture after fusion surgery, the recommendation is similar, utilizing a fabricated orthosis (expensive) or an off-the-shelf orthosis, i.e., Jewett (less expensive), for soft tissue healing (10–14 days). The contribution of engineering to develop better internal implant devices in other anatomic areas, such as the extremi-ties, has taken place in the spine allowing less external restriction for shorter time frames.

Apple and Perez [2] prospectively followed 138 patients for 2 years after surgery for thoracic or lumbar fractures and immobilization by a TLSO or Jewett brace for 4 weeks. The overall complication rate was 2%. The results, although not statistically significant, support the concept that decreased postoperative brace time has an acceptable complication rate and no increased risk of neurological complication

5.6 Summary

Use of orthoses in spinal column injuries has a place at three intervals in the continuum of fracture care. The first is in the acute period to immobilize the spine while awaiting definitive stabilization. The second is the pri-mary stabilization for the fracture in those few spa-tients where internal fixation is contraindicated. The third is in the postoperative period. The orthopedic texts continue to recommend 3–6 months of postoperative use, but the practice in the community is gradually to use less restrictive orthoses for a shorter period of time. This practice is due to better implants and improved surgical technique.

5.6.1 Cast Application for Burst Fracture

5.6.1.1 Equipment Needed

1. Large tubular stockinette
2. Six-inch cast padding and 1/8–1/4-in felt, 4 and 6-in fiberglass casting material
3. Two padded examining tables
4. Pain medication
5. Staff assistance to maintain patient position if needed

5.6.1.2 Technique

In preparation for casting, two padded examining tables are placed parallel to each other approximately separated by the truncal height of the patient. The patient is brought in on a gurney, having had the large tubular stockinette placed on his body with arms placed through previously cut armholes (Fig. 5.9). After pain medication is given intravenously, the patient is rolled from the gurney onto the padded examining tables to a prone posture. The tables can be adjusted to the appropriate width, with the arms extended above the head (Fig. 5.10). Legs are extended across the second parallel table using the Y ligament of the hips to create extension of the pelvis + lower spine, and thus help reduce the fracture. While the patient is suspended between the two examining tables, gradually the muscle spasm will relax and the patient will sage into more and more hyperextension. While this occurs, cast padding should be applied. All prominent bony areas should be padded, including anterior iliac crest, the posterior sacrum, and the sternum. The 1/4 in felt padding is torn in half to create 1/8 in thick pads with one irregular side that the fiberglass casting material will hold in place.

After sufficient padding is applied, the fiber glass casting material in 5- or 6-in rolls is then wrapped circumferentially on the patient for the first layer. This should go from high sternum to low pubic symphysis. Splints of 4- and 5-in fiberglass should be made to reinforce the lateral aspect of the cast, as well as the superior sternal region and the inferior circumferential edge of the cast. After the splints are applied, the final layers colored, if desired, are applied and smoothed with lotion.

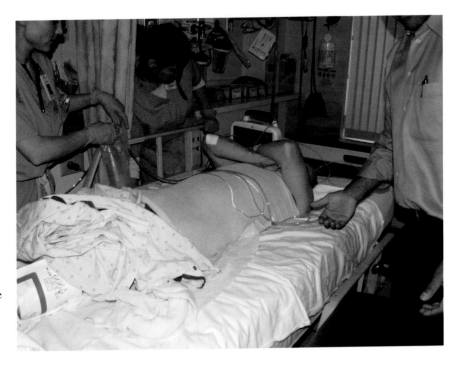

Fig 5.9 Thoracolumbar spine fracture prepared for hyperextension casting with stockenette (Courtesy of Courtney Brown, MD)

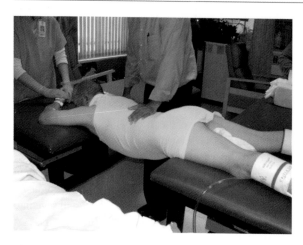

Fig 5.10 Patient is rolled from the bed and suspended between two exam tables to reduce the fracture and apply the cast (courtesy Courtney Brown, MD)

After about 10 min, the cast will harden sufficiently to allow the patient to be rolled back onto the gurney with a hyperextension pillow placed underneath the lordotic spine, so that while the cast finishes hardening, it will not crack (Fig. 5.11).

While the patient is lying on his back, an abdominal hole should be cut, and the cast is trimmed about the hips and the axilla. Final trimming and finishing of the cast can be performed the next day after the patient has been mobilized (Fig. 5.12).

Postcasting X-rays should be obtained to ascertain the amount of correction obtained with the hyperextension casting. The desire is to have posterior element loading, which requires a significant amount of lordosis.

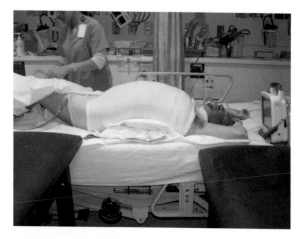

Fig 5.11 Hyper-extension cast applied with spine in hyperextended position (Courtesy of Courtney Brown, MD, Personal Communication)

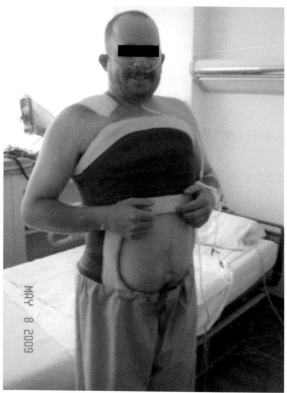

Fig 5.12 Standing in jacket finished with appropriate cut out and padding (Courtesy Courtney Brown, MD, Personal Communication)

It is common that these patients will require a second casting within 1–2 weeks as the abdominal swelling reabsorbs, and the hyperlordosis created by the cast may be lost. If this does occur, a second similar cast should be applied. Patients will require casting for a minimum of 6 weeks and sometimes longer. After cast removal, a Jewitt brace is used for another 4–6 weeks depending on the fracture status.

Pearls

- Application of stockinette and padding is as important as the application of cast material.
- Not all fractures are amenable to casting – there must be some internal stability to provide internal support in addition to the cast.
- Patient must be cooperative.
- Ensure adequate pain control for the procedure, but patients tolerate it surprisingly well.

Pitfalls

- Pressure sores can develop and progress quickly, monitor for them carefully and inform the patient to report such sores immediately.

Inadequate padding can lead to many more complications and complaints.

References

1. Anderson LD (1971) Fractures. In: Chrenshaw AH (ed) Campbell's operative orthopaedics. C.V. Mosby, London
2. Apple D, Perez M (2006) Prospective study of orthotic use after operative stabilization of traumatic thoracic and lumbar fractures. Top Spinal Cord Inj Rehabil 12(2):77–82
3. Axelsson P, Johnson R, Stromqvist B (1993) Lumbar orthosis with unilateral hip immobilization. Spine 18:876–879
4. Bible JE, Biswas D, Nhang PG et al (2008) Postoperative bracing after spine surgery for degenerative conditions; a questionnaire study. Spine J 9(4):309–316
5. Buchalter D, Kahanovitz N, Viola K et al (1989) Three dimensional spinal motion measurement. Part 2: non invasive assessment of lumbar brace immobilization of the spine. J Spinal Disord 1:284–286
6. Butler JS, Walsh A, O'Byrne J (2005) Functional outcome of burst fractures of the first lumbar vertebra managed surgically and conservatively. Int Orthop 29:51–54
7. Cholewicki J, Kashif A, Silfies SP et al (2003) Comparison of motion restriction and trunk stiffness provided by three thoracolumbar orthosis (TLSO). J Spinal Disord Tech 16:461–468
8. Davies WE, Morris JH, Hill V (1980) A Analysis of conservative (non-surgical) management of thoracolumbar fractures and fracture dislocations with neural damage. J Bone Joint Surg Am 62:1324–1328
9. Ferlic D (1962) The range of motion of the normal spine. Bull Johns Hopkins Hosp 2:59–65
10. Johnson RM, Hart DL, Simmons EF et al (1977) Cervical orthoses. A study company their effectiveness in restricting cervical motion in normal subjects. J Bone Joint Surg Am 59:332–339
11. Jones RF, Snowdon E, Coan J et al (1987) Bracing of thoracic and lumbar spine fractures. Paraplegia 25:386–393
12. Koivikko MP, Myllynen P, Karjalainen M et al (2000) Conservative and operative treatment in cervical burst fractures. Arch Orthop Trauma Surg 120:448–451
13. Lantz SA, Schultz AB (1986) Lumbar spine orthosis weaving 1. Restriction of gross body motions. Spine 11:834–837
14. Miller RA, Hardcastle P, Renwick SE (1992) Lower spinal mobility and external immobilization in the normal and pathologic condition. Orthop Rev 21:753–757
15. Nickel VL, Perry J, Garrett A et al (1960) Application of the halo. Orthop Prosthet App J 14:31–35
16. Norton PL, Brown T (1957) The Immobilizing efficiency of back braces; their effect on the posture and motion of the lambosacral spine. J Bone Joint Surg Am 39:111–220
17. Plasmans FMW (1983) The effect of four types of support on the segmental mobility of the lumbosacral spine. J Bone Joint Surg Am 65:943–947
18. Razak M, Basir T, Hyzan Y et al (1998) Treatment in traumatic cervical spine injury. Med J Malaysia 53:1–5
19. Seljeskog EL (1978) Non-operative management of acute upper cervical injuries. Acta Neurochir (Wien) 41:87–100
20. Vander Kooi D, Abad G, Basford JR et al (2003) Lumbar spine stabilization with a thoracolumbar sacral orthosis. Spine 29:100–104
21. Vieweg U, Schultheib R (2001) A review of halo rest treatment of upper cervical spine injuries. Arch Orthop Trauma Surg 121:50–53
22. Yi L, Jingping B, Gele J (2008) Operative versus non-operative treatment for thoracolumbar burst fractures without neurological deficit (review). Cochrane Database Syst Rev 4:1–14

The Halovest

Anthony Dwyer

6.1 Description [1]

The halovest (HV) is a form of spinal external fixation and as such plays a vital role in the damage control management of polytrauma. The halo is affixed to the skull in order to apply both traction to the spine (to reduce cervical dislocations and subluxations) as well as provide spinal stability (after reduction) with the connection to the vest.

6.2 Key Principles

The halo ring is securely affixed to the skull with pins placed in the safe anatomical areas of the skull (Figs. 6.1–6.22). Skull penetration is avoided by using appropriately designed pins and a [2] torque screwdriver set at a safe limit of 8 in./lbs (0.09 N-m).

Garfin and others have described the optimal features of a HV system:

- Titanium or carbon fibre rings with maximum screw holes and an open occipital area.
- Pin insertion at 90° to skull.
- Upright posts and connectors that allow multiplane adjustment and does not interfere with lateral X-rays or have the rods extending beyond the skull.
- Vests of lightweight plastic with sufficiently necessary rigidity and ready access for CPR.

6.3 Expectations

After safely affixing the halo to the skull, traction forces can be applied to the cervical spine to reduce fractures, subluxations and dislocations. These forces can be in excess of 100 lb with stainless steel pins and less than 100 lb with the commonly used titanium pins that provide MRI compatible external fixation.

6.4 Indications [4]

6.4.1 Trauma

- Reduction and fixation of cervical fractures, subluxations and dislocations.
- Restoration of the normal spinal canal capacity in both complete and incomplete spinal cord injury (SCI).
- Provision of sufficient spinal stability to allow the polytrauama patient to sit up or remain prone as needed to maximize management of pulmonary dysfunction.
- Provision of sufficient spinal stability to allow special and necessary positioning in the operating room for treatment of orthopaedic injuries.
- Provision of temporary stability until definitive treatment can be performed.
- Provision of definitive treatment for fractures that can be stabilized in the halo.

6.4.2 Other

Provision of stability in the management of infection, tumour, inflammation, degeneration, congenital malformation and after surgical procedures.

A. Dwyer
Department of Orthopaedic Surgery, Denver Health Medical Center, 777 Bannock Street, MC 0188, Denver, CO 80204, USA
e-mail: anthony.dwyer@dhha.org

V.V. Patel et al. (eds.), *Spine Trauma*,
DOI: 10.1007/978-3-642-03694-1_6, © Springer-Verlag Berlin Heidelberg 2010

A. Dwyer

Fig. 6.1 Select appropriate H/C

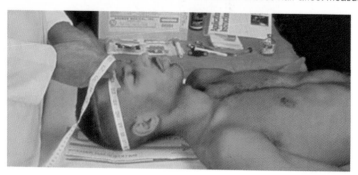

SELECT APPROPRIATE HALO CROWN
Measure patient's skull circumference at equator. Do not let excess hair affect measurement.

Small	17" to 22" (43-56cm)
Large	22" to 26" (58-66cm)

Note: Use smallest possible size

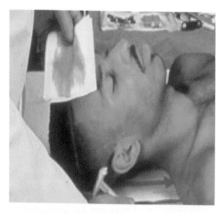

PREP PIN SITE AREAS

• Standard prep is used.

• Areas may be shaved if needed. Excess hair should be trimmed to avoid contact With the pin site or tangling With skull pins as they are inserted or removed.

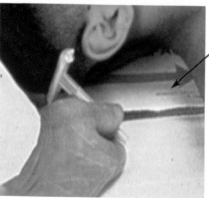

• Cardboard head support (included in kit) may be placed if additional head support is needed. Support may be folded for additional height.

Fig. 6.2 Preperation of pin sites

Fig. 6.3 H/C Position at 'skull equator'

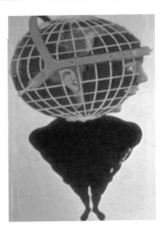

POSITION CROWN AT EQUATOR

- Place crown over patient's head as shown
  Care should be used as crown and pins are sterile.
- Plastic positioning pins are used to adjust crown position.

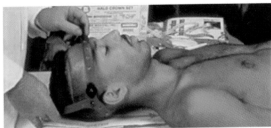

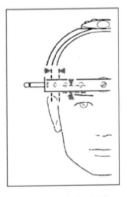

POSITIONING CROWN - DETAILS

- Bottom of crown is aligned with top of eyebrows putting pin holes no more than 1 cm above eyebrows.
- Crown 1 cm from head at anterior pin sites.

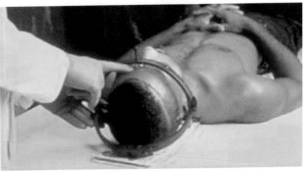

Fig. 6.4 H/C Position re ears and eyebrows

SELECT PIN SITES
Anterior Safe Zones

- Use the lateral 1/2 of the eyebrow as a landmark.
- Safe zones in red.
- Stay lateral to the supraorbital nerve.

SELECT PIN SITES
Posterior Safe Zones

- Posterior pin Sites Safe Zone below the equator.

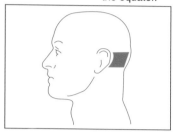

Fig. 6.6 Posterior pin sites

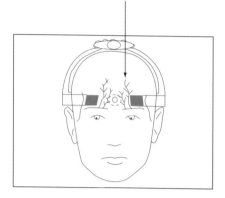

Fig. 6.5 Anterior pin sites

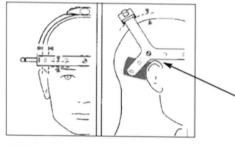

POSITIONING CROWN - DETAILS

- Posterior pin sites below equator of skull.
- Crown should be as low as possible without touching ears.
- Capital arch should not touch top of head.

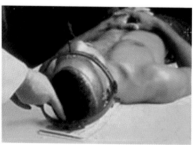

Fig. 6.7 H/C Position

Fig. 6.8 Application of local anaesthesia

ADMINISTER ANESTHESIA

- Anterior anesthesia is administered through the selected pin sites.

- Close patient's eyes to protect from stray anesthesia

- Infiltrate periosteum generously for best pain reduction.

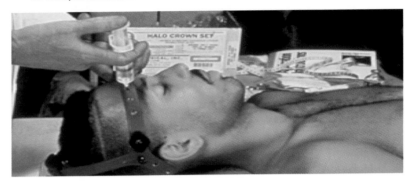

INSERT SKULL PINS

- Skull pins are inserted at the selected pin sites.
- Patient's eyes must be closed.
- Pins are hand tightened until skin is pierced.
- Make sure crown stays in proper position.

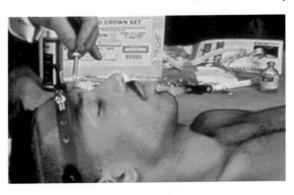

Fig. 6.9 Pin insertion

Fig. 6.10 Torque limiting pin insertion

APPLY TORQUE LIMITING CAPS

- Torque caps are placed over skull pin heads.
- Torque caps are preset to break off at 8 inch pounds.
- A properly set torque wrench may also be used.

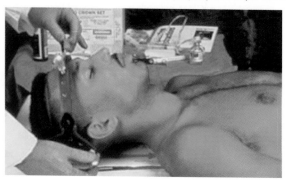

Fig. 6.11 Pin fixation to H/C

TORQUE SKULL PINS

- In order not to shift crown, slowly and sequentially tighten opposing pins, untill proper torque is reached or torque caps break off.
- Lock nuts should be up near head of pin.
- Not down near crown.
- Remove positioning pins and pads.

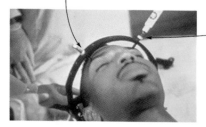

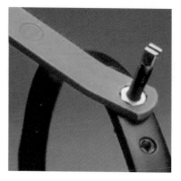

Fig. 6.12 Pin locking

CAUTION:

Before applying traction or moving a patient on whom an AirFlo® or Classic II Vest has been applied, **after approximately 15 minutes, retorque the skull pins using the four remaining torque limiting caps as previously shown** - then secure the locking nuts on all four pins against the Halo crown with the 7/16" (11mm) wrench.

Note : lock nuts should be tightened only until they feel firm. Over tightening could damage threads on the crown, pin or lock nut.

Fig. 6.13 Applying traction

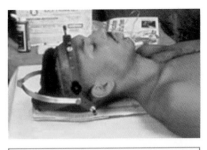

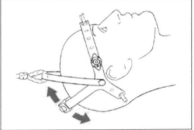

APPLYING TRACTION

- Traction hoop, (included with kit) is attached at juncture of crown and capital arch.

- Carefully adjust head position.

- Tighten bolts and apply desired traction.

- Traction is at the discretion of the surgeon; however, it is suggested not to exceed 70 lbs.

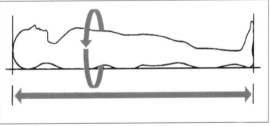

SELECT THE APPROPRIATE VEST

- Measure patient height.

    Tall*   Over 5'7"

    Short*   Under 5'7"

    (*AirFlo®only see catalogue for Classic II sizes)

- Measure patient circumference at zyphoid process.

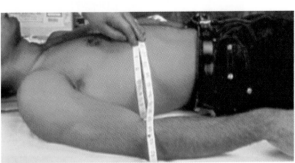

Fig. 6.14 Select appropiate vest

Fig. 6.15 Position posterior shell – 'log roll technique'

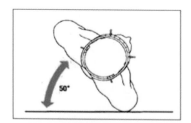

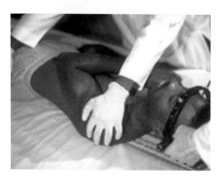

POSITION POSTERIOR SHELL
Log roll technique

- Patient is carefully rolled to one side.
- Shell is placed under patient.
- Patient is lowered.
- Maintain relative position of head and body at all times.
- Do not tangle leads or wires.

Fig. 6.16 Position posterior shell – 'lift technique'

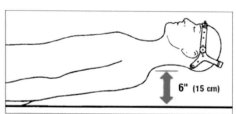

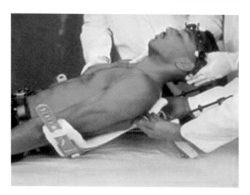

POSITION POSTERIOR SHELL
Lift technique

- Patient is carefully lifted at shoulders.
- Shell is placed under patient.
- Patient is lowered.
- Maintain relative position of head and body at all times.
- Do not tangle leads or wires.

FINAL POSITIONING, ANTERIOR SHELL

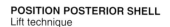

- Ensure superior half of vest is tight against patient's upper chest by pressing firmly on superior edge of vest.
- While holding, tighten universal and vest joints.

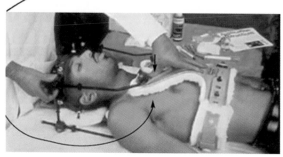

Fig. 6.17 Position anterior shell

Fig. 6.18 Final steps

FINAL STEPS

- Check all bolts, thoracic bands and shoulder straps for security and proper tightness.

- If second skull pin torquing (as noted in crown application) has not been completed, do it now using last four torque caps or torque wrench set at 8 in. lbs.

LONG TERM FOLLOW UP

- **8 in/lbs** <u>24 to 48</u> hours after initial application.
- **2 to 3 in/lbs** every <u>2 to 3 weeks </u>or on patient complaint of pain at pin sites.

Important: Be sure lock nuts are loosened before checking. pin torque and retightened before patient is moved.

Fig. 6.19 Pin care

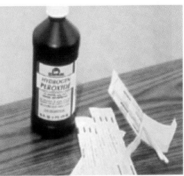

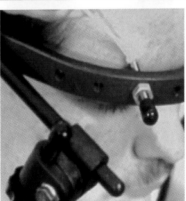

PIN CARE

Daily cleaning with Hydrogen Peroxide or water and sterile Q-tip. No ointments.

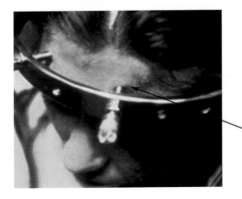

PIN CARE

To check for pin migration:
- Listen for patient complaint of pain at pin site.

- Look for skin build up on top of pin.

- Look for a pin track under the pin.

Fig. 6.20 Pin care

Fig. 6.21 Pin site infection

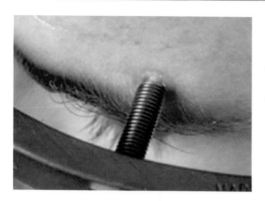

INFECTION

- Administer oral antibiotics until resolved.
- If does not reolve in appropriate time:
  1. Insert and torque a new, sterile, pin in an adjacent pin site.
  2. Then, remove and discard old pin.

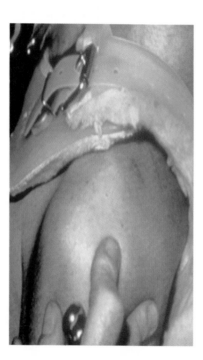

SKIN CARE

- Patients should be checked often for signs of a developing problem.
- Wash daily.
- Neurologically compromsied patients are at increased risk for Skin complications. Their skin Should be examined daily.

Fig. 6.22 Skin care

6.5 Contraindications

Skull fractures involving safe anatomical areas.

6.6 Special Considerations [3]

Osteopenia/osteoporosis, thin cranial bone, and paediatric skulls require special consideration, and the dangers of poor bone fixation and skull penetration can be avoided with the use of multiple pins and reduction of the torque screwdriver settings.

6.7 Special Instructions, Positions and Anaesthesia [5, 6]

Preliminary measurement of the circumference of the skull and chest, and the distance between the shoulders and xiphoid, and the shoulders and iliac crest is ideal for obtaining the appropriate size of halo and vest.

A head support is needed to allow appropriate positioning of the patient over the head of the bed to provide access to the posterior pin sites. The head support can be of proprietary design or by the use of a paediatric size trauma board and, less ideally, by a forearm or IV splint. These can be placed under the patient after gently log rolling the patient, with the trauma collar on.

The hair behind and above the ear may need cutting to allow appropriate access for povidone–iodine skin cleaning, injection of local anaesthetic and posterior pin placement.

The anterior pin sites should be located above the eyebrow and in the lateral half of the supraorbital ridge to avoid the supraorbital nerve.

Four 25-gauge spinal needles and two 10 cc syringes are needed for the injection of 1% lidocaine hydrochloride, which should be first injected into the skin of the pin target area and finally into the skull periostium.

A CPR crash cart should be available at all times.

6.8 Tips and Pearls

- If possible, place the halo ring below the "equator" of the skull to avoid pin displacement with traction.
- Ideally, three people should be available to affix the halo efficiently; one to hold the halo centred, parallel to the eyebrows, equidistant from the forehead and above the ears, while the other two insert the pins.
- Some halo devices come with blunt capped pins to aid in the positioning. Place one anterior and one each laterally.
- For traction in extension, place the posterior pin anterior to the external meatus.
- For traction in flexion, place the posterior pin anterior to the external meatus.
- Position the locking nuts at the end of the thread to avoid their contact with the ring, which would lock and prevent adequate pin travel and penetration.
- Position all the four pins just past the internal surface of the ring prior to insertion.
- If the patient is conscious, ask them to tightly close their eyes (if unconscious, tape the eyes and eyebrows), to avoid anterior skin stretching and elevation of the eyebrows.
- To prevent anterior pin insertion driving the ring away from the skull, the insertion of one anterior pin must be simultaneously matched with the insertion of the opposite posterior pin.
- Have two halo torque screwdrivers available.
- Initially, insert the pins by hand as quickly as possible and when tight, continue the insertion with two torque screwdrivers set at 8 in. per lbs.

- Lock each pin to the halo with the nut, tightening with the wrench, while holding the ring with the other hand, to avoid twisting the head.
- Unlock the nuts and re-torque the pins (8 in. lbs) after 24 h.
- Educate the patient and their family on recommended skin and pin site care, as well as advice on sleeping position.
- Tape wrenches to the vest for use in emergency.

6.9 Pitfalls

Hair can entangle the posterior pins binding them and preventing pin advancement.

Placing pins in the holes needed for the rod holder attachment.

Inadequate skin preparation and placement of the local anaesthetic.

Nerve injury

Arterial injury

6.10 Challenges

Lacerations and skull and facial fractures.

6.11 Complications [2]

Infected skin sites and pin loosening can be prevented by adequate skin and pin site care and managed with replacing the loose pin in an adjacent appropriate pin site.

Garfin and others have listed the associated complications:

- Pin loosening 36%
- Pin infection 20%
- Severe pin discomfort 18%
- Pressure sores 11%
- Severe scars 9%
- Nerve injury 2%
- Dysphagia 1%
- Bleeding pin sites 1%
- Dural puncture 1%

References

1. Botte J, Garfin SR, Byrne TP, Woo S, Nickel V (1989) The halo skeletal fixator, principles of application and maintenance. Clin Orth Rel Res 239:12–18

2. Garfin SR, Botte MJ, Nickel VL, Waters RL (1986) Complications in the use of the halo fixation device. J Bone Joint Surg 68A:320

3. Kopits SE, Steingass MH (1970) Experience with the "halo cast" in small children. Surg Clin North Am 50:935

4. Kostuik JP (1981) Indications for the use of the halo immobilization. Clin Orthop 154:46

5. Thompson H (1962) Halo traction apparatus. A method of external splinting of the cervical spine after surgery. J Bone Joint Surg 44B:655

6. White R (1966) Halo traction apparatus. J Bone Joint Surg 48B:592

Direct Anterior Screw Fixation of Odontoid Fractures

7

Andrew T. Dailey, Todd D. McCall, and Ronald I. Apfelbaum

7.1 Case Example

A 76-year-old woman with no known significant medical issues had a ground-level fall in which her head struck the ground. She immediately had upper neck pain, for which she went to an emergency room. She had no neurological deficits on examination. A computed tomography (CT) scan demonstrated a type II odontoid fracture without significant displacement (Fig. 7.1). Direct anterior odontoid screw fixation was recommended to the patient for treatment, but she refused to undergo surgical intervention. The patient was, therefore, treated initially with a hard cervical collar. She returned to clinic at 1 week's time with continued severe neck pain, and a lateral radiograph demonstrated anterior displacement of the dens fragment (Fig. 7.2). The patient chose to proceed with surgery for odontoid screw fixation (Fig. 7.3). At 1-month follow-up examination, her neck pain had completely resolved, and at 6 months, she had no motion at the fracture site on flexion-extension views of the spine.

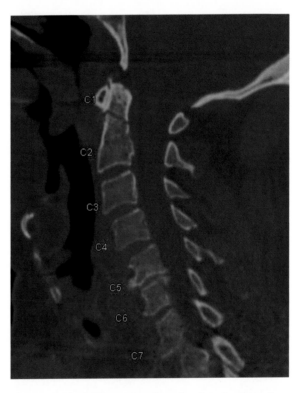

Fig. 7.1 Sagittal CT reconstruction of patient showing a fracture across the base of the dens, representing a Type II odontoid fracture

7.2 Background

A.T. Dailey (✉) and R.I. Apfelbaum
Department of Neurosurgery, University of Utah,
175 N. Medical Drive East, Salt Lake City, UT 84132, USA
e-mail: andrew.dailey@hsc.utah.edu

T.D. McCall
Department of Neurosurgery, Illinois Neurological Institute,
University of Illinois, College of Medicine at Peoria,
530 N.E. Glen Oak, Peoria, 61637, USA

Fractures of the odontoid comprise 10–15% of all cervical fractures [36]. In 1974, Anderson and D'Alonso described a classification system for odontoid fractures, which remains the standard today [3]. Sixty percent of all fractures of the dens are classified as type II using this classification system, indicating that they involve the base of the odontoid process. Many type III fractures,

V.V. Patel et al. (eds.), *Spine Trauma*,
DOI: 10.1007/978-3-642-03694-1_7, © Springer-Verlag Berlin Heidelberg 2010

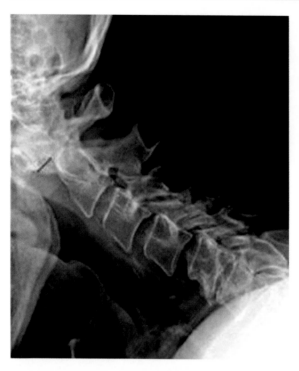

Fig. 7.2 Lateral flexion radiograph demonstrating the inherent instability in a Type II odontoid fracture with 6-7 mm of subluxation in flexion

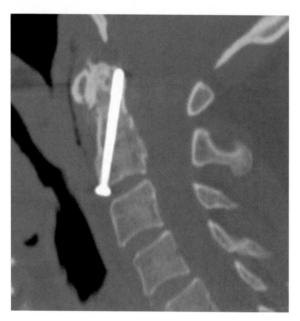

Fig. 7.3 Sagittal CT recontruction of patient with one year post-operative CT showing good position of the odontoid screw and healing of the bone across the base of the dens

which extend into the body of C2 will heal with immobilization, but the overall fusion rate for type II fractures remains lower with immobilization alone. The

traditional treatment of rigid immobilization in a halo can lead to nonunion in more than 50% of cases, with a recent study showing only a 46% fusion rate using rigorous radiographic criteria [13, 34]. Factors that increase the nonunion rate for type II fractures, even with rigid immobilization, include age greater than 50, displacement greater than 6 mm, posterior displacement, angulation of the fracture, and smoking [22, 23, 35]. In addition, rigid immobilization with a halo can be cumbersome and uncomfortable. Cranial, pulmonary, and even cardiac complications have all been reported in patients who have been placed in a halo device [37, 46].

C1–2 arthrodesis was the traditional alternative to rigid immobilization, leading many surgeons to at least attempt stabilization with a halo or other rigid orthosis [19, 24, 42]. Although the success rates of arthrodesis before the advent of C1–2 transarticular screws reported in the literature varied from 60 to 95%, fusion at this area limited motion, had potentially catastrophic complications, and did not eliminate the need for a postoperative orthosis. Although the use of C1–2 transarticular screw placement has increased fusion rates above 95%, the technique is technically demanding and still eliminates rotation about the C1/C2 joint, limiting overall head rotation by more than 50% [10, 15, 17, 30].

As a result, direct fixation of the odontoid process was viewed as a method to provide direct fixation of the fracture fragment and eliminate the need for more extensive C1–2 arthrodesis techniques. The procedure was reported independently by Bohler [8] and Nakanishi [39]. In this procedure, a screw is placed from the base of C2, across the fracture fragment, all the way to the distal tip of the dens. This allows the fracture fragments to be directly realigned and the distal tip to be lagged into approximation with the C2 body (Fig. 7.3). Either one or two screws can be placed with this method, which allows for immediate stabilization of the odontoid to approximately one-half the strength of the intact dens [18, 43]. Since the initial application of this technique, the authors of many case series have reported good fusion rates in the range of 80–90% [1, 6, 11, 21, 27, 31, 32, 38, 45].

7.3 Indications

Meticulous preoperative planning and careful patient selection are the keys to successful placement of an anterior odontoid screw. Any patient with a type II or shallow type III odontoid fracture is a potential candidate for anterior fixation, regardless of age. However, relative and absolute contraindications for the use of a direct anterior approach to C2 must be reviewed before taking the patient to the operating room. In addition, preoperative discussion should include informing the patient of the possibility that direct anterior screw fixation may not yield a successful result, in which case a posterior arthrodesis will need to be performed.

The orientation of the fracture is an important consideration when selecting appropriate candidates for anterior odontoid screw fixation. Posterior oblique fractures, in which the fracture line is in an anterocephalad-to-posterocaudal direction, are ideally suited for this technique because the screw is placed in a trajectory almost perpendicular to the fracture. Conversely, anterior oblique fractures (anterior caudal to posterior cephalad) are in a more parallel orientation in relation to the screw, which places the screw at a mechanical disadvantage to resist shear forces. The screw may also tend to pull the distal fragment anteriorly and inferiorly with anterior oblique fractures [1]. Consequently, anterior oblique fractures are associated with a significantly lower fusion rate than posterior oblique fractures. In a large cohort of 147 patients treated with anterior odontoid screw fixation, anterior oblique fractures obtained a successful bony fusion in only 50% of cases, compared with an overall rate of 88% in recent fractures [6].

7.4 Potential Contraindications

Absolute contraindications to the procedure include pathologic fracture of C2, incompetence of the transverse atlantal ligament resulting in C1–2 instability, and a chronic nonunion of an odontoid fracture. Relative contraindications include severe osteoporosis, comminution of the fracture, a fracture that cannot be completely reduced preoperatively, or patients with a barrel chest or severe thoracic kyphosis in whom it is difficult to obtain a clear trajectory for drill and screw placement.

7.4.1 Age of the Fracture

Remote fractures are known to be at increased risk for nonunion compared with recent fractures. For example, in one study of odontoid fractures treated with anterior screw fixation, recent fractures (<6 months) had a bony fusion rate of 88% compared with only 25% for remote fractures (>18 months) [6]. In a contemporary study, Agrillo et al. [2] found that type II odontoid fractures between 6 and 12 months of age had a 77% bony fusion rate. Thus, it appears that the rate of successful bony fusion declines over time, with an acceptable rate of success when surgery is performed within 1 year.

7.4.2 Age of the Patient

The influence of patient age on the fusion rate of anterior odontoid screw fixation has received considerable attention. Historically, advanced age has been considered very detrimental to the successful healing of type II dens fractures. Indeed, the rate of nonunion for type II dens fractures treated with halo immobilization was 21 times higher in patients over 50 years of age than in those under 50 years [35]. However, studies evaluating fusion after odontoid screw fixation in the elderly have yielded mixed results. In a case-control study of 27 patients, Börm et al. [9] found no significant difference in bony fusion rates between patients above 70 years of age (73%) and those under 70 years (75%). The authors of other studies have found similar fusion rates in elderly patients after odontoid screw fixation, ranging from 73 to 89% [4, 14, 25]. A large retrospective study of 110 patients treated with odontoid screw fixation found a nonunion rate of 12% for patients at least 65 years old, compared with 4% for those under 65 years [41]. While this difference between age groups was significant, the fusion rate of 88% in the elderly group is quite tolerable. Overall, data suggest that elderly patients with type II dens fractures should not be excluded from anterior screw fixation based on their age alone.

7.5 Procedure

Equipment needed

1. OR Bed with radiolucenthead/shoulder region
2. Towel roll under shoulders
3. Rigid head positioner such as Mayfield head holder
4. Anterior cervical access instruments
5. Fluoroscopy – biplanar
6. Anterior cervical/odontoid screw system
7. Anterior cervical/odontoid retractor system
8. Neuromonitoring if desired

Patients are intubated with an awake fiberoptic technique. We do not routinely use neuromonitoring for these procedures for several reasons. Firstly, fluoroscopy is used extensively to assure reduction and guide screw trajectory, so that drastic changes in alignment are not performed. Secondly, the generous space available for the cord at C1 and the dens makes spinal cord compression unlikely without drastic changes in position. Finally, the set-up for biplanar fluoroscopy at the head of the table makes the technical aspects of establishing and maintaining scalp leads quite cumbersome and may lead to technically inadequate motor and sensory evoked potentials, which gives misleading information.

The technique described in this section has been developed by the senior author and uses a complete system with retractors and drill guides designed to accurately and safely reapproximate and fixate the fracture fragments [5, 6]. After intubation, proper patient positioning and radiographic exposure of the C2 vertebral body must be confirmed. Anatomic reduction of the fragment must be confirmed and can usually be performed with gentle flexion and extension maneuvers of the head. If necessary, direct manual transoral manipulation of a ventrally displaced dens fragment can help with reduction [7, 20]. The patient is placed supine with halter, halo, or tong traction used to stabilize the head.

To optimize the extended position of the neck and provide the best trajectory for placement of the screw, we place a folded sheet or blanket under the patient's shoulders. Biplanar fluoroscopy must be used for all procedures, so that simultaneous anterior-posterior (AP) and lateral images can be obtained and immediate confirmation of changes in fracture alignment or instrumentation placement is obtained. To obtain a direct AP image, a radiolucent bite block is used to open the jaw.

After the neck is prepped and draped, a transverse incision is made using a skin crease at approximately the C5 vertebral body level. The platysma muscle is identified, opened transversely, and then undermined to allow rostral exposure. Blunt dissection is then performed down to the precervical fascia, and lateral fluoroscopy is used to confirm the level of the exposure. The blunt dissection is carried up until the anterior inferior surface of the C2 vertebral body is identified and confirmed radiographically.

Once the precervical fascia is identified over the C5 body, it is opened sharply, and the longus colli muscles are dissected laterally. A two-piece retractor system with both transverse and longitudinal blades (Fig. 7.4 a, b) has been designed for this approach, and the Caspar retractor blades can be placed under the edges of the longus muscle medially and laterally. From this transverse retractor

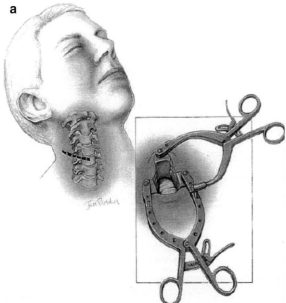

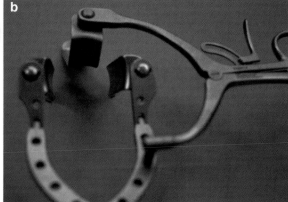

Fig. 7.4 (**a**) Drawing depicting the typical location of the skin incision at the C5-6 level and then the two piece retractor system in place with the medial and lateral blades seated beneath a cuff of longus colli muscle. (**b**) Ex vivo view of the retractor showing extra blade that provides cephalad retraction (top of page) and how it locks to the medial/lateral portion of the retractor

base, the space anterior to the precervical fascia is opened and retracted by the longer longitudinal blades. This protects the esophagus and allows the surgeon a working portal to the anterior inferior border of the C2 body.

A K-wire is used to define an entry point in AP and lateral trajectories. Care must be taken to define an entry point under the anterior lip of C2 (Fig. 7.5a,b) and not on the anterior body of C2 as the latter entry

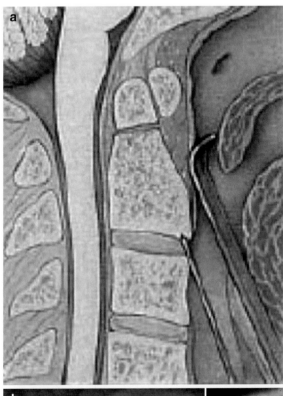

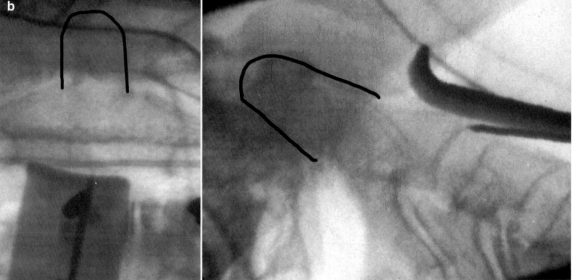

Fig. 7.5 (**a**) Drawing depicting the selection of an entry point in the inferior portion of C2 using a K-wire. (**b**) AP (*left*) and lateral (*right*) fluoroscopic images with the tip of the odontoid outlined in black. The K-wire is seen entering the inferior border of C2 with the trajectory towards the tip of the odontoid carefully selected prior to drilling

point predisposes to screw breakout or pullout, loss of fracture reduction, and subsequent nonunion. K-wire or screw breakout through the anterior cortex prevents adequate screw purchase and, in most instances, requires conversion of the surgery to a posterior fusion. To further recess the screw entry point into the inferior edge of the C2 vertebral body, a larger 8-mm drill is placed over the K-wire, and a trough is created along the trajectory line in the C2–3 disk space (Fig. 7.6), a technique that assures positioning of the screw head so that it does not sit on the anterior body of C2.

Once the entry point has been determined, the drill guide is placed over the K-wire and secured into position along the anterior border of the C3 vertebral body (Fig. 7.7). The drill guide we use can be secured to the C3 body and thus allows manipulation of the proximal C2–C3 vertebral body complex. This technique can be useful in final reduction of the fracture fragments, particularly if the distal fragment (tip of the odontoid) is displaced posteriorly. The K-wire is removed, and a 2.7-mm drill is used to drill through the cortex at the tip of the odontoid (Fig. 7.8). We prefer a noncannulated drill bit so that breakage of the K-wire is avoided and the K-wire cannot be captured by the drill and driven through the distal cortex and beyond. It is important to drill through the distal cortex so that a screw will engage the cortex and lag the distal

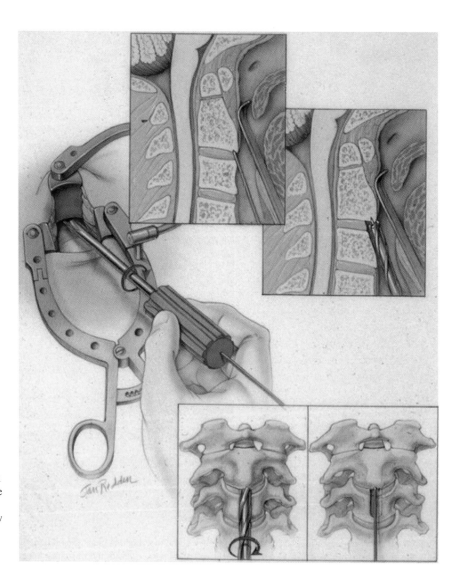

Fig. 7.6 Drawing showing the AP and lateral views with the 7-mm overdrill to create and an entry site in the C2-3 disc space and adjacent vertebral body. This helps ensure that the screw is not placed too anteriorly along the front of the C2 vertebral body

Fig. 7.7 Drawing depicting placement of the drill guide over the K-wire. The drill guide has two pieces with the outer portion having spikes that can be affixed to the C3 vertebral body. The inner drill guide can be advanced so that the tip is directly against the inferior portion of the C2 body

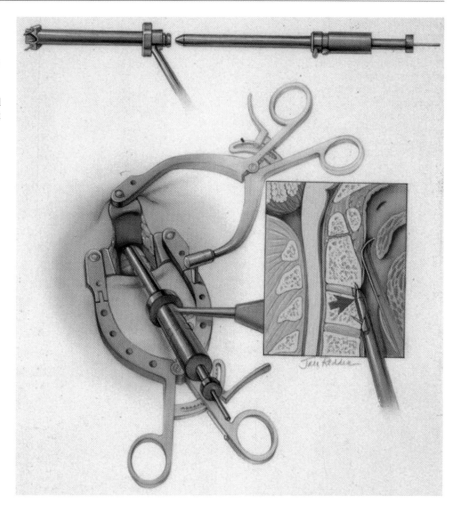

fragment into tight approximation with the proximal C2 body. After drilling, the length of the screw can be determined, and the entire screw tract including the distal cortex is tapped (Fig. 7.9). We use one or two 3.5-mm screws. The first screw placed is a partially threaded lag screw that provides approximation of the fracture fragments. If the surgeon chooses to place a second screw (see discussion below), a fully threaded screw can be used at this time.

Several modifications have been proposed using tubular retractors to accomplish the esophageal retraction [12, 28, 44]. However, these minimally invasive or minimal access techniques do not allow drill guides that can be affixed to the spine and thus do not allow manipulation of the proximal portion of the C2 body. The drill guide described in this technique allows the surgeon to manipulate the C2 body and thus perfectly align the fracture fragments. In

addition, many of the minimal access techniques describe the use of cannulated drill over a drill guide, the limitations and dangers of which have already been outlined.

7.6 Technical Pearls and Pitfalls

7.6.1 Surgical Technique

As previously mentioned, preoperative radiographs must be carefully evaluated to determine whether there are any absolute contraindications to direct fixation of the odontoid. All patients must be counseled about potential complications from hoarseness or swallowing difficulties. Furthermore, all patients are advised

Fig. 7.8 Drawing depicting the drill placed across the fracture fragment. We use the K-wire only to assess the entry point for the drill. The drill is a 2.7mm drill and is not cannulated so that the K-wire can not be inadvertenly driven through the tip of the odotoid

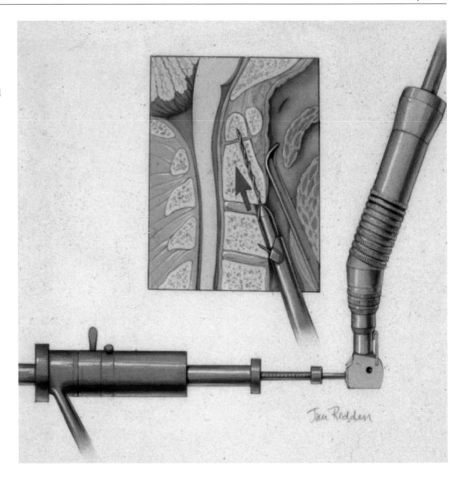

that direct fixation may not be possible for anatomical regions. For example, men with barrel chests or older patients with a significant thoracic kyphosis often present difficult trajectories for placement of the drill. To determine whether the patient's chest will prevent placement of the drill to the tip of the dens, an intraoperative lateral fluoroscopic image is obtained with a long K-wire to determine drill trajectory [5, 6].

If direct fixation is not possible or the fracture does not unite, posterior C1–2 fusion is the salvage option. Various techniques are available, including C1–2 transarticular screws or C1 lateral mass–C2 pedicle/lateral mass fixation, all of which provide similar biomechanical strength [29, 33]. The new posterior cervical modular fixation systems have led to a variety of surgical options, which often make fusion to the occiput unnecessary unless there is instability of the condylar–C1 joint. Posterior C1–2 fusion rates as high as 95% have been reported.

7.6.2 One or Two Screws

Conceptually, the use of two screws, instead of one, to prevent rotation of the distal dens fragment and add more strength to resist shear forces is appealing. However, the space needed for successful anatomic placement of the two 3.5-mm screws has been estimated to be at least 9 mm [40], and many patients do not have a dens this large in diameter [21, 26]. Some authors have suggested using different screws, such as a 4.5-mm Hebert screw [11] or two smaller 2.7-mm screws, in order to get two screws into every fractured dens [21]. The use of two screws, instead of one, also reduces the surface area available for a bony fusion to occur.

Available evidence suggests that there is little difference in fusion outcome between one- and two-screw constructs. In cohorts of patients treated with anterior odontoid screw fixation, there have been no significant differences in the rate of union between fractures

Fig. 7.9 Lateral radiographs showing the drill (*left*) followed by the tap (right) placed to the distal cortex of the odontoid tip. Following tapping, a screw is placed to this distal cortex, with a partially threaded screw placed first to allow the screw to lag the distal fragment to the C2 vertebral body (Figure 3)

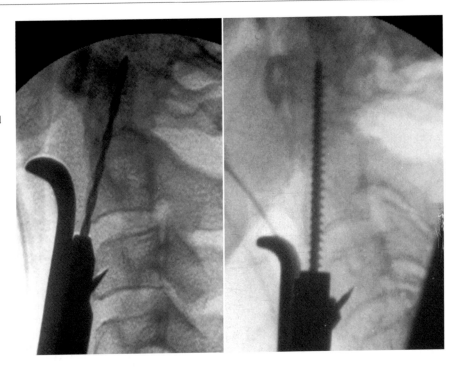

treated with one screw and those treated with two screws [6, 31]. A biomechanical study found no difference between one and two screws for loading to failure, although two screws did provide superior stiffness in extension loading [43]. However, a recent clinical series found that placement of two screws did lead to a higher fusion rate in patients over the age of 70, suggesting that extra fixation may be beneficial as C2 becomes progressively osteopenic [16].

7.7 Postoperative Considerations

7.7.1 Postoperative Bracing

We do not routinely place patients in a collar after anterior screw fixation. However, if an elderly patient is found to have poorer bone quality or if additional fractures, particularly of the C1 vertebra, are noted in the cervical spine, a collar is provided for additional postoperative stability. Typically, we have the patients use the collar for 10–12 weeks. One rationale for the use of a collar in patients with less than optimal bone is provided by the biomechanical study of Doherty et al. [18], in which the authors suggested that odontoid

screws only reestablish half the original strength of the dens after initial placement. Although we have not found a need for bracing in the patient with healthy bone, the use of a collar in older patients with osteoporosis should not be ruled out. The patient should be encouraged to walk whether or not a brace is used.

7.7.2 Follow-up Monitoring

Follow-up monitoring consists of sequential radiographs to confirm that reduction of the fracture is maintained, proper bone healing is occurring, and the odontoid screw remains in proper position. Generally, we obtain radiographs at 1, 3, 6, and 12 months after surgery, with dynamic radiographs at 3, 6, and 12 months.

7.7.3 Potential Complications

The most common complication after surgery is a nonunion of the fracture, in which case we advocate a posterior C1–2 fusion. Less commonly, the screw can back out. If the initial screw was not long enough to properly engage the distal cortex of the fracture segment, the anterior screw can likely be salvaged with replacement by a longer screw that has bicortical purchase. If the initial screw placement was adequate, screw back-out must be addressed with a posterior fusion. Breakout of the screw head through the anterior cortex of C2 will lead to nonunion and should be salvaged with a posterior C1–2 fusion.

Approach-related complications occur more frequently in the elderly and include dysphagia, hoarseness, and postoperative hematoma. Dysphagia places the patient at risk for aspiration pneumonia and may require the temporary placement of a nasogastric feeding tube. A recent series of patients over the age of 70 years revealed an incidence of dysphagia of 35%, with 25% of patients requiring a temporary feeding tube for 2 days to 4 months [16].

7.8 Conclusions

Anterior screw fixation for type II odontoid fractures is very successful with proper patient selection. Pathological fractures, fractures over 18 months old, incompetence of the transverse atlantal ligament resulting in C1–2 instability, and anterior oblique fractures are all situations we consider to be strong contraindications for this technique. Patient characteristics including the presence of osteoporosis and body habitus must also be carefully weighed. On the other hand, advanced age and the possibility that only one screw may be placed instead of two should not be considered deterrents. In appropriate patients, odontoid screw fixation should be considered a first-line treatment for type II dens fractures.

References

1. Aebi M, Etter C, Coscia M (1989) Fractures of the odontoid process. Treatment with anterior screw fixation Spine 14:1065–1070
2. Agrillo A, Russo N, Marotta N, Delfini R (2008) Treatment of remote type ii axis fractures in the elderly: feasibility of anterior odontoid screw fixation. Neurosurgery 63:1145–1150, discussion 1150–1141
3. Anderson LD, D'Alonzo RT (1974) Fractures of the odontoid process of the axis. J Bone Joint Surg Am 56: 1663–1674
4. Andersson S, Rodriquez M, Olerud C (2000) Odontoid fractures: high complication rate associated with anterior screw fixation in the elderly. Eur Spine J 9:56–60
5. Apfelbaum R (1992) Anterior screw fixation for odontoid fractures. In: Rengachary SS, Wilkins RH (eds) Neurosurgical Operative Atlas, vol 2. American Association of Neurological Surgeons, Park Ridge, IL, pp 189–199
6. Apfelbaum RI, Lonser RR, Veres R, Casey A (2000) Direct anterior screw fixation for recent and remote odontoid fractures. J Neurosurg 93:227–236
7. Ben-Galim P, Reitman CA (2008) Direct transoral manipulation to reduce a displaced odontoid fracture: a technical note. Spine J 8:818–820
8. Bohler J (1982) Anterior stabilization for acute fractures and non-unions of the dens. J Bone Joint Surg Am 64:18–27
9. Borm W, Kast E, Richter H, Mohr K (2003) Anterior screw fixation in type II odontoid fractures: is there a difference in outcome between age groups? Neurosurgery 52:1089–1092
10. Campanelli M, Kattner KA, Stroink A, Gupta K, West S (1999) Posterior C1-C2 transarticular screw fixation in the treatment of displaced type II odontoid fractures in the geriatric population - a review of seven cases. Surg Neurol 51: 596–601
11. Chang KW, Liu YW, Cheng PG, Chang L, Suen KL, Chung WL, Chen UL, Liang PL (1994) One Herbert double-threaded compression screw fixation of displaced type II odontoid fractures. J Spinal Disord 7:62–69
12. Chi Y, Wang X, Xu H, Lin Y, Huang Q, Mao F, Ni W, Wang S, Dai L (2007) Management of odontoid fractures with percutaneous anterior odontoid screw fixation. Eur Spine J 16: 1157–1164
13. Clark CR, White AA 3rd (1985) Fractures of the dens. A multicenter study. J Bone Joint Surg Am 67:1340–1348
14. Collins I, Min WK (2008) Anterior screw fixation of type II odontoid fractures in the elderly. J Trauma 65:1083–1087
15. Coyne TJ, Fehlings MG, Wallace MC, Bernstein M, Tator CH (1995) C1-C2 posterior cervical fusion: long-term evaluation of results and efficacy. Neurosurgery 37:688–692, discussion 692–683
16. Dailey A, Finn M, Hart D, Schmidt M, Apfelbaum R (2008) Difference in fusion rate for one versus two screws in elderly odontoid fractures. Cervical Spine Research Society, Austin, TX
17. Dickman CA, Sonntag VK (1998) Posterior C1-C2 transarticular screw fixation for atlantoaxial arthrodesis. Neurosurgery 43:275–280, discussion 280–271
18. Doherty BJ, Heggeness MH, Esses SI (1993) A biomechanical study of odontoid fractures and fracture fixation. Spine 18:178–184
19. Dunn ME, Seljeskog EL (1986) Experience in the management of odontoid process injuries: an analysis of 128 cases. Neurosurgery 18:306–310
20. Elias WJ, Ireland P, Chadduck JB (2006) Transoral digitally manipulated reduction of a ventrally displaced Type II odontoid fracture to aid in screw fixation. Case illustration. J Neurosurg (Spine) 4:82
21. ElSaghir H, Bohm H (2000) Anderson type II fracture of the odontoid process: results of anterior screw fixation. J Spinal Disord 13:527–530, discussion 531
22. Hadley MN, Browner C, Sonntag VK (1985) Axis fractures: a comprehensive review of management and treatment in 107 cases. Neurosurgery 17:281–290
23. Hadley MN, Dickman CA, Browner CM, Sonntag VK (1989) Acute axis fractures: a review of 229 cases. J Neurosurg 71:642–647

24. Hanssen AD, Cabanela ME (1987) Fractures of the dens in adult patients. J Trauma 27:928–934

25. Harrop JS, Przybylski GJ, Vaccaro AR, Yalamanchili K (2000) Efficacy of anterior odontoid screw fixation in elderly patients with Type II odontoid fractures. Neurosurg Focus 8:e6

26. Heller JG, Alson MD, Schaffler MB (1992) Qunatitative internal dens morpholgy. Spine 17:861–866

27. Henry AD, Bohly J, Grosse A (1999) Fixation of odontoid fractures by an anterior screw. J Bone Joint Surg Br 81: 472–477

28. Hott J, Henn J, Sonntag V (2003) A new table-fixed retractor for anterior odontoid screw fixation: technical note. J Neurosurg (Spine 3) 98:294–296

29. Hott J, Lynch J, Chamberlain R, Sonntag V, Crawford N (2005) Biomechanical comparison of C1-2 posterior fixation techniques. J Neurosurg (Spine) 2:175–181

30. Jeanneret B, Magerl F (1992) Primary posterior fusion C1/2 in odontoid fractures: indications, technique, and results of transarticular screw fixation. J Spinal Disord 5:464–475

31. Jenkins JD, Coric D, Branch CL Jr (1998) A clinical comparison of one- and two-screw odontoid fixation. J Neurosurg 89:366–370

32. Julien TD, Frankel B, Traynelis VC, Ryken TC (2000) Evidence-based analysis of odontoid fracture management. Neurosurg Focus 8:e1

33. Kim S, Lim T, Paterno J, Hwang T, Lee K, Balabhadra R, Kim D (2004) Biomechanical comparison of anterior and posterior stabilization methods in atlantoaxial instability. J Neurosurg (Spine) 100:277–283

34. Koivikko MP, Kiuru MJ, Koskinen SK, Myllynen P, Santavirta S, Kivisaari L (2004) Factors associated with nonunion in conservatively-treated type-II fractures of the odontoid process. J Bone Joint Surg Br 86:1146–1151

35. Lennarson PJ, Mostafavi H, Traynelis VC, Walters BC (2000) Management of type II dens fractures: a case-control study. Spine 25:1234–1237

36. Maak TG, Grauer JN (2006) The contemporary treatment of odontoid injuries. Spine 31:S53–S60

37. Majerik S, Tashijan RZ, Biffl WL, Harrington DT, Cioffi WG (2005) Halo vest immobilization in the elderly: A death sentence? J Trauma 60:199–203

38. Moon MS, Moon JL, Sun DH (2006) Treatment of dens fracture in adults: A report of thirty-two cases. Bull Hosp Jt Dis 63:108–112

39. Nakanishi T (1980) Internal fixation of the odontoid process. Cent Jap J Orthop Trauma 23:399–406

40. Nucci RC, Seigel S, Merola AA (1995) Computed tomographic evaluation of the normal odontoid. Implications for internal fixation. Spine 20:264–270

41. Platzer P, Thalhammer G, Ostermann R, Wieland T, Vecsei V, Gaebler C (2007) Anterior screw fixation of odontoid fractures comparing younger and elderly patients. Spine 32: 1714–1720

42. Polin RS, Szabo T, Bogaev CA, Replogle RE, Jane JA (1996) Nonoperative management of Types II and III odontoid fractures: the Philadelphia collar versus the halo vest. Neurosurgery 38:450–456, discussion 456-457

43. Sasso R, Doherty BJ, Crawford MJ, Heggeness MH (1993) Biomechanics of odontoid fracture fixation. Comparison of the one- and two-screw technique. Spine 18:1950–1953

44. Shalayev S, Mun I, Mallek G, Palmer S, Levi A, Lasner T, Kantrowitz A (2004) Retrospective analysis and modifications of retractor systems for anterior odontoid screw fixation. Neurosurg Focus 16:E14,1–4

45. Subach BR, Morone MA, Haid RW Jr, McLaughlin MR, Rodts GR, Comey CH (1999) Management of acute odontoid fractures with single-screw anterior fixation. Neurosurgery 45:812–819, discussion 819–820

46. Tashjian RZ, Majercik S, Biffl WL, Palumbo MA, Cioffi WG (2006) Halo-vest immobilization increases early morbidity and mortality in elderly odontoid fractures. J Trauma 60:199–203

Occiput–Cervical Fixation

8

Ciro G. Randazzo, Bryan LeBude, John Ratliff, and James Harrop

8.1 Case Example

A 37-year-old male presents as an unrestrained passenger in a high speed motor vehicle accident. Cardiopulmonary resuscitation has been performed by fire rescue. He is resuscitated, immobilized,and transferred to the Emergency Department. The patient arrives intubated and immobilized on a long board.

On examination in the Emergency Department, he is intubated, opens his eyes spontaneously and appears to be localizing with the left upper extremity and withdrawing the left lower extremity.

Patients may present, after high energy injuries, with hemodynamic and respiratory instability as a result of atlantooccipital or atlantoaxial dislocation due to neuronal injury in the brainstem and/or proximal spinal cord. Due to the mechanism and high energy, there is an associated high incidence of traumatic brain injuries and long bone or visceral trauma. Management strategies consist of immobilization of the dislocation and fusion, so as to limit further neuronal injury and potentiate recovery.

Remember, preliminary films may be read as no fracture, and atlantoaxial dislocation can easily be overlooked (Figs. 8.1 and 8.2).

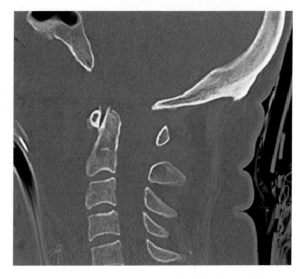

Fig. 8.1 Craniocervical dislocation. Note the increased distance between the dens and the clivus (greater than 12 mm). Also note that there is no associated bony injury

8.2 Background

Occiput to cervical fixation (OCF) has undergone significant evolution due to advances in operative techniques and instrumentation techniques, most recently, with the development of modern titanium plates, screws, and rod systems. This procedure has evolved from simple autograft onlay fusion techniques to sublaminar wiring techniques, and, most recently, rigid occipital plating with midline bicortical screws connected via rods to atlantoaxial or subaxial screw fixation [1, 2]. Currently, the most rigid of fixation systems utilizes subaxial rod-plate systems and subaxial rod-independent plate systems [4–6, 8]. The advantage of this technique is that it provides immediate rigid fixation without the need for

J. Harrop (✉), C.G. Randazzo, B. LeBude, and J. Ratliff
Department of Neurosurgery, Thomas Jefferson University,
909 Walnut Street, Philadelphia, PA 19107, USA
e-mail: james.harrop@jefferson.edu

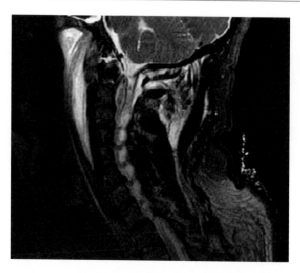

Fig. 8.2 MRI of craniocervical dislocation (T2-weighted image). Note the significant ligamentous injury, edema, and swelling in the prevertebral and soft tissues of the neck and posterior paraspinal muscles, interspinous regions, and ligamentum nuchae

prolonged external halo-vest immobilization [9, 10]. Thus the new techniques yield a higher fusion rate while reducing the morbidity of halo-vest orthoses.

8.3 Indications and Advantages for Procedure

Common indications for occipital–cervical fusion include traumatic instability across the craniocervical junction, e.g., atlanto-occipital dislocation from high impact trauma and Type III Anderson and Montesano occipital condyle fractures. Nontraumatic causes of instability across the craniocervical junction include rheumatoid arthritis, oncologic destruction, infection, and congenital abnormalities.

8.4 Contraindications for Procedure

There are relatively few contraindication s prohibiting occipital–cervical fusion. Generally, however, absence or hypoplasia of the occipital bone would prohibit fusion to the occiput. Also, patients with medical or traumatic comorbidities that would prevent an operative procedure or the prone positioning required for this procedure are not appropriate candidates.

8.5 Procedure

8.5.1 Equipment

- Chest rolls, gel pads for arms, multiple pillows for leg positioning
- Three inch tape for securing patient to bed
- Hair clippers – do not use a razor
- Mayfield three point head fixation equipped operating room table (assuming skull fractures do not preclude this)
- Halo attachment for Mayfield and/or operating room bed if the patient is to be positioned while in a Halo orthosis
- Traction apparatus and weights if the patient is to be maintained/positioned in traction
- Occipital–cervical fixation system of choice (Figs. 8.3–8.5)
- Iliac crest bone graft harvest instruments
- Cervical collar or Halo-vest orthosis
- Neuromonitoring
- Fluoroscopy

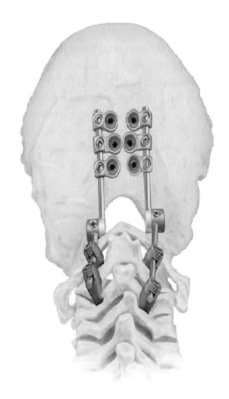

Fig. 8.3 Commonly used fixation systems for occipital–cervical fusion

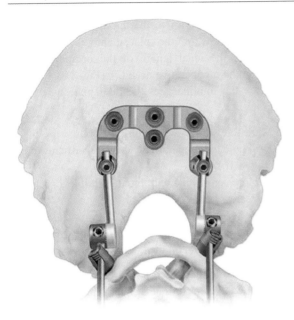

Fig. 8.4 Commonly used fixation systems for occipital–cervical fusion

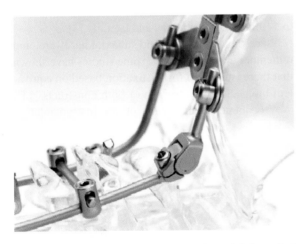

Fig. 8.5 Commonly used fixation systems for occipital–cervical fusion

8.6 Anesthetic and Neuromonitoring Considerations

Review with the patient and family the possibility of not obtaining baseline neuromonitoring after anesthesia is induced (if neuromonitoring is utilized). If this happens, a decision will have to be made whether to proceed with the fixation or not. Also, remember to avoid long-acting paralytics and inhalational agents as these will interfere with neuromonitoring.

Maintain the mean arterial pressure (MAP) >85 mmHg to sustain spinal cord perfusion throughout the case including induction of anesthesia. All patients should have an arterial line placed to monitor blood pressure.

Awake fiber optic or in line traction intubation minimizes neck motion with intubation. Fiber optic is preferred when possible.

Check the postintubation MEPs and SSEPs as a baseline and then again after final positioning, to make sure that they are maintained. A change in neurophysiologic monitoring should prompt the following steps:

- Assure that MAPs >85 mm Hg.
- Undo any recent changes in head or neck position.
- Assure that it is not a technical or neuromonitoring equipment problem.
- If signals do not return to baseline, consider waking up the patient and doing a neurologic exam.

8.7 Patient Positioning and Room Setup

Position the patient in Mayfield three point fixation, assuming that skull fractures do not preclude this. Position the body on chest or laminectomy rolls or a Wilson frame. A long draw sheet and tape can be used to secure the patient to the OR bed. The shoulders do not require taping, if they do not preclude X-ray imaging of the upper cervical spine. Be sure to check the OR bed and Mayfield head frame and draw sheet appropriateness before commencing the placement of the patient prone. After turning, assure that the patient's face and chin have adequate clearance from the bed and there is no pressure on the eyes. Assure that all the intravenous lines and neuromonitoring are functional before finally securing the patient prone. Maintain the head in a neutral position.

Remember: The stretcher should not leave the OR until the patient is secured safely to the bed, IVs and neuromonitoring are working appropriately, respiration and oxygenation are adequate, and MEPs and SSEPs are satisfactory.

Do not forget to prep for posterior ICBG harvest.

8.8 Surgical Approach

Hair should be clipped to above the inion. The entire cervical spine should be draped off. Remember to prep the iliac crest for bone graft harvest as needed. Appropriate antibiotics should be administered within 1 h of the skin incision (Figs. 8.6 and 8.7).

Make a midline incision from the inion far enough caudal to include the predetermined level of the distal end of the fusion. In OCF for trauma, we prefer to fuse to the first one to two levels of normal ligamentous anatomy, at minimum down to C2. Starting the exposure at the level of the inion and working caudally facilitates exposure in the midline raphe. Also maintain subperiosteal dissection to minimize blood loss.

Occipital exposure should be above the superior nuchal line to facilitate plate placement. Choose a plate

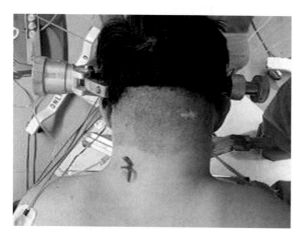

Fig. 8.6 Hair clipped to above inion, head in Mayfield

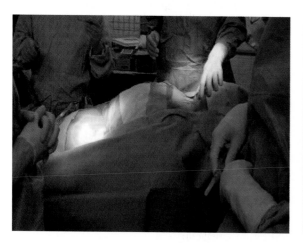

Fig. 8.7 Inion to cervico–thoracic junction and posterior ICBG bone harvest site prepped into field

such that it is inferior to the inion, but allows distal bone exposure for the placement of bone graft. Determine the ideal length of the occipital screws based on the preoperative head CT (Fig. 8.8).

Place the midline keel occipital plate as follows (Fig. 8.9):

- Mark screw holes with high speed burr.
- Drill hole to preoperatively determined screw depth (Fig. 8.10).
- Explore screw hole with blunt ball tipped probe.
- Tap screw hole.
- Place screw of preoperatively determined length.
- The inion can be burred down such that the occipital plate fits flush on the cranium.

Note that midline unicortical screws have pullout strength equivalent to that of lateral bicortical screws [7]; however, placing midline and lateral screws increases the stiffness of the construct and reduces the risk of rotational pullout. Remember that the thickness of the occipital bone varies. It is thickest in the midline (11–17 mm males, 10–12 mm females) and the thickness decreases radially from the occipital prominence to as thin as 0.3 mm below and laterally [3].

Place the atlantoaxial and subaxial hardware, and remember that if fusing C2, some studies have shown that there is no need for C1 fixation based on equivalent biomechanical strength of both constructs [11]. We recommend placement of all instrumentation

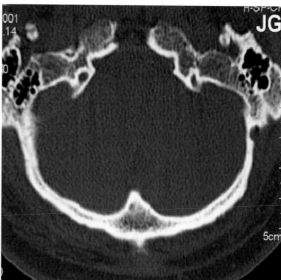

Fig. 8.8 Measurement of occipital keel thickness on preoperative head CT

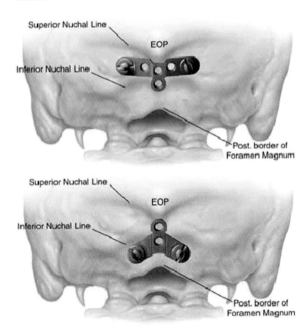

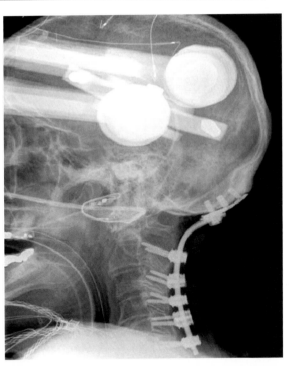

Fig. 8.9 Placement of midline keel plate – inferior to inion, but distal bone present for the placement of bone graft

Fig. 8.11 Final intraoperative lateral X-ray prior to closing the wound

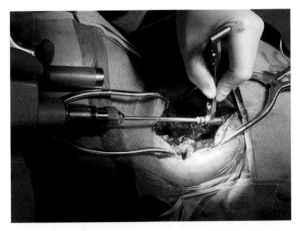

Fig. 8.10 Drilling hole to preoperatively determined screw depth

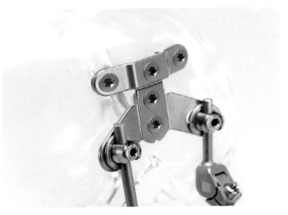

Fig. 8.12 Midline keel plate with midline bicortical screws and lateral unicortical screws

prior to any decompression to reduce the risk of iatrogenic neurologic injury. Also, burr the facet joints and fusion surfaces prior to the placement of the rods. Subsequently, bend the rods carefully to match the contour of the hardware for optimal fixation and strength. When placing the cap screws, do not force the rods into place; they should lay in the screw heads and plate without tension. Rod contouring can be very difficult; plan extra time for this.

After final tightening, copiously irrigate the wounds with antibiotic solution before placing the bone graft in the lateral gutters (Fig. 8.11). Place drains (if desired) and close in a watertight fashion in layers. If there is a cerebrospinal leak, you can patch with dural substitute or biological glue and close fascia with both interrupted suture followed by running suture and close the skin with running locked suture for a watertight seal.

Fixation technique

Occiput – Midline Keel plate with midline bicortical screws and lateral unicortical screws (Fig. 8.12).

C1/Atlas – Lateral mass screws, may not be necessary if there is adequate fixation at C2 or below [11]; can also use posterior arch screws (Fig. 8.13).

C2/Axis – Pars screws, pedicle screws, transarticular screws from C2 into C1 (Fig. 8.14).

C3 to C7/Subaxial spine – Lateral mass screws (Fig. 8.14).

C7 – Option of pedicle screws rather than lateral mass screws.

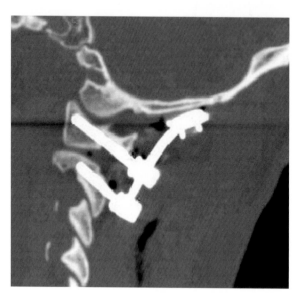

Fig. 8.13 C1 lateral mass screws and C2 pars screws

8.9 Technical Pearls and Pitfalls

8.9.1 Pearls

- Review with the patient and family, the possibility of not obtaining baseline neuromonitoring after anesthesia is induced (if neuromonitoring is utilized).
- Stretcher should not leave the OR room until the patient is secured safely to bed, IVs and monitoring are working appropriately, respirations and oxygenation are adequate and MEPs and SSEPs are satisfactory.
- Beginning incision at level of inion and working caudally facilitates exposure in the midline raphe.
- Midline unicortical screws have pullout strength equivalent to that of lateral bicortical screws [7].
- Placing midline and lateral screws increases stiffness of construct and reduces the risk of rotational pullout.
- Thickness of occipital bone varies.

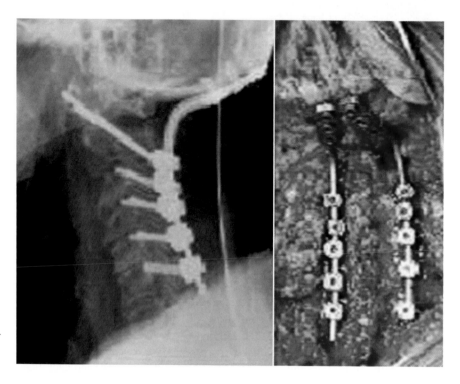

Fig. 8.14 C2–C1 transarticular screws and subaxial lateral mass screws

- Place all instrumentation prior to any decompression to reduce the risk of iatrogenic neurologic injury.
- If there is cerebrospinal leak, you can patch with dural substitute or biological glue and close fascia with both interrupted suture followed by running suture and close the skin with running locked suture. Occiput–cervical injuries are often associated with cranial nerve injuries – assess carefully preoperatively and postoperatively.

8.9.2 Pitfalls

- Be sure to check OR bed and Mayfield head frame and draw sheet appropriateness before commencing the placement of the patient in prone position.
- Do not forget to prep for posterior ICBG harvest.
- Do not force rods into place; they should lay in screw heads and plate without tension.

8.10 Potential Intraoperative Complications

- Changes in neuromonitoring.
- Drilling or placing occipital screws into dural venous sinuses or into brain parenchyma (Figs. 8.15 and 8.16).
- Drilling or placing cervical spine screws into spinal canal or vertebral artery (Figs. 8.17 and 8.18).
- Cerebrospinal fluid leakage or spinal cord injury from overzealous use of electrocautery near interspinous and interlaminar spaces and particularly at occiput–axial junction.

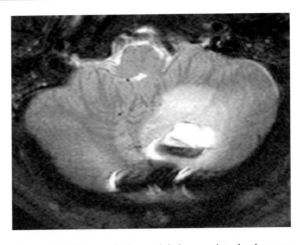

Fig. 8.16 Drilling or placing occipital screws into dural venous sinuses or into brain parenchyma

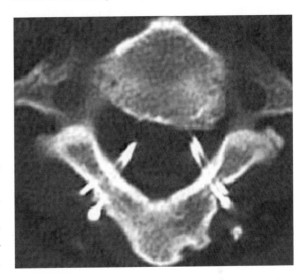

Fig. 8.17 Placement of cervical spine sublaminar wires into spinal canal

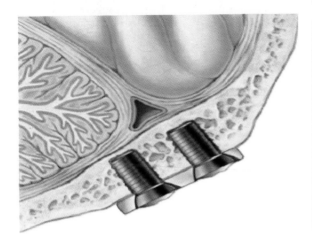

Fig. 8.15 Drilling or placing occipital screws into dural venous sinuses or into brain parenchyma

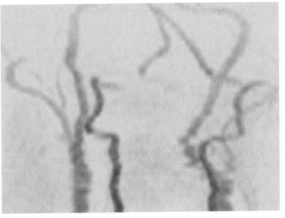

Fig. 8.18 Drilling or placing cervical spine screws into vertebral artery with resultant vertebral occlusion

8.11 Bailout/Salvage
for Procedure Failure

- Halo-vest orthosis.
- C1 lateral mass screws and subaxial spine fixation, if not able to fixate to C2.

8.12 Postoperative Considerations

8.12.1 Bracing

If the patient has good bone quality without osteopenia, there is no need for Halo-vest orthosis, and such patients may use a Philadelphia, Aspen, or Miami J collar until there is evidence of bony fusion.

8.12.2 Activity

Early activity
   Out of bed with assistance on postoperative day #1.

8.12.3 Follow-up

Wound/incision check at week one. Clinic visit at two weeks with AP and lateral cervical spine X-rays. Ideally, follow with regular X-rays until a solid fusion is noted.

8.12.4 Potential Complications

Pseudoarthrosis/Failure of hardware (Fig. 8.19)
   Infection (Fig. 8.20)
   Wound breakdown
   Occipital neuralgia

8.12.5 Treatments/Rescue
for Complications

Infection/wound breakdown – if the patient demonstrates radiographic evidence of fusion, it may be

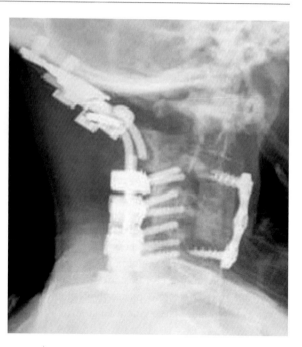

Fig. 8.19 Pseudoarthrosis/failure of hardware

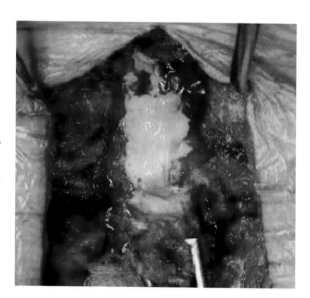

Fig. 8.20 Infection

appropriate to wash out/revise the wound and remove all instrumentation; otherwise, instrumentation should be maintained until there is a solid fusion. Multiple washouts and rebone grafting may be needed.

   Occipital neuralgia may be from irritation of C2 nerve root by a C1 screw or may be a sign of pseudoarthrosis with motion. Check radiographs. Options for the resolution of pain include nerve blocks and removal of C1 screws if adequate fixation is present distally. Pseudoarthrosis/failure of hardware – placement in Halo vest vs. reoperation with reinstrumentation; pseudoarthrosis may be a sign of indolent infection – assess CBC, ESR, and CRP.

References

1. Baskin JJ, Dickman CA, Sonntag VKH (2004) Occipitocervical fusion. In: Winn HR (ed) Youmans neurological surgery. Saunders, Philadelphia, PA
2. Ebraheim NA, Elgafy H, Xu R (2001) Bone graft harvesting from iliac and fibular donor sites: techniques and complications. J Am Acad Orthop Surg 9:210–218
3. Ebraheim NA, Lu J, Biyani A, Brown JA, Yeasting RA (1996) An anatomic study of the thickness of the occipital bone: implications for occipitocervical instrumentation. Spine 21:1725–1729
4. Inamasu J, Kim DH, Klugh A (2005) Posterior instrumentation for craniocervical junction instabilities: an update. Neurol Med Chir 45:439–447
5. Lee SC, Chen JF, Lee ST (2004) Complication of fixation to the occiput – anatomical and design implications. Br J Neurosurg 18:590–597
6. Levene JR, Jallo JI (2008) Occipital cervical fusion. In: Vaccaro AR, Baron EM (eds) Spine surgery. Saunders Elsevier, Philadelphia, PA
7. Papagelopoulos PJ, Currier BL, Stone J, Grabowski JJ, Larson DR, Fisher DR, An KA (2000) Biomechanical evaluation of occipital fixation. J Spinal Disord 13:336–344
8. Smucker JD, Sasso RC (2006) The evolution of spinal instrumentation for the management of occipital cervical and cervicothoracic junctional injuries. Spine 31:S44–S52
9. Vaccaro AR, Lim MR, Lee JY (2005) Indications for surgery and stabilization techniques of the occipito-cervical junction. Injury, Int J Care Injured 36:S-B44–S-B53
10. Vender JR, Rekito AJ, Harrison SJ, McDonnell DE (2004) Evolution of posterior cervical and occipitocervical fusion and instrumentation. Neurosurg Focus 16:E9
11. Wolfla CE, Salerno SA, Yoganandan N, Pintar FA (2007) Comparison of contemporary occipitocervical instrumentation techniques with and without C1 lateral mass screws. Neurosurgery 61:ONS87–ONS93

C1–2 Fixation: Transarticular Screws

Sohail Bajammal and R. John Hurlbert

9.1 Case Example

This 35-year-old lady sustained a whiplash-type injury in a motor vehicle accident 1 month prior to assessment. Since then she has been complaining of neck pain. Physical examination revealed painful limitation of neck movement and a normal neurological examination. Flexion and extension lateral X-rays and MRI of the cervical spine confirmed the diagnosis of long-standing atlantoaxial instability (Fig. 9.1a–c). Options of treatment were discussed with the patient who agreed to undergo internal fixation and arthrodesis.

9.2 Background

The atlantoaxial joint is a complex articulation between the C1 (atlas) and C2 (axis) vertebrae. The complexity of this articulation is due to multiple reasons: (1) The unique morphology of C1 and C2 compared to the rest of the spine; C1 has no body and no spinous process. Instead, it is a ring-like structure with an anterior and posterior arch connecting two lateral masses. C2, on the other hand, has the dens (odontoid) to form a pivot around which C1 rotates.

(2) The stability of C1–C2 articulation is dependent on multiple ligaments (e.g., the transverse ligament of the cruciform ligament, the alar ligament, tectorial membrane, and C1–C2 joint capsules). (3) The close proximity of the vertebral artery to C1–C2 articulation: After emerging from the subclavian artery, the vertebral artery typically enters the transverse foramen at C6 and ascends rostrally. As the artery exits the transverse foramen of C2, it courses laterally and rostrally to enter the transverse foramen of C1. At this area, the artery is at risk of injury during surgical dissection. After exiting the transverse foramen of C1, the artery courses posteromedially along the superior aspect of the posterior ring of C1 before entering the dura near the midline to pass through the foramen magnum. (4) The fact that more than half of the head rotation on the spine occurs at the C1–C2 articulation makes this joint very unstable and not amenable to external immobilization alone to achieve fusion.

Atlantoaxial instability can occur due to either traumatic or nontraumatic causes that disrupt the bony articulation and/or ligaments between C1 and C2 vertebrae. The traumatic causes of atlantoaxial instability include odontoid fractures (especially type II and III) and traumatic ligamentous injury (e.g., transverse and alar ligament). The nontraumatic causes include: rheumatoid arthritis, congenital anomalies (e.g., os odontoideum and odontoid agenesis), infection, and malignancy.

Treatment of atlantoaxial instability includes operative and nonoperative techniques. Nonoperative external immobilization using a Halo-vest is associated with high nonunion rate. Hence, its use as a sole method of treatment is rarely indicated. The operative options for atlantoaxial stabilization include posterior, and more recently, anterior procedures. The posterior techniques include: posterior wiring (e.g., Gallie's [4] and Brooks-Jenkins' [2] techniques), interlaminar clamps [7], C1–C2 transarticular

S. Bajammal (✉)
Department of Surgery, Umm Al-Qura University,
PO Box 7607, Makkah, Saudi Arabia
e-mail: ssbajammal@uqu.edu.sa

R.J. Hurlbert
Department of Neurosciences, Division of Neurosurgery,
University of Calgary, 1403 - 29th Street NW,
Calgary, Alberta T2N 2T9, Canada

V.V. Patel et al. (eds.), *Spine Trauma*,
DOI: 10.1007/978-3-642-03694-1_9, © Springer-Verlag Berlin Heidelberg 2010

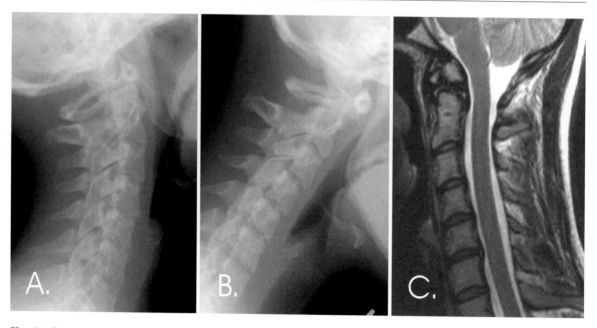

Fig. 9.1 Preoperative images of the case example. (**a**) Extension lateral C-spine X-ray. (**b**) Flexion lateral C-spine X-ray. (**c**) Midsagittal T2 MRI of the cervical spine. The images show atlantoaxial instability

screws (Magerl's technique [9]), C1 lateral mass – C2 pars screws-rods fixation (Harms modification [6] of Goel's technique [5]), and C1 lateral mass – C2 laminar screws-rods fixation (Wright's technique [17]). Apart from anterior screw fixation of acute type II odontoid fractures, anterior procedures for C1/2 stabilization have not been widely adopted nor are long-term results available; hence, currently, they should be considered only on a case-by-case basis [14, 15].

Posterior wiring for C1/2 stabilization was first described by Gallie in 1939 [4]. Multiple modifications of the technique were subsequently published. However, the fact that these constructs do not control rotation and thus require postoperative Halo-vest immobilization to improve their biomechanical stability and long-term success rate is common to all. Similarly, the interlaminar clamps provide excellent stability for flexion and extension movement, but they are inferior in controlling rotation compared to the posterior wiring technique. In 1986, Magerl described the posterior transarticular screw technique for C1/2 fixation and fusion [9]. This technique achieved high fusion rates and superior biomechanical stability than the posterior wiring and interlaminar clamps techniques. It has subsequently gained popularity and become a gold standard against which other procedures are compared. However, the procedure may not

be feasible because of either vertebral artery anomalies or unfavorable bony anatomy, reportedly in up to 20% of patients [1]. As a result of perceived technical difficulties and potential complications of the Magerl technique (e.g., injuries to the vertebral artery, dura, spinal cord, hypoglossal nerve, and internal carotid artery), Harms [6] popularized a modification of Goel's technique [5] to fuse the atlantoaxial joint using C1 lateral mass screws and C2 pars interarticularis screws and rods construct. His rationale in proposing this method was less risk of injury to the vertebral artery and ease of application in patients with persistent mal-alignment of C1/C2. More recently, Wright has published a new technique for fusing the atlantoaxial articulation using C1 lateral mass screws and C2 laminar screws and rods constructs [17] to further lower the risk of injuring the vertebral artery.

Multiple studies have compared the biomechanical characteristics of these different constructs [8, 10–13] and concluded that biomechanical stability of the Harms lateral mass/pars method was similar to the Magerl C1–C2 transarticular screws. Superiority over wired constructs has also been established. The decision to choose between these two procedures is based on the experience of the surgeon, the anatomy of the vertebral artery, the local bone anatomy of C1 and C2, and whether the C1–C2 articulation is reducible.

9.3 Indications and Advantages for Procedure

9.3.1 Indications

(1) Atlantoaxial instability due to trauma, rheumatoid arthritis, malignancy, infection, congenital anomalies, or postoperative iatrogenic causes. Traumatic causes of atlantoaxial instability include: odontoid fractures (type II and III) and traumatic disruption of the transverse ligament. (2) Can be used as part of occipitocervical fusion.

9.3.2 Advantages

(1) Greater biomechanical stability than posterior wiring techniques. (2) Does not require intact posterior arch of C1 unlike the posterior wiring techniques. (3) Does not require postoperative halo immobilization if supplemented with posterior wiring technique.

9.4 Contraindications and Disadvantages for Procedure

9.4.1 Contraindications

(1) Irreducible atlantoaxial subluxation. (2) Anomalous vertebral artery. (3) Narrow C2 isthmus will not accommodate a 3.5 mm screw. (4) Collapsed lateral masses of C1 secondary to comminuted fracture, malignancy, or advanced cranial settling. (5) Severe osteoporosis.

9.4.2 Disadvantages

(1) Technically more challenging than posterior wiring techniques. (2) Should optimally include the supplemental use of posterior wiring technique.

9.5 Procedure

9.5.1 Equipments Needed

1. C-arm fluoroscope.
2. Cell saver.
3. Sugita head holder, ideally, or Mayfield head holder (Mizuho Ikakogyo Co., Tokyo, Japan).
4. Bolsters or Jackson Table.
5. Cannulated or regular cervical spine instrumentation screw system.
6. High-speed drill (e.g., Midas Rex®, Medtronic Sofamor Danek, Minneapolis, MN).
7. Braided titanium cable (e.g., Atlas Cable System®, Medtronic Sofamor Danek, Minneapolis, MN).
8. Bone harvesting instruments (oscillating saw, osteotomes, gouges, curettes).
9. Posterior cervical spine dissection tools (curettes, rongeurs, self-retaining retractors, etc.).
10. Fine cut CT scan of C-spine to evaluate bony and vascular structures.

9.5.2 Anesthetic and Neuromonitoring Considerations

Awake intubation is recommended to prevent excessive flexion or extension during intubation. Electrophysiological neuromonitoring can help protect against inadvertent spinal cord compression. Recycling of lost blood through cell saver technology is important, because blood loss in this procedure can be substantial in some cases. We avoid the use of the cell saver when we are using local thrombotic agent in the wound.

9.5.3 Patient Positioning and Room Setup

Midmark radiolucent table with Sugita head holder connection (Mayfield pin fixation is not ideal, and is prone to intraoperative failure.): The bed is positioned with the patient's head 180° opposite to the anesthetic cart enabling elevation of the head to decrease venous engorgement, C-arm access, and uninhibited surgical visualization. After awake intubation and attachment of neuromonitoring needles, alcohol solution is used to sterilize the skin in preparation for the Sugita head holder (Fig. 9.2a, b). Baseline neuromonitoring signals are obtained. The patient is carefully log rolled from the stretcher into a prone position on the Midmark table keeping the neck neutral. Longitudinal bolsters are

centered under the patient from the shoulder to the waist and bony prominences are protected. The arms are kept along the sides of the body and tucked with the bed sheet under the body. Once trunkal position is secure, the patient's head is carefully flexed and distracted into a military tuck position and the Sugita head holder tightly secured to the table. This position ensures a favorable trajectory for screw insertion (Fig. 9.2c). Neuromonitoring signals are checked to ensure continued spinal cord function. In addition, C-arm fluoroscopy is undertaken at this point to verify atlantoaxial alignment and attempt further reduction if necessary. It is of paramount importance that a perfect lateral projection of the C1–C2 complex is obtained as obliquity in the image will negatively affect screw trajectory. A free K-wire can be superimposed with fluoroscopy on the side of the patient's head and neck to judge the trajectory of the C1–C2 transarticular screw with respect to the shoulders and thoracic kyphosis (Fig. 9.3a, b).

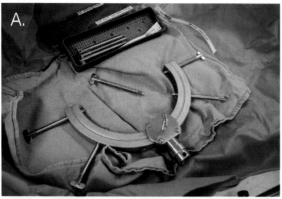

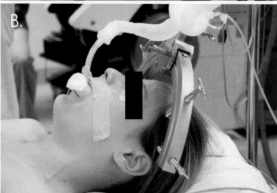

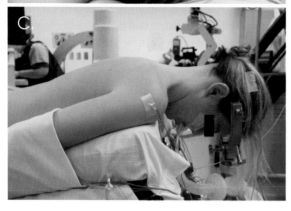

Fig. 9.2 Sugita head holder application. (**a**) Assembly of the Sugita holder. (**b**) Application of the Sugita head holder with the patient supine. (**c**) The patient was turned prone with the military tuck position of the head to ensure a favorable trajectory for screw insertion. Notice the neuromonitoring needles around the tip of the shoulder and in the scalp

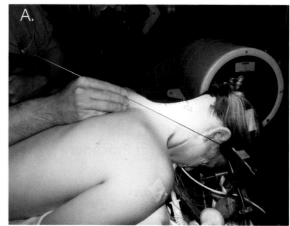

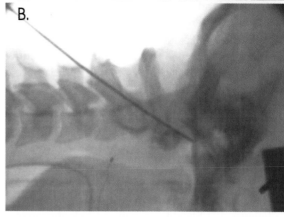

Fig. 9.3 Preoperative confirmation of the reducibility of the C1–C2 articulation. (**a**) A K-wire is positioned along the side of the neck to check the trajectory of the screw. (**b**) A C-arm image corresponding to Fig. 9.3a

9.5.4 *Surgical Approach*

Hair is shaved from the external occipital protuberance to the C7 area. Similarly, the area of posterior iliac crest bone graft is shaved. An incision is marked from the external occiput protuberance to the tip of C7 process, and from the posterior superior iliac spine (PSIS) approximately 10–15 cm laterally following the curve of the iliac crest (Fig. 9.4a, b). Both the areas are prepped and draped according to the sterile technique. A local anesthetic is injected into the subcutaneous tissue of the planned incisions. Skin is incised with a scalpel from the external occipital protuberance to C7. Although the approach can be made by limiting the midline incision from the external occipital protuberance to C3, division of the ligamentum nuchae more inferiorly with exposure of C3–7 spinous processes

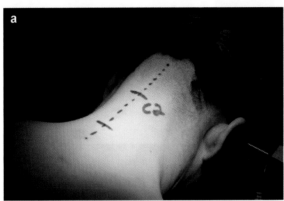

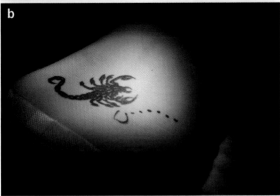

Fig. 9.4 Proposed skin incisions. (**a**) The incision extends from the external occipital protuberance to the tip of C7 spinous process. As mentioned in the text, an alternative shorter incision to C3 can be made to expose the C1–C2 facet with separate stab incisions for inserting the screws. (**b**) The skin incision over PSIS. Either longitudinal or curved incision can be made. Incision should never extend beyond 5cm lateral to the PSIS to avoid injuring the superior cluneal nerves

greatly facilitates screw trajectory and control. Percutaneous stab techniques can be used instead, but are more limiting. Monopolar electrocautery is used for dissection in the midline through the ligamentum nuchae remaining in the avascular plane between the posterior cervical muscles (Fig. 9.5a). The dissection is carried along the midline to the posterior arch of C1 and C2 spinous process and laminae. Dissection continues laterally over the posterior arch of C1 using a small blunt dissector (e.g., Penfield No. 1) and bipolar cautery. The extent of lateral dissection over the posterior arch of C1 should be limited to approximately 15–20 mm on each side of the midline to avoid injuring the vertebral artery along its normal course (Fig. 9.5b). Careful assessment of preoperative X-rays and thin 1 mm cuts of CT images should be made to rule out vertebral artery anomalies and the presence of ponticulus posticus (congenital arcuate foramen) [18]. This bony variant occurs in 20% of patients and might be confused with C1 lamina. Failure to recognize it can result in injury to the vertebral artery. As a part of the exposure of C1, the superior and inferior edge of the posterior arch are dissected free of the posterior atlanto-axial and atlantooccipital membranes to enable passing sublaminar cables. Muscle attachments to C2 spinous process are preserved if possible, but if more exposure is needed, the muscles are carefully reattached at the end of the procedure using intraosseous sutures. Care must be taken to avoid disrupting the C2–C3 facet joint as the lateral mass of C2 is exposed and self-retaining retractors inserted.

Exposure of the C1–C2 facet joint is undertaken by first following the C2 lamina laterally and superiorly to the pars interaticularis. Careful dissection along the posterior aspect of the pars in a cephalad direction will bring exposure to the C1/2 facet joint (Fig. 9.5c, d). *We expose the medial border of the C2 pars interarticularis to guide the screw trajectory and ensure that the screw does not breach the medial cortex towards the spinal cord.* Even if a small medial breach is noted, it is not necessary to reposition the screw. When approaching the C1–C2 facet joint along the pars the perivertebral venous plexus must be negotiated. Bleeding can be extensive and is not readily controlled with bipolar cautery because of the large varicose nature of the veins. Careful dissection along the subperiosteal corridor afforded by the pars helps to avoid disruption of the veins. When bleeding is encountered, patience, and tamponade from neuro patties on top of a coagulating material such as microfibrillar collagen

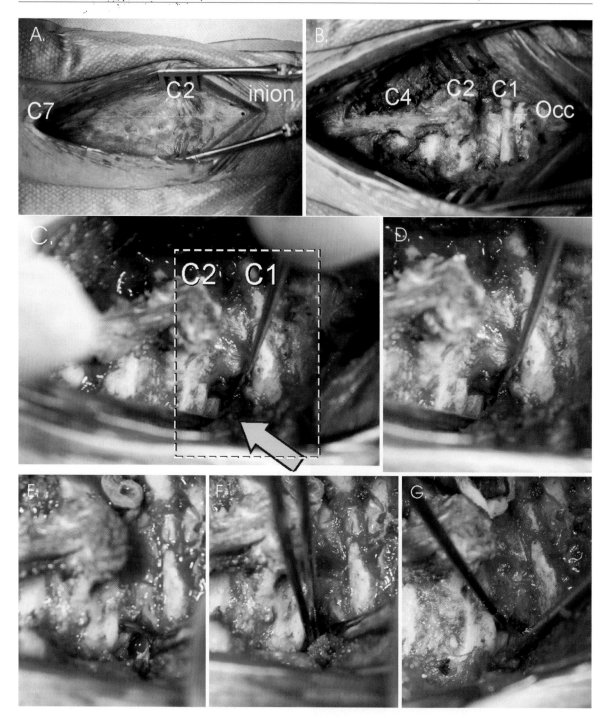

Fig. 9.5 Surgical exposure of the occipitocervical junction. In all the intraoperative images in this chapter, the head of the patient is to the right of the pictures. (**a**) Superficial dissection through the skin and subcutaneous tissue. The midline avascular ligamentum nuchae is identified. (**b**) The posterior arch of C1 and the spinous process and laminae of C2 are exposed. (**c**) The right C1–C2 joint is exposed with a Penfield No. 4 (*yellow arrow*) and retraction of the C2 nerve root rostrally. (**d**) Close-up picture of Fig. 9.5c showing the C1–C2 joint. (**e**) A picture of the C1–C2 joint after curettage and decortication. (**f**) Morcelated cancellous bone graft obtained from the posterior superior iliac spine is packed in the right C1–C2 facet. (**g**) A picture of the C1–C2 after packing the morcelated cancellous bone graft

(Instat Collagen Absorbable Hemostat, Ethicon, New Brunswick, NJ), or floseal (Baxter Healthcare, Deerfield, IL) is very helpful. Occasionally, when torrential bleeding is encountered, Gelfoam® (Pfizer, New York, NY) can be of use despite the inflammatory response and subsequent scar formation accompanying it. The C2 nerve root should be protected during the approach and retracted rostrally using a Penfield No. 4 as it is located immediately posterior to, and directly overlying the C1/2 facet joint. Keeping the dissection in this area in the subperiosteal plane will also avoid injuries to the dura and spinal cord. Dissection lateral to the lateral border of the pars and C1–C2 facet is dangerous because of the close proximity of the vertebral artery. Once the C1–C2 facet joint is exposed, the joint capsule is entered from the medial to lateral edge with a blunt oblique nerve hook. Then the C1 and C2 articular surfaces are prepared using the smallest cervical curette (e.g., size 000 Karlin Cervical Curette, Codman, Raynham, MA). Care must be taken to avoid curettage too medially, potentially compressing the spinal cord, or too laterally, possibly violating the vertebral artery. Facet articular surface decortication is completed with a high-speed drill (e.g., AM-8 tip Midas Rex®), being careful to always have two-hands on the drill to prevent accidental slipping (Fig. 9.5e). Morcelated cancellous bone graft obtained from the posterior iliac crest is packed in the joint space (Fig. 9.5f, g).

9.5.5 Reduction Technique

Most of any attempt to reduce C1/C2 subluxation should have been attempted and achieved with halo or tong traction prior to general anesthesia and surgery. A small degree of reduction can also be realized with head positioning prior to neck incision. Intraoperative reduction is possible to a degree, particularly, if C1 is anterolisthesed with respect to C2. In this circumstance, downward pressure can be applied on a sharp towel clip piercing a thick part of the C2 spinous process, pushing C2 anteriorly with respect to C1. This should be performed only under fluoroscopic guidance, at the time guide when wires are being inserted across the C1/2 joint space (see Fixation Technique below). The guide wires are sequentially driven through the pars of C2, approaching, but not entering, the C1/2 joint space.

The surgical assistant can then apply downward force on the towel clip maintaining reduction fluroscopically as the K-wires are driven into and through the lateral masses of C1, securing the reduction in place.

In more rare circumstances when C1 is retrolisthesed on C2, a similar technique may be used to "pull back" on the spinous process of C2. However, this can compromise the C1/2 transarticular trajectory driving it down somewhere into the patient's shoulders rendering it difficult to drive the guide wires and place screws. Partial insertion of the guide wire up to but not through the C1/2 joint is important in preserving this trajectory *prior* to manual reduction of C2. Translation of C1 is always unsatisfactory because of the strong atlantooccipital joints combined with pin fixation of the head.

9.5.6 Fixation Technique

The starting point and trajectory for the screw depend on the individual patient's anatomy. Typically, the entry point is approximately 2.5 mm above the tip of the inferior C2 facet and 2.5 mm lateral to the medial border of C2 lamina (Fig. 9.6a, b). In almost all cases, the starting point will be in the transition zone or "corner" between the horizontal facet/lateral mass inferiorly and the vertical ascent of the lamina medially. A 1 mm deep starting point is created in the bone with the Midas Rex® drill to receive the guide wire, preventing slippage during guide wire positioning. With an assistant exposing the medial border of the C2 pars interarticularis, medial–lateral angulation is determined by aiming the guide wire straight down the length of the exposed pars interarticularis. Typically, this results in a trajectory angled somewhere between 0 and 10° medial to the sagittal plane. Too much lateral angulation will miss the lateral mass of C1 and might potentially injure the vertebral artery. Too much medial angulation will breach the medial cortex of the pars risking spinal cord injury. Rostral–caudal angulation of the screw path is determined using C-arm fluoroscopy (Fig. 9.6c–e). The intended tip of the guide wire should be just above or cephalad to the anterior tubercle of the anterior arch of C1 and about 1–2 mm posterior to its anterior cortex as seen on fluoroscopy. *Note: Some surgeons prefer to use a drill without a guide wire to prevent inadvertent advancement of the wire and to provide better control of the trajectory of the desired hole. Also, some surgeons will start with a drill*

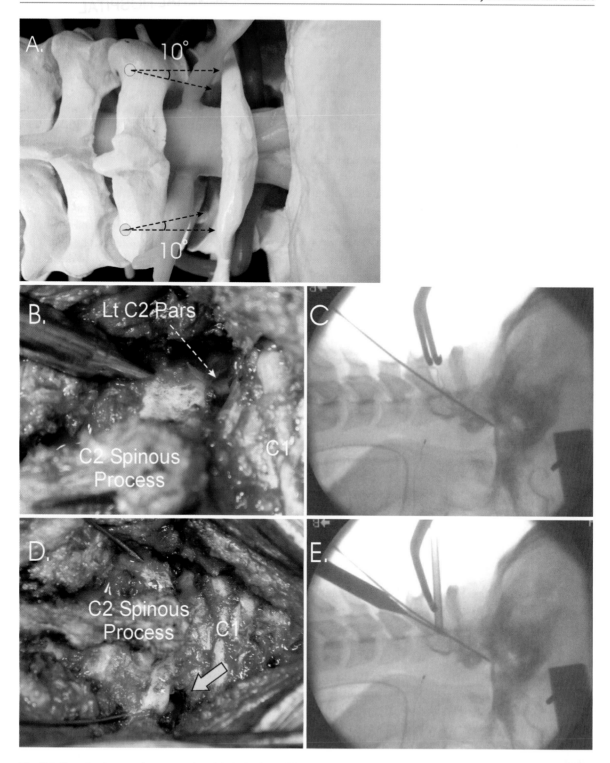

Fig. 9.6 Cannulated screws instrumentation. (**a**) A plastic model illustrating the entry point of C1–C2 transarticular screw depicted by the yellow circle and the 10° medial trajectory depicted by the dotted line. (**b**) Pointed awl to localize the entry point of the screw which is 2.5 mm above the tip of the inferior C2 facet and 2.5 mm lateral to the medial border of C2 lamina. (**c**) A C-arm image to confirm the acceptable trajectory of the screw. In this image, the tip of the guide wire is slightly superior than the ideal position. (**d**) A threaded guide wire is inserted across each C1–C2 joint. The *yellow arrow* shows the trajectory of the guide wire in relation to the C2 pars. (**e**) A C-arm image of two threaded guide wires inserted across the C1–C2 joint. The *yellow arrow* points towards the C1–C2 joint

for the initial trajectory followed by the placement of the guide wire for the rest of the screw placement. Prior to guide wire insertion, checking and double-checking of medial–lateral angulation (visually sighting down the pars interarticularis) and rostro–caudal angulation (fluoroscopy) should be done. Avoid adversely biasing the trajectory by keeping the guide wire driver supported, not allowing the tip of the guide wire to pierce the lateral mass of C2 until insertion has commenced. During insertion, the trajectory should be reexamined visually and fluroscopically every 5–10 mm of advancement. There is usually a feel of less resistance or "give" when the threaded guide wire leaves the endplate of C2 entering into the C1/2 joint space followed by renewed resistance as it advances into the endplate of C1. The guide wire is carefully advanced under fluoroscopic guidance and by feel, until the anterior cortex of C1 is breached resulting in another "give" sensation. The overall trajectory of the guide wire is assessed clinically and radiographically. Then the screw length is estimated by comparing the discrepancy in the length of a fresh guide wire held adjacent to the exposed segment of the inserted guide wire. Keeping the guide wire in situ, a cannulated 2.5 mm drill bit is used to overdrill the guide wire. For this step, it is important that the surgical assistant uses a snap to make sure that the guide wire does not migrate and advance with drilling (Fig. 9.7a). Frequent fluoroscopy images will ensure that advancement of the guide wire does not happen (Fig. 9.7b). Overdrilling of the guide wire is continued to within 5 mm of the C1 anterior cortex. A cannulated tap advanced to the same position completes the preparation for screw insertion. Self-tapping partially threaded cannulated titanium (lag) screws are used to secure C1 against C2 (outer diameter 4.0 mm, inner diameter 2.5 mm – DePuy ACE small fragment set; DePuy Spine Inc., Raynham, MA). A washer can be used against the screw head in cases where softer bone may allow it to cut through the lateral mass of C2 (Fig. 9.7c). The same process is repeated on the other side (Fig. 9.7d–f).

The next step is to carry out the modified Brooks posterior wiring technique [16]. This is optional, based on the quality of the screw fixation and the preference of the surgeon. With the high-speed drill, the inferior aspect of C1 and the superior aspect of C2 are contoured perpendicular to the spinal canal and parallel to each other (Fig. 9.8a). Optimally bleeding cancellous bone should be visualized at the raw surfaces of these posterior elements. The resulting space between C1

posterior arch and the top of C2 spinous process is measured (Fig. 9.8b) and a rectangular bone graft harvested from the posterior iliac crest to match the measurement (Figs. 9.4b and 9.9a). Titanium cables are passed from caudal to rostral under the lamina of C2 and posterior ring C1 on both sides. A blunt nerve hook can be used to dissect through the ligamentum flavum between C2 and C3 into the epidural space. The malleable leader of the braided titanium cable shaped like a lazy "S" is then gently inserted in the epidural space from C2/3 rostrally into the C1/2 interspace (Fig. 9.8b). Passage of the cable under the C1 lamina is facilitated by the "reverse-suture" technique where the needle of a 0-Vicryl suture is inserted hilt first under the C1 posterior arch from rostral to caudal (Fig. 9.8c). After cutting the malleable leader to within 1 mm of the braided cable, the cable is looped through the Vicryl suture. Maintaining opposing tension on the suture loop and the braided cable, the surgeon gently pulls the suture and the cable under the C1 posterior arch from caudal to rostral. Meanwhile, the assistant makes sure that the cable is laid flat against the dura between C1 and C2 as the surgeon pulls the loop under C1, thus preventing inadvertent injury to the spinal cord (Fig. 9.8d). The same steps are repeated on the contralateral side (Fig. 9.8e). The rectangular piece of the bone graft is fitted between the posterior arch of C1 and the upper laminae of C2. The leading edge of each cable is passed through the ring of the cable. A tensioning device is applied on each cable and tensioned simultaneously to gently compress the bone graft between C1 and C2 (Fig. 9.9a, b). In elderly patients with osteopenic bone, gentle tensioning should be applied to avoid fracturing the posterior ring of C1 (Fig. 9.9b). The neck of the cable is crimped using the crimping tool. The cable is then cut flush (Fig. 9.9c). A final C-arm image is taken to document the position of the graft and hardware (Fig. 9.9d).

If the deep muscles were detached from C2 spinous process, they should be reattached with absorbable intraosseous sutures. Deep muscles are reapproximated with absorbable interrupted sutures positioned between the spinous processes (0-Vicryl). The deep fascia of the neck is repaired in three subsequent layers with absorbable sutures (0-Vicryl). The first layer is brought together overlying the spinous processes with a running throw. The second layer is reconstructed in an interrupted manner bringing the laterally displaced trapezius muscles together at the midline. The most

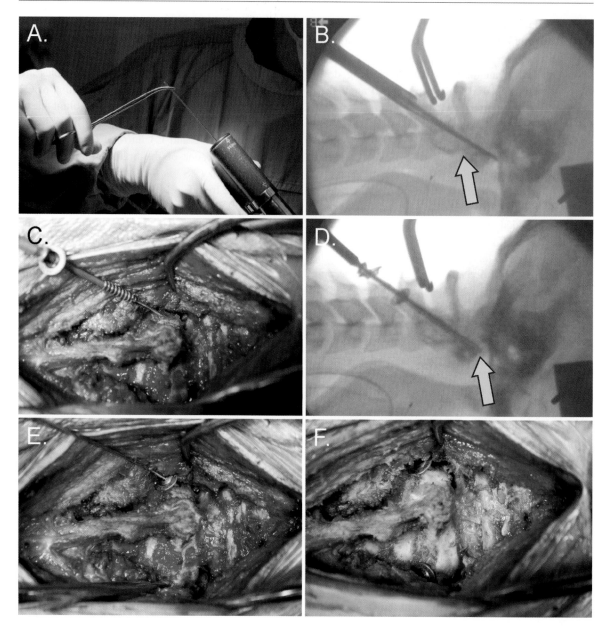

Fig. 9.7 Screw insertion. (**a**) An assistant is holding the tip of the threaded guide wire with a snap while the surgeon is disassembling the pneumatic drill from the guide wire. This is to prevent the advancement of the guide wire into the anterior neck neurovascular bundle and soft tissue. (**b**) A C-arm image to confirm that the guide wire was not moved during disassembling the pneumatic drill. The *yellow arrow* indicates that the C1–C2 articulation remained reduced. (**c**) Cannulated partiallythreaded screw with a washer is inserted. (**d**) A C-arm image to confirm the position of the screw. In this case, as indicated in Fig. 9.6c and shown here, the tip of the screw is slightly superior than ideal (*yellow arrow*). (**e**) The same steps are repeated on the right side. (**f**) The two screws are well seated across the C1–C2 articulation

superficial layer is closed with a running locking stitch. Subcutaneous tissues are repaired with inverted absorbable sutures (2–0 Vicryl). Skin is closed with absorbable sutures (3–0 Monocryl) in a subcuticular fashion. Steri-strips are applied to protect the subcuticular suture. A sterile dressing is applied followed by a rigid cervical collar with a foam liner (Aspen collar, Aspen Medical Products, Irvine, CA). The patient is

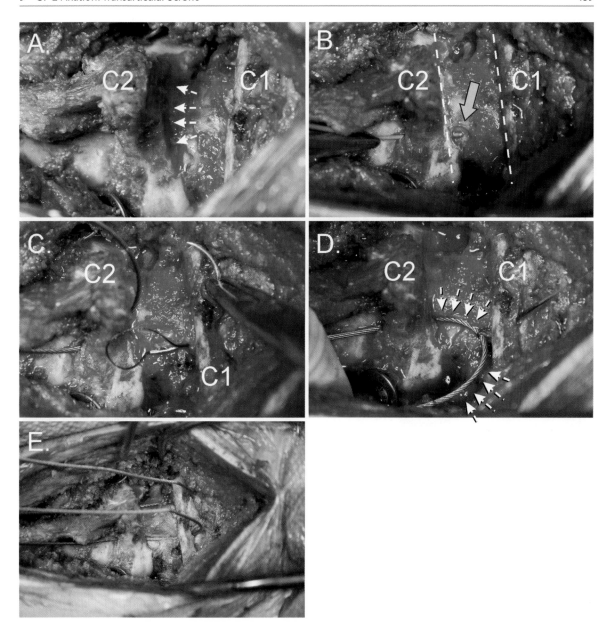

Fig. 9.8 The modified Brooks posterior wiring technique [16]. (a) The inferior margin of the posterior arch of C1 and the superior surface of C2 spinous process and laminae are decorticated in preparation for the bone graft. The superior surface of C2 spinous process is recessed (*small arrows*) to increase the stability of seating the bone graft. The distance between the inferior edge of C1 posterior arch and C2 lamina is measured to prepare the bone graft. (b) The leading edge of the cable is passed under the right lamina of C2 from caudal to rostral. (c) The "reverse-suture" technique. A large Vicryl needle is passed under the posterior arch of C1 from rostral to caudal by feeding the hilt first.

The tip of the needle should be protected and under direct vision throughout this step to avoid injury to the dura. (d) The leading edge of the cable is passed through the loop of the suture. The surgeon (on the right side of the picture) is applying tension while pulling the suture to prevent redundancy of the cable and potential damage to the dura. The assistant (on the left side of the picture) is making sure that the cable is laid flat (*white arrows*) parallel to the dura and to the undersurface of the posterior arch of C1 to ease its passage under the arch. (e) The process was repeated on the left side. One cable on each side is shown passing under the posterior arch of C1 and the lamina of C2

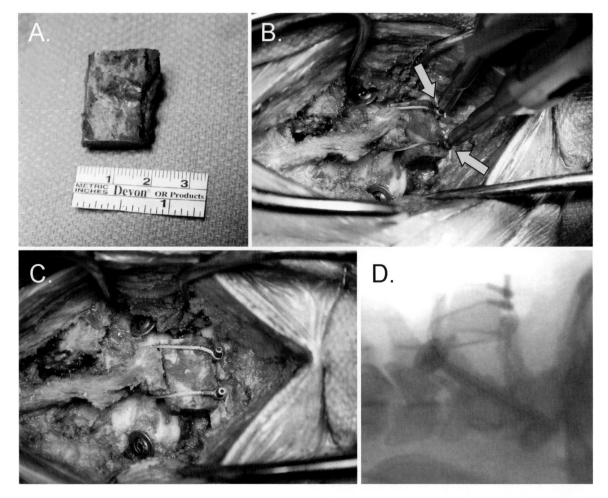

Fig. 9.9 Bone graft preparation and completion of the modified Brooks posterior wiring technique [16]. (**a**) A rectangular piece of tricortical bone graft was shaped to fit the space between C1–C2 posterior articulation. (**b**) The bone graft is secured in place. The cables are simultaneously tightened using the tensioning device to ensure a snug fit around the bone graft. The collar of the cable is crimped before cutting the cable flush. The *yellow arrows* indicate the appropriate position of the tensioning devices and the location where the crimping device is applied. (**c**) Intraoperative image of the construct at the conclusion of the procedure. (**d**) A C-arm image corresponding to Fig. 9.9c

log rolled to the supine position in a hospital bed. The Sugita head holder is removed. The patient is extubated and transferred to the recovery room.

9.6 Technical Pearls and Pitfalls

9.6.1 Pearls

(1) Assess the reducibility of atlantoaxial subluxation using flexion/extension lateral C-spine X-rays, unless contraindicated. If it is reducible, then C1–C2 transarticular screw is technically feasible only after confirming the vertebral artery route and the favorable size of C2 isthmus. If atlantoaxial subluxation is irreducible during passive range of motion, then transarticular screw fixation is relatively contraindicated and C1 lateral mass-C2 pars screws fixation is an option. If partial reduction occurs during passive range of motion, complete intraoperative reduction may be possible. (2) Review preoperative 1 mm thin cuts CT scan of the cervical spine in both the axial and sagittal planes. Specifically, look for: (a) anatomy of the vertebral artery and whether there is anomaly, (b) width of the C2 isthmus and whether the C2 transverse foramen is high-riding, (c) absence

of ponticulus posticus, (d) status and quality of C1 and C2 bone for the intended path of the screw. A cadaveric study estimated that 20% of the specimens had unfavorable anatomy that precluded the insertion of C1–C2 transarticular screws [1]. A single screw (i.e., one side only) can be combined with a posterior wiring technique such as the modified Brooks procedure and managed postoperatively in a collar with essentially the same good to excellent postoperative outcomes.

9.6.2 Potential Intraoperative Complications

Complications from this procedure occur due to either improper trajectory of the guide wire/screw or an unrecognized anatomic variant of the vertebral artery. If the screw is directed *too medial*, breach of the medial cortex of the pars interarticularis of C2 could occur, with potential risk of dural tear, cerebrospinal fluid leak, and spinal cord injury. If the screw is directed too lateral, there is increased risk of injury to the vertebral artery. If the screw is too long, the internal carotid artery [3], the hypoglossal nerve, and the pharynx are at risk. Torrential bleeding from the perivertebral venous plexus around the C2 nerve root can be encountered during the exposure of the C2 pars and the C1/2 facet joint. A cell saver system should be employed in all cases of C1/2 transarticular screw fixation. If venous bleeding persists despite repeated attempts to enter and curette the C1/2 facet joint, this part of the procedure should be abandoned, at least on the problematic side.

9.6.3 Bailout/Salvage for Procedure Failure

The management of intraoperative complications is discussed in Section 5.7.5. If C1–C2 transarticular screw fixation cannot be completed intraoperatively, the surgeon has the options of performing either a posterior wiring technique with postoperative Halo immobilization, a C1 lateral mass-C2 pars screw fixation if the anatomy is favorable, or a C1 lateral mass – C2 intralaminar screw fixation.

9.7 Postonsiderations

9.7.1 Bracing

Following stabilization of the C1–C2 junction using C1–C2 transarticular screws and Brooks posterior wiring technique, the patient is immobilized in a hard cervical collar (e.g., Aspen Collar, Aspen Medical Products, Irvine, CA) for 12 weeks and then weaned off the collar if there is evidence of bony fusion. If only transarticular screws are used (e.g., incompetent or absent posterior C1 arch), Halo-Vest immobilization is considered for 12 weeks instead of an Aspen collar, depending on the quality of bone and screw purchase.

9.7.2 Activity

Upright AP and lateral X-rays of the cervical spine are ordered on the first postoperative day. If the X-rays show maintenance of the reduction, the patient is allowed to ambulate as tolerated with the cervical orthosis. Weight lifting is limited to 10 pounds for the first 6 weeks. By 3 months, if there is good evidence of fusion, all restrictions are removed with the exception of advice against organized contact sports.

9.7.3 Follow-Up

In addition to the immediate postoperative X-rays, follow-up is needed with X-rays at appropriate intervals such as 6 weeks scheduled for 3 months, 6 months, and 12 months with serial X-rays (AP, lateral, open mouth, and flexion/extension) of the cervical spine to assess for evidence of fusion (Fig. 9.10a–d).

9.7.4 Potential Complications

In addition to the intraoperative complications discussed earlier (injuries of the vertebral artery, dural tear, spinal cord, internal carotid artery, hypoglossal

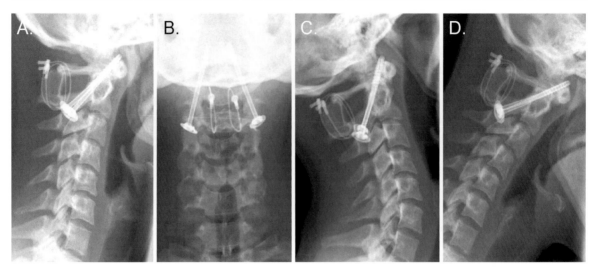

Fig. 9.10 Postoperative imaging. (**a**) Lateral. (**b**) AP. (**c**) Extension. (**d**) Flexion

nerve), postoperative complications include postoperative infection, chronic occipital pain and dysthesia (due to C2 nerve root injury or irritation), nonunion, fibrous union, and hardware failure.

9.7.5 Treatments/Rescue for Complications

Unfavorable angle of the guide wire can be salvaged by carefully using a Penfield 4 or similar dissector to repack the surrounding cancellous bone from just inside the entry point to cover or block the old guide wire trajectory. The tip of the dissector can be used to produce a fresh contact site for the guide wire within the same cortical bone entry point. Alternatively, if necessary, the high-speed drill can be used to "move" the cortical entry point slightly (1 mm) more medially or laterally to provide a new contact site for the guide wire avoiding the old tunnel and trajectory. Medial breach of the screw on the C2 pars interarticularis can be left alone if the dura has not been violated and <1 mm of the screw thread is within the spinal canal. However, if cerebrospinal fluid leakage is noticed, the screw should be withdrawn and the hole sealed with bone wax. As long as no more leakage is noticed, no further treatment is required. No further screw insertion is attempted on that side. The procedure should continue on the opposite side and with the posterior wired construct as planned.

If vertebral artery injury is encountered intraoperatively, the anesthesiologist is immediately alerted and the angiography suite is notified of the need to do an urgent postoperative vertebral artery angiogram. The screw hole is packed with bone wax to control the active bleeding and when appropriate, the screw is inserted in through the drilled trajectory and its final position confirmed with the fluoroscopy imaging. With a known vertebral artery violation, it is, however, contraindicated to subsequently insert a screw on the contralateral side (unless it has already been placed) to prevent the risk of bilateral vertebral artery injury and brainstem stroke or death.

References

1. Abou MA, Solanki G, Casey AT, Crockard HA (1997) Variation of the groove in the axis vertebra for the vertebral artery. Implications for instrumentation. J Bone Joint Surg Br 79:820–823
2. Brooks AL, Jenkins EB (1978) Atlanto-axial arthrodesis by the wedge compression method. J Bone Joint Surg Am 60:279–284
3. Currier BL, Todd LT, Maus TP, Fisher DR, Yaszemski MJ (2003) Anatomic relationship of the internal carotid artery to the C1 vertebra: A case report of cervical reconstruction for chordoma and pilot study to assess the risk of screw fixation of the atlas. Spine 28:E461–E467
4. Gallie W (1939) Fractures and dislocations of the cervical spine. Am J Surg 46:495–499

5. Goel A, Desai KI, Muzumdar DP (2002) Atlantoaxial fixation using plate and screw method: a report of 160 treated patients. Neurosurgery 51:1351–1356
6. Harms J, Melcher RP (2001) Posterior C1-C2 fusion with polyaxial screw and rod fixation. Spine 26:2467–2471
7. Holness RO, Huestis WS, Howes WJ, Langille RA (1984) Posterior stabilization with an interlaminar clamp in cervical injuries: technical note and review of the long term experience with the method. Neurosurgery 14:318–322
8. Kuroki H, Rengachary SS, Goel VK, Holekamp SA, Pitkanen V, Ebraheim NA (2005) Biomechanical comparison of two stabilization techniques of the atlantoaxial joints: transarticular screw fixation versus screw and rod fixation. Neurosurgery 56:151–159
9. Magerl F, Seemann P (1986) Stable posterior fusion of the atlas and axis by transarticular screw fixation. In: Kehr P, Wiedner A (eds) Cervical spine. Springer-Verlag, Berlin, pp 322–327
10. Melcher RP, Puttlitz CM, Kleinstueck FS, Lotz JC, Harms J, Bradford DS (2002) Biomechanical testing of posterior atlantoaxial fixation techniques. Spine 27:2435–2440
11. Puttlitz CM, Melcher RP, Kleinstueck FS, Harms J, Bradford DS, Lotz JC (2004) Stability analysis of craniovertebral junction fixation techniques. J Bone Joint Surg Am 86-A:561–568
12. Richter M, Schmidt R, Claes L, Puhl W, Wilke HJ (2002) Posterior atlantoaxial fixation: biomechanical in vitro comparison of six different techniques. Spine 27:1724–1732
13. Rocha R, Sawa AG, Baek S, Safavi-Abbasi S, Hattendorf F, Sonntag VK, Crawford NR (2009) Atlantoaxial rotatory subluxation with ligamentous disruption: a biomechanical comparison of current fusion methods. Neurosurgery 64:137–143
14. Sen MK, Steffen T, Beckman L, Tsantrizos A, Reindl R, Aebi M (2005) Atlantoaxial fusion using anterior transarticular screw fixation of C1-C2: technical innovation and biomechanical study. Eur Spine J 14:512–518
15. Vaccaro AR, Ring D, Lee RS, Scuderi G, Garfin SR (1997) Salvage anterior C1-C2 screw fixation and arthrodesis through the lateral approach in a patient with a symptomatic pseudoarthrosis. Am J Orthop 26:349–353
16. Vecil GG, Chan CF, Hurlbert RJ (2001) Modified Brooks posterior wiring technique for three-point C1-C2 arthrodesis. Can J Neurol Sci 28:125–129
17. Wright NM (2004) Posterior C2 fixation using bilateral, crossing C2 laminar screws: case series and technical note. J Spinal Disord Tech 17:158–162
18. Young JP, Young PH, Ackermann MJ, Anderson PA, Riew KD (2005) The ponticulus posticus: implications for screw insertion into the first cervical lateral mass. J Bone Joint Surg Am 87:2495–2498

C1–2 Fixation: Lateral Mass/Pars Screw-Rod Fixation

10

Jeffery A. Rihn, David T. Anderson, Ravi Patel, and Todd J. Albert

10.1 Case Example

A 70-year-old woman presented with complaints of neck pain after she tripped and fell down five stairs. She was immobilized at the scene of the accident in a rigid cervical orthosis and transported to the emergency department by ambulance. On physical examination, she was awake, alert, and oriented. She had evidence of facial trauma with abrasions and ecchymosis. Her motor and sensory examination was intact. She had normal rectal tone and no evidence of hyperreflexia in her upper and lower extremities. Her past medical history was significant for hypertension, osteoporosis, and mild COPD. She smoked about 10 cigarettes per day and had a 25-pack-year history of smoking.

Initial plain radiographs, CT scan, and MRI of the cervical spine revealed a type II odontoid fracture with approximately 2 mm displacement and 5° of angulation (Fig. 10.1a–c). The MRI revealed no evidence of spinal cord compression and no evidence that this fracture could be due to a tumor.

The patient was given the option of halo-vest immobilization vs. C1–2 fusion. After explaining all the risks and benefits of each type of treatment, the patient chose the surgical option. The decision was made to perform a C1–2 fusion with a rod/screw construct, using C1 lateral mass screws and C2 pars screws.

Autogenous iliac crest bone graft was used given the patient's smoking history. An initial postoperative lateral radiograph of the cervical spine can be seen in Fig. 10.2a, and a flexion, extension, and open mouth odontoid obtained 3 months postoperatively can be seen in Fig. 10.2b–d. The patient was immobilized in a rigid cervical orthosis for 6 weeks and then placed into a soft collar for comfort, which was weaned over a period of 3 weeks. The patient had an uncomplicated postoperative course.

10.2 Background

The atlantoaxial spinal segment is a complex system composed of the upper two cervical vertebrae, their articular surfaces, and several crucial ligaments (i.e., transverse, apical, and alar ligaments). The orientation and architecture of this spinal segment allow for high levels of movement under normal physiological circumstances, particularly in rotation. Atlantoaxial instability may result from trauma, malignancy, congenital malformation, or inflammatory diseases, such as rheumatoid arthritis. Instability at this segment can lead to pain, progressive neurological deficit, and potentially death. Many traumatic injuries of C1–2 that are relatively stable can be effectively managed in either a rigid cervical orthosis or a halo-vest; however, the transverse ligament, which is the primary restraint to C1–2 subluxation, does not reliably heal once injured. Furthermore, type II fractures of the odontoid, which are relatively common, have a high nonunion rate and can be associated with atlantoaxial instability. Jefferson fractures of the C1 ring can also be associated with transverse ligament injury and significant atlantoaxial instability. These types of injuries typically require surgical stabilization.

J.A. Rihn (✉), D.T. Anderson, and T.J. Albert
Department of Orthopaedic Surgery, The Rothman Institute, Thomas Jefferson University Hospital, 925 Chestnut Street, Philadelphia, PA 19107, USA
e-mail: jrihno16@yahoo.com

R. Patel
Jefferson Medical College, 1020 Walnut Street, Philadelphia, PA 19107, USA

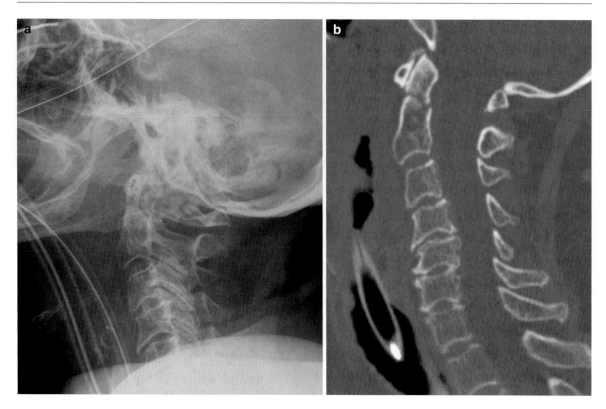

Fig. 10.1 A lateral cervical radiograph (**a**) and sagittal reconstruction of the cervical CT scan (**b**) demonstrating a type II odontoid fracture that is slightly displaced and posteriorly angulated

Several techniques of C1–2 stabilization have been described, including the use sublaminar wires, clamps, screws, rods, or some combination thereof. Many of these techniques are of historical interest only. This chapter will focus on the technique of C1–2 stabilization using a screw/rod construct, with C1 lateral mass screws and C2 pars screws.

10.3 Indications and Advantages for Procedure

Atlantoaxial instability usually requires surgical treatment. Certain traumatic conditions that affect the C1–2 spinal segment, including fracture of the C1 ring, type III odontoid fracture, and rotatory subluxation, may be amenable to external immobilization using either a rigid cervical orthosis or a halo-vest. Type II odontoid fractures are infamous for a high nonunion rate. Treatment of this fracture pattern remains controversial. Nondisplaced type II odontoid fractures may be amenable to halo-vest immobilization; however, it is important that the patient understands the risk of nonunion, which is reported to be as high as 50% [9]. Up to half of the patients with an odontoid fracture treated in a halo-vest for 3 months will require surgical stabilization for a nonunion. Furthermore, halo-vest immobilization of odontoid fractures in elderly patients has been shown to increase morbidity and mortality and provide inferior outcomes when compared to C1–2 fusion [5, 9, 10, 19]. Halo-vest immobilization is also poorly tolerated in this patient population. Acute trauma that results in a transverse ligament injury, with an atlantodens interval of greater than 5 mm in an adult patient should be treated surgically. More chronic conditions that cause atlantoaxial instability, including rheumatoid arthritis, also often require surgical stabilization. Patients with rheumatoid atlantoaxial instability who have a space available for the cord of less than 14 mm have been shown to benefit from surgical treatment [2].

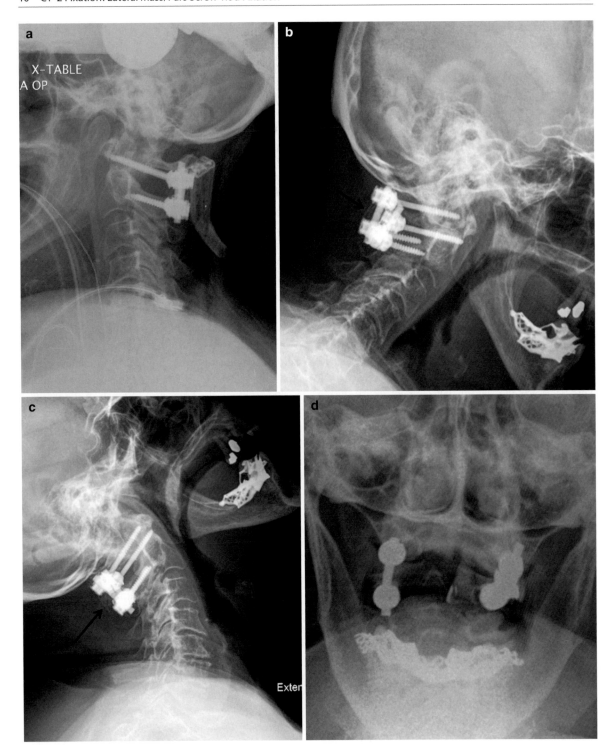

Fig. 10.2 An intraoperative lateral cervical radiograph (**a**) following a C1–2 fusion using a screw/rod construct with C1 lateral mass and C2 pars screws and autogenous iliac crest bone graft. Lateral flexion (**b**), lateral extension (**c**), and open mouth odontoid radiographs (**d**) taken 3 months postoperatively are shown. There is no atlantoaxial motion seen when comparing the flexion and extension radiographs, and a fusion mass can be seen in both the flexion and extension views (*solid black arrow*)

Atlantoaxial stabilization and fusion using a screw/rod construct is indicated in most situations in which stabilization of this spinal segment is required. This includes transverse ligament injury, rheumatoid arthritis with significant atlantoaxial instability, pathological processes (i.e., infection or tumor), rotatory subluxation, acute type II odontoid fracture, unstable type III odontoid fracture, and odontoid nonunion. Type II odontoid fractures that have a superior-anterior to inferior-posterior obliquity and are minimally displaced or can be adequately reduced may be amenable to anterior odontoid screw fixation [6]. Odontoid screw fixation is advantageous because, unlike C1–2 fusion, it does not theoretically limit atlantoaxial motion. The indications for odontoid screw fixation, however, are somewhat limited. This procedure cannot be performed for acute fractures with significant comminution and/or a superior-posterior to inferior-anterior obliquity or for the treatment of odontoid nonunion [6].

The use of lateral mass/pars screws is advantageous over sublaminar wires or interlaminar clamps because the implants are not passed within the spinal canal. This decreases the risk of neurological injury during instrumentation. Furthermore, screw fixation can still be obtained when the C1 and/or C2 lamina have to be removed for decompression purposes or are not structurally sound due to the presence of a pathological process (infection or tumor) or the nature of the trauma (i.e., lamina fracture). C1–2 transarticular screw fixation is a possible alternative to the C1 lateral mass/C2 pars screw technique [8, 12]. Placement of the C1–2 transarticular screw is, however, technically demanding and may be associated with increased risk of vertebral artery injury [7]. Although there is clinical evidence that it is not necessary [22], transarticular screw fixation is often supplemented with sublaminar wiring to increase the stability of the construct, which further increases the risk of this technique.

10.4 Contraindications and Disadvantages for Procedure

Atlantoaxial stabilization is contraindicated when either the bony or vascular anatomy precludes the placement of the C1 lateral mass and/or the C2 pars screw. Thus preoperative understanding of the vascular anatomy is essential. Alteration of bony anatomy can be the result of a congenital malformation, pathological processes (infection or tumor), or trauma. It is important to review the preoperative imaging studies to ensure that the bony anatomy is sufficient to accommodate C1 and C2 screws. In cases of severe osteoporosis, the poor quality of bone may preclude adequate C1–2 stabilization due to inadequate screw purchase. In cases where bony anatomy and/or quality is insufficient, it is often necessary to perform an occipitocervical fusion to ensure adequate screw fixation proximal and distal to the unstable atlantoaxial segment. The level to which the fusion is extended caudally into the subaxial cervical spine is dictated by the extent of pathology and instability and the quality of the patient's bone.

Fortunately, the incidence of vertebral artery injury during screw placement is low [15]. Abnormal vertebral artery anatomy, however, may preclude the use of the C1 lateral mass/C2 pars screw construct. C1 lateral mass screw placement is usually safe with regard to the vertebral artery; however, the ability to place a C2 pars screw can be significantly compromised by anomalous vertebral artery anatomy. The vertebral artery normally ascends through the transverse foramen of the cervical vertebrae, beginning at the C6 level. After exiting the C2 transverse foramen superiorly, the vessel courses acutely laterally within the vertebral artery groove prior to passing through the transverse foramen of C1. The vessel then continues posteromedially along the superior aspect of the atlas midline before entering the foramen magnum near the midline. The left and right vertebral arteries are dominant (i.e., larger) in 36 and 23% of patients, respectively [13, 20] (Fig. 10.3a, b). Equivalent right and left vertebral arteries are present in only 41% of patients [13, 20]. An anomalous or dominant vertebral artery can erode into or change the bony anatomy of the vertebral artery groove and/or the C2 transverse foramen in such a way that there is less isthmus bone available to place the C2 screw (Fig. 10.4a–c). Paramore et al. [16] reviewed 94 fine-cut axial CT scans of the C1–C2 spinal segment to indirectly evaluate the vertebral artery anatomy by studying the C2 transverse foramen and vertebral artery groove. These authors found that 18% of patients had a "high-riding" C-2 transverse foramen on at least one side that would compromise C2 screw placement. An additional 5% of patients were considered to have anatomy in which screw placement would be feasible but high-risk [16]. It is imperative that the preoperative CT scan be studied carefully to determine if the C2 isthmus on both sides can accommodate a screw.

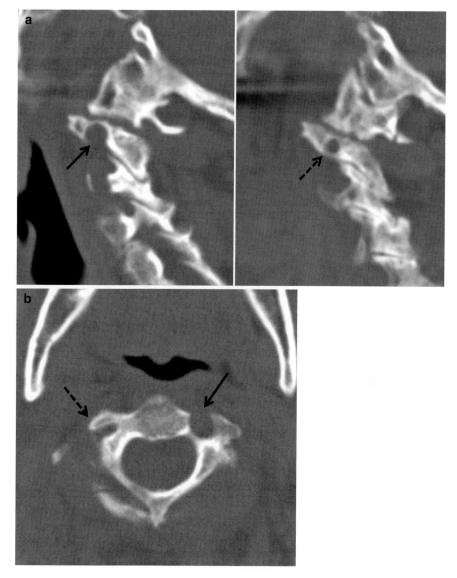

Fig. 10.3 Sagittal (**a**) and axial (**b**) cervical CT scan of a patient who has a dominant left vertebral artery (*solid black arrow*) and hypoplastic right vertebral artery (*interrupted black arrow*). Note how the dominant vertebral artery erodes into the lateral mass and pars of C2 and decreases the amount of bone available for safe screw placement

10.5 Procedure

Although C1–2 fusion can be a technically challenging and risky surgery, many of the pitfalls of this surgical procedure can be avoided by adequate preoperative preparation. This includes ensuring that all of the necessary equipment are present and easily accessible, that all persons involved (i.e., nursing staff, surgical assistants, and anesthesiologists) are educated as to the nature and goals of the procedure, and that special attention is given to proper setup of the room and positioning of the patient.

10.5.1 Anesthetic and Neuromonitoring Considerations

A large percentage of patients who require C1–2 fusion are elderly, have significant medical comorbidities, and/or have degenerative, inflammatory, or traumatic spinal pathology at contiguous levels of the cervical spine. It is important to communicate with the anesthesiologist any concerns regarding the patient's general or spine-specific health. Most patients with atlantoaxial instability require special consideration when undergoing anesthesia. *It is important not to*

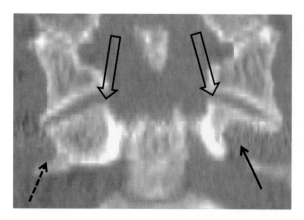

Fig. 10.4 A coronal reconstruction image of a cervical CT scan in a patient with a left sided dominant vertebral artery. This image demonstrates the extent to which the dominant left vertebral artery (*solid black arrow*) erodes into the C2 lateral mass (*open black arrows*). This can be compared to the normal or hypoplastic right vertebral artery (*interrupted black arrow*), that does not erode into the C2 lateral mass. Placement of a left C2 pars screw in this patient would put the vertebral artery at risk for injury

hyperextend patients with an unstable C1–2 segment due to the risk of spinal cord injury. These patients will often require an awake, fiberoptic intubation to avoid the potential for neurological complications [14]. For patients who have evidence of spinal cord compression and are myelopathic, it is important that the anesthesiologist maintain a relatively high mean arterial blood pressure (i.e., greater than 85 mmHg) [11, 21]. Adequate intravenous access and continuous blood pressure monitoring via an arterial line are essential. It is important to communicate to the anesthesiologist that the patient will be turned 180° from the anesthesiologist during that procedure. In order to accommodate this position, the anesthesiologist will have to organize the access lines and EKG leads appropriately and will need a long extension for the endotracheal tube. Prophylactic antibiotics are given at the time of induction, within an hour of making incision. Sequential compression devices are used throughout the procedure for deep venous thrombosis prophylaxis.

All patients at our institution who undergo atlantoaxial fusion are monitored using both somatosensory evoked potential (SSEPs) and motor evoked potentials (MEPs). The neurophysiologist applies the monitoring leads and obtains baseline readings prior to intubation. Subsequent readings are obtained after intubation prior to positioning, after positioning, and throughout the

procedure. It is important to maintain communication with the person performing the neuromonitoring during the procedure to ensure that any change from baseline is detected and the potential causes for this change are investigated and addressed.

10.5.2 Patient Positioning and Room Setup

After anesthesia is administered and the patient's airway is secured, a Mayfield 3-pin head-holder is applied to the patient in standard fashion. The patient is then positioned prone on a well-padded spinal frame with a Mayfield attachment. All vital and bony areas are carefully padded and protected. The Mayfield 3-pin head-holder is secured to the Mayfield attachment. In order to facilitate intraoperative fluoroscopy, the operating table is turned 180° from the anesthesiologist after the patient is positioned and secured on the table. It is important to make sure that the patient is square on the table and that the head is pointed straight down relative to the body to prevent excessive lateral rotation or bending of the cervical spine. Following final positioning, a lateral fluoroscopic image of the upper cervical spine is obtained to ensure that an acceptable view can be obtained. Fluoroscopy is also used, in cases of odontoid fracture and C1–C2 instability, to ensure that adequate fracture alignment and an adequate C1–2 reduction are achieved prior to fusion. Both odontoid fracture alignment and C1–2 alignment can be altered by adjusting and holding the position of the head and neck (i.e., flexion/extension, anterior/posterior translation) with the Mayfield attachment. The C-arm should be positioned in the operating room above the patient's head and out of the way of the surgical field during the approach. It should be positioned in a way that allows the radiology technician to bring the C-arm into the field for a lateral image of the upper cervical spine in a sterile fashion.

10.5.3 Surgical Approach

Sterile preparation and draping of the posterior cervical region and posterior iliac crest area (i.e., if iliac crest autograft is going to be used for fusion) is performed.

A 10 cm incision is made in the midline, from the base of the skull to the upper-level of the subaxial cervical spine. Dissection is carried down through the subcutaneous tissue, the ligamentum nuchae, and down to the posterior C1 arch proximally and the C2 spinous processes distally. Subperiosteal dissection down the C2 spinous process and onto the C2 lamina and lateral mass is accomplished using electrocautery. Electrocautery can carefully be used for subperiosteal dissection near the midline and on the inferior aspect of the posterior C1 arch. Blunt subperiosteal dissection is used further from the midline and closer to the lateral mass of C1 to avoid injury to the venous plexus surrounding the C2 nerve root inferior to the C1 ring and the vertebral artery superior to the C1 ring. Soft tissue dissection should extend to the level of C3 caudally to ensure that the cephalad angulation required for screw placement can be achieved. Although it is usually obvious, an intraoperative lateral fluoroscopic image can be used to confirm the cervical level if there is any question.

Care must be taken to avoid aggressive dissection too far laterally on the posterior arch of C1. The vertebral artery runs along the superior surface of the posterior arch of C1 until it pierces the atlantooccipital membrane. Dissection that extends more than 1.5 cm lateral to the midline, particularly along the superior aspect of the posterior arch of C1, places the vertebral artery at risk for injury. If bleeding is encountered from the cavernous venous sinus between C1 and C2, hemostasis can usually be obtained by packing this area off with thrombin-soaked gelfoam or oxycel cotton.

10.5.4 C1 Lateral Mass Screw Fixation

Harms and Melcher [7] originally described the technique of C1–2 fusion with a screw/rod construct, using C1 lateral mass screws and C2 pars screws. When placing the C1 lateral mass screw, blunt dissection is continued along the inferior aspect of the posterior C1 pedicle down to the lateral mass. This can be accomplished using a 1/2 × 1/2 in. cottonoid and a number 4 Penfield. While doing so, the C2 nerve root gets pushed caudally, taking care not to injure the enveloping venous plexus, which can bleed profusely if violated. If this happens, gelfoam and thrombin with packing are usually sufficient to control the bleeding while you work on the other side. With blunt dissection, the medial and lateral borders of the lateral mass can be identified with the number 4 Penfield. Once these borders have been identified, a 2 mm burr is used to create a starting point for the screw at the superior-most aspect of the lateral mass, where the lateral mass meets the posterior arch of C1. In the medial-lateral plane, the starting point is right at the middle of the lateral mass(Fig. 5a). The 2 mm burr hole prevents the drill from slipping off of the lateral mass when drilling. The drill is placed in the starting hole and its position and orientation are confirmed on a lateral fluoroscopic image. The drill should be aimed directly at the anterior arch of C1 on the lateral fluoroscopic view, which usually requires the surgeon to direct the drill cephalad approximately 5°. In the medial-lateral direction, the drill should be oriented directly straight anterior or angulated slightly medial [7] (Fig. 10.5a, b). After

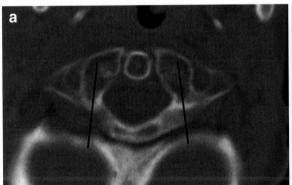 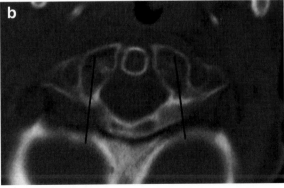

Fig. 10.5 The starting point and trajectory for C1 lateral mass screw placement are depicted (*solid black line*) on an axial CT image (**a**) and sagittal CT image (**b**) of the C1 vertebra. The C1 lateral mass (*open black arrow*) and posterior arch (*solid black arrow*) are labeled on the sagittal view

confirming the orientation on the lateral fluoroscopic image, the drill is advanced under fluoroscopic guidance. One should be careful not to advance the drill past the anterior edge of the odontoid and not go all the way to the anterior edge of C1 on the fluoro views because the curvature of the vertebral body anteriorly would put the tip of the drill bit in the precervical space and near the carotid artery. The drill hole is then tapped and an appropriate sized screw is placed (usually a 28 mm or 30 mm screw) [18]. We prefer to use a 3.5 mm polyaxial screw that has a smooth shank proximally, near the screw head, in order to avoid irritation of the C2 nerve root [7].

10.5.5 C2 Pedicle/Pars Screw Fixation

As part of their C1–2 fixation construct, Harms and Melcher [7] also described placement of the C2 pedicle screw. The C2 pedicle screw has a starting point located in the cranial, medial quadrant of the C2 pars. From this starting point, the screw is directed 20° medial and 20° cephalad. It is placed through the pars, through the C2 pedicle, and into the lateral aspect of the C2 vertebral body. The C2 pedicle screw is usually 20–22 mm in length and 3.5 mm in diameter. It is a longer screw than the C2 pars screw and may provide stronger fixation. Because its staring point is closer to the vertebral artery, however, we prefer to use C2 pars screws for C2 fixation.

The C2 pars screw can usually be safely placed using anatomical landmarks as a guide, but intraoperative fluoroscopy can be used to confirm screw position. Blunt, subperiosteal dissection can be accomplished using a number 4 Penfield. The number 4 Penfield is slid laterally along the superior surface of the C2 lamina to its junction with the isthmus of C2 and can be used to feel the rounded, medial border of the C2 isthmus. The starting point for the C2 pars screw is caudal and lateral to the C2 pedicle screw starting point, just proximal to the C2–3 articulation [7]. A 2 mm burr is used to create a starting point for the drill. The medial border of the C2 isthmus should be used as a guide during drilling and screw placement. The drill should be directed cephalad, in line with the angle of the C2 pars, which is approximately 40–45° from the starting point (Fig. 10.6). The drill should be directed just lateral to the medial border of the C2 isthmus without breaching the medial wall of the isthmus into the spinal canal. From the position of

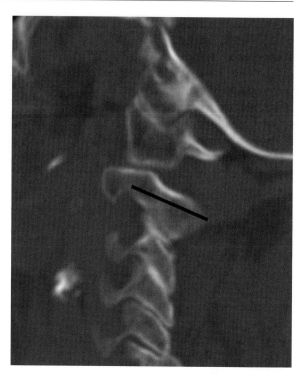

Fig. 10.6 The starting point and trajectory for C2 pars screw placement are depicted (*solid black line*) on a sagittal CT image

the starting point, medial angulation is usually 10–15°. After drilling, the hole is tapped and a 3.5 mm fully threaded polyaxial screw of appropriate length is placed. The length of this screw is usually 16–18 mm [23]. A lateral fluoroscopic view can be obtained to assist in screw placement.

As part of the preoperative planning, it is important to review the sagittal reconstructions of the cervical CT scan to ensure that the isthmus of C2 is of adequate size on both the left and right side of the patient. Screw placement on the side of a dominant or anomalous vertebral artery can lead to vertebral artery injury. The vertebral artery is most at risk if drilling, tapping, or screw placement is off in the lateral and caudal direction [24]. If, preoperatively, it is noted that there is anomalous vertebral artery anatomy, a shorter screw can be used. This can be measured preoperatively on the sagittal CT reconstruction (Fig. 10.7).

Following screw placement bilaterally, rods are cut to an appropriate length and contoured using a rod bender. There is usually only a slight degree of lordosis at this spinal segment. The rods are placed into the polyaxial screw heads and the screw caps are inserted and tightened. If autograft is to be used, a piece of

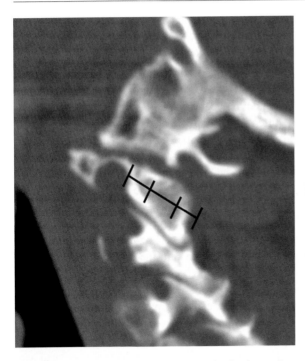

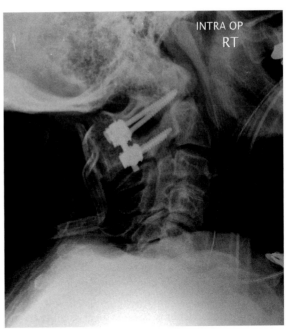

Fig. 10.7 A sagittal CT image of the cervical spine in a patient with a dominant vertebral artery on the left side. This figure demonstrates how to measure the safe length of a C2 pars screw

Fig. 10.8 An intraoperative lateral cervical radiograph following a C1–2 fusion using a screw/rod construct with C1 lateral mass and C2 pars screws and a cortical autogenous iliac crest bone graft. The cortical bone graft is seen dorsal to the posterior C1 arch and is placed between the posterior C1 arch and the C2 spinous process

cortical bone from the superior aspect to the iliac crest and the outer iliac table that measures approximately 3.5 cm in length × 2 cm in width is harvested (measure distance between the C1 arch and C2 spinous process before harvesting), in addition to some cancellous bone. The cortical bone is contoured in such a way that the surgeon can position it dorsal to and between the posterior C1 arch and the C2 spinous process. A notch can be fashioned in the inferior aspect of the cortical graft to accommodate the superior aspect of the C2 spinous process. The same cortical graft can be fashioned from either a piece of allograft iliac crest or an allograft patella. Prior to inserting the bone graft, the posterior arch and lateral mass of C1 and the spinous process, lamina, and lateral mass of C2 are decorticated using a high-speed burr. If possible, the C2 nerve root is retracted and the C1–2 joint is decorticated bilaterally using a high-speed burr. This is often easier to accomplish before the instrumentation is inserted. Autograft cancellous bone or the bone graft substitute is placed over the decorticated bone of C1 and C2, followed by the placement of the contoured cortical piece of bone dorsal to and between the posterior arch of C1 and the

C2 spinous process. We prefer to thread and tie a number one Vicryl suture ventral to the rods and dorsal to the cortical bone graft to ensure that a significant displacement of the graft does not occur during the closure or early postoperative period (Fig. 10.8).

A deep drain can be placed to avoid hematoma formation, although some prefer not to use a drain if adequate hemostasis is achieved and if there was no decompression performed. A careful closure of the posterior cervical wound is essential, as the posterior cervical wound is infamous for complications, including persistent drainage, infection, and dehiscence. The closure is performed in layers, starting with the ligamentum nuchae. This fascial layer tends to retract into the musculature during the case and can be difficult to identify when performing the closure. Care must be taken to identify and close this fascial layer. Failure to adequately close the ligamentum nuchae can lead to splaying of the paraspinal muscles postoperatively, which can in turn lead to neck pain and prominence of the spinous processes that were exposed. Closure of the ligamentum nuchae is followed by the closure of the subcutaneous tissue and the skin, in two separate layers.

10.6 Technical Pearls and Pitfalls

Atlantoaxial fusion using a screw/rod construct can be a technically challenging procedure. Several measures can be taken before and during the procedure, however, to minimize the risk of complications.

- It is essential to carefully review the preoperative imaging studies, particularly the CT scan, for the evidence of abnormal vertebral artery anatomy in the upper cervical spine. Understanding the vertebral artery anatomy prior to screw placement will minimize the risk of vertebral artery injury. The reported incidence of vertebral artery injury during C2 pars screw placement is less than 1% [15].
- It is important to turn the operating room table 180° from anesthesia. This enables the use of intraoperative C-arm to visualize the upper cervical spine and ensure accurate and safe screw placement. Because the table is turned away from anesthesia, there is adequate room to manipulate the C-arm into and out of the surgical field while minimizing the risk of inadvertent field contamination.
- Intraoperatively, it is important to use blunt dissection along the lateral aspect of the C1 ring and the C2 lamina. Care should be taken as blunt dissection will prevent injury to the large venous plexus that surrounds the C2 nerve root, which can bleed profusely. If this venous complex is violated and profuse bleeding is encountered, it is best to pack the area with thrombin-soaked gelfoam or oxycel cotton until hemostasis is achieved. Screw placement in the face of significant bleeding from this plexus can be extremely challenging. Bipolar cauterization of this venous plexus can actually make the bleeding more profuse and more difficult to control.
- Intraoperatively, if C1–2 fixation is achieved but is tenuous (e.g., poor bone quality), the patient can be immobilized in a halo-vest postoperatively for added stability until the bone graft begins to incorporate. Again, however, the halo-vest is not very well tolerated in the elderly population. If adequate fixation cannot be achieved in either C1 or C2, the decision must be made whether an alternative means of fixation (i.e., using a sublaminar wiring technique, e.g., modified Gallie [4] or Brooks [3]) can be achieved or whether the fusion has to be extended to the occiput and/or distally into the subaxial cervical spine. Sublaminar wiring tech-

niques require an intact C1 posterior arch and C2 lamina and require an extended period of postoperative halo-vest immobilization, which may not be tolerated.
- Extending the fusion to the occiput adds considerable morbidity to the procedure. The patient's motion would be significantly decreased postoperatively, often prohibiting the patient from driving and making many daily activities more challenging. If, however, it is discovered intraoperatively that the fracture or pathological process involved more of C1 than originally thought, and adequate C1 lateral mass screw fixation cannot be achieved, extension of the fusion to the occiput may be necessary. Adequate C1 fixation with inadequate C2 fixation may require extension of the fusion into the subaxial cervical spine, using lateral mass screws for fixation at the subaxial levels. The caudal extent of the fusion will be dictated by the extent of pathology, instability, and/or bone quality. Extension of the fusion into the subaxial cervical spine does not add much time or morbidity to the procedure, and the motion loss associated with fusion of an additional caudal level should be minimal. The technique of occipital cervical fusion and lateral mass screw fixation in the subaxial cervical spine is beyond the scope of this chapter.

10.7 Postoperative Considerations

Postoperatively, the patients are immobilized in a rigid cervical orthosis, which typically is continued for a period of 6–8 weeks. The majority of patients, especially those who are elderly and/or have significant medical comorbidities, should be sent to a monitored setting postoperatively for at least a 24 h period. Patients should be out of bed on the first postoperative day and early ambulation should be encouraged to prevent deep venous thrombosis and to facilitate rehabilitation. Antibiotics are continued for 24 h postoperatively. The drain is discontinued on the first postoperative day or when the drainage is less than 30 ml per 8 h.

Aerobic conditioning, including the use of a treadmill and/or stationary bike, can begin 2–3 weeks after surgery, while the patient it still in a rigid cervical orthosis. Six to eight weeks postoperatively, the rigid orthosis is replaced by a soft collar, which is used for comfort and can be weaned over a period of the 3 weeks. After the rigid cervical orthosis is removed, the patient can begin physical therapy, which consists of gentle cervical range of motion and strengthening exercises. Patients are seen in the office 2 weeks postoperatively for a wound check, then at 6 weeks, 12 weeks, 6 months, and 12 months postoperatively, followed by annual visits. Cervical radiographs, including anteroposterior, lateral, and flexion/extension views, are obtained at every postoperative visit to check the position of the instrumentation and the status of the fusion. Dynamic radiographic studies are not performed at the 2-week postoperative appointment.

The reported incidence of instrumentation failure and/or nonunion following the procedure is remarkably low. Reported rates of solid fusion range from 98 to 100% [1, 7, 17]. The rate of postoperative wound infection is reported to be 3–4% [1, 7]. If a wound infection is encountered, it should be treated with irrigation and debridement and long-term (i.e., 6 weeks) administration of culture-guided intravenous antibiotics. Removal of the instrumentation is not necessary, unless the infection persists despite multiple debridement procedures and antibiotic treatment. Removal of the instrumentation necessitates halo-vest immobilization until the infection is adequately treated and a solid fusion is obtained. Consultation with a musculoskeletal infectious disease specialist and a plastic surgeon is important when treating patients who develop complicated postoperative wound infections. Revision surgery, with more extensive instrumentation and fusion, may be necessary if nonunion is encountered.

References

1. Aryan HE, Newman CB, Nottmeier EW et al (2008) Stabilization of the atlantoaxial complex via C-1 lateral mass and C-2 pedicle screw fixation in a multicenter clinical experience in 102 patients: modification of the Harms and Goel techniques. J Neurosurg Spine 8:222–229
2. Boden SD, Dodge LD, Bohlman HH et al (1993) Rheumatoid arthritis of the cervical spine. A long-term analysis with predictors of paralysis and recovery. J Bone Joint Surg Am 75:1282–1297
3. Brooks AL, Jenkins EB (1978) Atlanto-axial arthrodesis by the wedge compression method. J Bone Joint Surg Am 60:279–284
4. Dickman CA, Sonntag VK, Papadopoulos SM et al (1991) The interspinous method of posterior atlantoaxial arthrodesis. J Neurosurg 74:190–198
5. Frangen TM, Zilkens C, Muhr G et al (2007) Odontoid fractures in the elderly: dorsal C1/C2 fusion is superior to halo-vest immobilization. J Trauma 63:83–89
6. Grauer JN, Shafi B, Hilibrand AS et al (2005) Proposal of a modified, treatment-oriented classification of odontoid fractures. Spine J 5:123–129
7. Harms J, Melcher RP (2001) Posterior C1-C2 fusion with polyaxial screw and rod fixation. Spine 26:2467–2471
8. Jeanneret B, Magerl F (1992) Primary posterior fusion C1/2 in odontoid fractures: indications, technique, and results of transarticular screw fixation. J Spinal Disord 5:464–475
9. Kuntz C, Mirza SK, Jarell AD et al (2000) Type II odontoid fractures in the elderly: early failure of nonsurgical treatment. Neurosurg Focus 8:e7
10. Lennarson PJ, Mostafavi H, Traynelis VC et al (2000) Management of type II dens fractures: a case-control study. Spine 25:1234–1237
11. Levi L, Wolf A, Belzberg H (1993) Hemodynamic parameters in patients with acute cervical cord trauma: description, intervention, and prediction of outcome. Neurosurgery 33:1007–1016, discussion 16-7
12. Magerl F, Seemann PS (1987) Stable posterior fusion of the atlas and axis by transarticular screw fixationed. Springer-Verlag, Berlin
13. Menendez JA, Wright NM (2007) Techniques of posterior C1-C2 stabilization. Neurosurgery 60:S103–S111
14. Mulder DS, Wallace DH, Woolhouse FM (1975) The use of the fiberoptic bronchoscope to facilitate endotracheal intubation following head and neck trauma. J Trauma 15:638–640
15. Ondra SL, Marzouk S, Ganju A et al (2006) Safety and efficacy of C2 pedicle screws placed with anatomic and lateral C-arm guidance. Spine 31:E263–E267
16. Paramore CG, Dickman CA, Sonntag VK (1996) The anatomical suitability of the C1-2 complex for transarticular screw fixation. J Neurosurg 85:221–224
17. Stulik J, Vyskocil T, Sebesta P et al (2007) Atlantoaxial fixation using the polyaxial screw-rod system. Eur Spine J 16:479–484
18. Tan M, Wang H, Wang Y et al (2003) Morphometric evaluation of screw fixation in atlas via posterior arch and lateral mass. Spine 28:888–895
19. Tashjian RZ, Majercik S, Biffl WL et al (2006) Halo-vest immobilization increases early morbidity and mortality in elderly odontoid fractures. J Trauma 60:199–203
20. Tokuda K, Miyasaka K, Abe H et al (1985) Anomalous atlantoaxial portions of vertebral and posterior inferior cerebellar arteries. Neuroradiology 27:410–413
21. Vale FL, Burns J, Jackson AB et al (1997) Combined medical and surgical treatment after acute spinal cord injury: results of a prospective pilot study to assess the merits of aggressive medical resuscitation and blood pressure management. J Neurosurg 87:239–246
22. Wang C, Yan M, Zhou H et al (2007) Atlantoaxial transarticular screw fixation with morselized autograft and without additional internal fixation: technical description and report of 57 cases. Spine 32:643–646
23. Xu R, Ebraheim NA, Yeasting RA et al (1995) Morphometric evaluation of the first sacral vertebra and the projection of its pedicle on the posterior aspect of the sacrum. Spine 20:936–940
24. Yoshida M, Neo M, Fujibayashi S et al (2006) Comparison of the anatomical risk for vertebral artery injury associated with the C2-pedicle screw and atlantoaxial transarticular screw. Spine 31:E513–E517

Closed Reduction of Unilateral and Bilateral Facet Dislocations

11

Thomas J. Puschak and Paul A. Anderson

11.1 Case Example

EM is 41-year-old woman in a rollover motor vehicle accident. She presented to another hospital 5 h prior and was reported to have tingling in her left hand. On presentation to our ER, she had only 3/5 strength of grip and wrist dorsiflexion on the left, and 3/5 right EHL and tibialis anterior. CT scan showed bilateral facet dislocation (Fig. 11.1).

Due to neurologic progression, she was taken to the OR for closed reduction under controlled traction. Mayfield head holder was applied and weight was gradually increased. At 40 lbs she noted a shift in her neck and weights were reduced. Fluoroscopic images showed only partial reduction with likely continued unilateral subluxation. Weights were increased again to 60 lbs and she noted another shift. Weights were again reduced; however the patient lost all function of her bilateral lower extremities and upper extremity weakness increased (Fig. 11.2).

She was anesthetized with immediate fiber-optic intubation and emergent anterior decompression was performed. Herniated disc material was removed from the canal taking care not to over distract the disc space. A 7-mm spacer was placed, again avoiding over distraction, and anterior an plate was placed. Post surgical CT showed facet reduction (Fig. 11.3). The patient gradually regained near full strength and function in all extremities.

T.J. Puschak (✉) and P.A. Anderson
Department of Orthopaedic Surgery and Rehabilitation, University Hospital, 600 Highland Avenue, Madison, WI, USA
e-mail: tpuschak@panoramaortho.com

11.2 Introduction

Spinal deformity from cervical facet subluxation and dislocation can cause spinal cord and nerve root injury not only from the original trauma, but can lead to ongoing neurologic worsening from continued mechanical compression and vascular compromise. Although manipulation of cervical dislocations is dangerous and not recommended, closed reduction with cranial tong traction is a safe and effective tool in the initial treatment of cervical dislocations. The goals of closed reduction are to restore normal spinal alignment and stabilize and immobilize the cervical spine. Closed reduction may decompress the spinal cord, enhance neurologic recovery, and minimize worsening of neurologic deficits.

11.3 Indications/Contraindications

In lower cervical injuries, cranial tong traction is most commonly used for unilateral and bilateral facet subluxation and dislocations as well as cervical burst fractures. Some upper cervical injuries such as C1 burst fractures, traumatic spondylolisthesis of the axis, and odontoid fractures are also amenable to closed reduction with cranial traction.

Contraindications to cranial traction include skull fractures with patterns that could result in depressed skull fractures or propagation of the fracture lines due to proximity of the pin placement. Not all skull fracture patterns preclude the application of cranial tongs; however, a thorough understanding of the fracture lines is required if tongs are to be used in the setting of a skull fracture. Distractive spinal injuries such as an atlantooccipital dissociation are an absolute contraindication to cranial traction. Severe soft tissue injuries such as scalping injuries

V.V. Patel et al. (eds.), *Spine Trauma*,
DOI: 10.1007/978-3-642-03694-1_11, © Springer-Verlag Berlin Heidelberg 2010

Fig. 11.1 Bilateral
facet dislocation with
minimal fracture

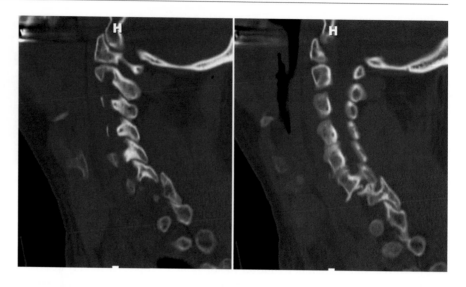

Fig. 11.1 Bilateral
facet dislocation with
minimal fracture

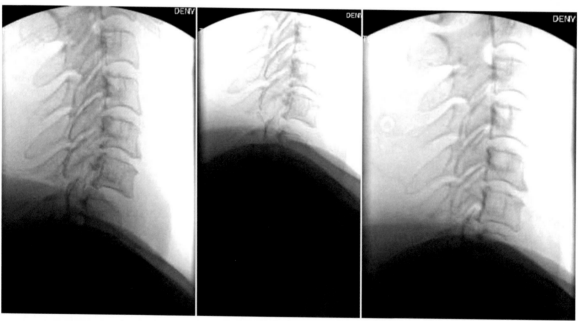

Fig. 11.2 Fluroscopy images showing unilateral reduction (**a**), bilateral reduction with traction still on (**b**) and reduction after traction was removed (**c**)

can provide a relative contraindication from logistic difficulty in safe placement of cranial tongs.

11.4 Timing

Although there is no clear consensus, evidence exists that suggests that rapid closed reduction improves neurologic recovery. Continued cord compression can lead to irreversible changes after 6–8 h. Early closed

reduction of cervical dislocations with neurologic deficits is widely accepted.

Controversy does exist over the timing of closed reduction with regard to obtaining MRI imaging. Several case reports reported neurologic deterioration after closed reduction due to displacement of a disc herniation into the spinal canal. The incidence of neurologic worsening in these reports ranges from 1.5 to 35%. Based on these reports, it has been suggested that MRI scans should be routinely acquired before closed

Fig. 11.3 CT images after reduction

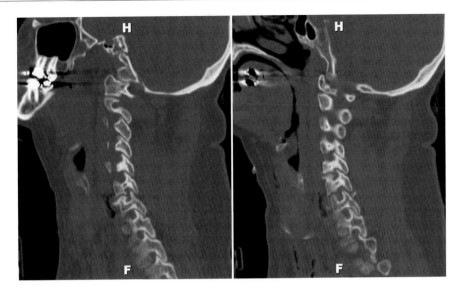

11.5 Equipment Required

Required resources for cranial tong reduction include C-arm fluoroscopy, a bed setup with a strong pulley and frame at the head end, and the ability to provide trendelenburg, reverse trendelenburg, and height adjustment, conscious sedation with pulse oximeter and rhythm strip EKG monitoring, and Gardner-Wells tongs with spring loaded threaded bolts or Mayfield head holder. Ideally, access to MRI and the operating room should be secured in the event of neurologic worsening and/or failed reduction. In a rural setting, the timing and location of reduction should be determined between the referring and accepting physician and will likely be determined by factors such as severity of injury, resources at the outlying facility, and experience of the physician. In our experience the emergency department trauma bay, ICU, or OR are all adequate locations to perform closed reductions. From a timing standpoint, the trauma bay is most often the best choice.

reduction in patients who are neurologically normal and cognitively impaired. Disadvantages to routinely obtaining MRI scans prior to reduction include critical time delays to obtain the imaging, manipulation of an unstable spinal column during transfers, and decreased monitoring of the patient during the scan.

Grant et al. reported on a prospective series of 82 patients with lower cervical fracture dislocations who underwent early closed reduction. Eighty patients were successfully reduced and average time to reduction was 2.5 h. Postreduction, MRI scans identified disc herniations in 23% of the patients with unilateral facet dislocations and 13% of the patients with bilateral facet dislocations. Neurologic improvement 24 h after reduction was seen in 64% of the Frankel grade A patients and 98% of the incomplete cord injury patients. One patient worsened neurologically; however, no causation was established to the reduction. Vaccaro et al. prospectively obtained pre and postreduction MRI scans in 11 cervical dislocations and found no neurologic worsening in their series.

These studies show the safety and efficacy of closed reduction of cervical dislocations prior to obtaining MRI scans in awake, alert cooperative patients. Reduction of dislocations in cognitively impaired patients without MRI imaging is controversial. Prolonged delays due to unavailability of MRI should be avoided.

If an awake patient deteriorates neurologically after reduction, one should be prepared to perform an emergent decompression via ACDF or laminectomy based on pathology.

11.6 Reduction Technique

The patient is placed supine on the bed with the frame and pulley setup at the head of the bed. A folded sheet is placed between the scapulae to improve head position. The shoulders are gently taped down to the bottom of the bed to aid in radiographic visualization of the spine as well as to act as a counterforce to prevent the patient from being pulled up in the bed as the reduction weights increase. Reverse trendelenburg positioning can also assist in resisting migration of the patient toward the head of the bed. Wrist straps allow intermittent application of downward traction to the arms, which is helpful in viewing the injury level in lower level injuries and in patients with broad shoulders or thick necks.

When applying the Gardner-Wells tongs, shaving the pin site can be helpful in patients with longer hair. I recommend palpating the skull at the pin sites to make sure there are no defects such as a previous craniotomy flap, old burr holes, or an unstable skull fracture. The pin sites are disinfected, and the skin, subcutaneous tissue, and periosteum are infiltrated with 2% lidocaine. A sterile set of tongs are placed a fingerbreadth above the pinna of the ear in line with the external auditory meatus. In individual situations the pins can be placed slightly posterior or anterior to this spot to affect a flexion or extension moment, respectively. Flexion or extension moments can also be applied by raising or lowering the pulley to change the vector of the traction or by placing pads under the patient's head or scapulae. The pin should be below the equator of the skull and the bolts are simultaneously advanced engaging the skin and skull until the spring loaded pressure indicator protrudes. The locking nuts on the bolts are advanced until they are seated against the tong frame to prevent inadvertent advancement of the pins.

Stainless steel tongs have a pull-out strength of 300 lbs in cadaver bone, while carbon fiber and titanium tongs have a pull-out strength of 75 lbs. Also, tongs have lower pull-out strength with repeated use due to spring or pin wear. Carbon fiber and titanium tongs have the benefit of being MRI compatible; however, if reduction weights exceed 70 lbs, a relatively new set of stainless steel tongs should be used.

Conscious sedation and muscle relaxation will aid in expedient reduction. Vital signs and pulse oximetry are monitored throughout. The patient must be conscious enough to remain responsive to repeated neurologic assessments.

At the start of the reduction, a lateral baseline radiograph is obtained. Next, 10 lbs is added and a radiograph is obtained to rule out occult distractive ligamentous injuries. More than 1.5 mm increase in widening from baseline at any interspace with only 10 lbs of traction suggests a ligamentous distraction injury and the closed reduction should be abandoned. One should check these gaps at all levels from occiput to T1 as possible with each addition of weight.

Weights are added in 5 or 10 lbs increments every 5–10 min with repeat lateral radiographs and neurologic reassessment with each change in weight. Placing a pad under the patient's head and/or raising the height of the pulley can provide a flexion moment to help unhinge the locked facet joints. Manual manipulation of the spine during traction has been reported, is controversial, and dangerous, and should not be performed by surgeons with little experience in this technique. The patient can be placed in reverse trendelenburg to avoid the patient getting pulled up to bed.

Weights up to 140 lbs may be required for reduction. If the reduction is not successful by 140 lbs or if there is greater than 1 cm distraction at the injury level, the procedure should be abandoned. Prolonged high weight traction should be avoided due to the potential for pin site complications. If the neurologic status worsens, the reduction is abandoned and the patient is transferred immediately to the MRI scanner and then to the OR for emergent open reduction and decompression.

Once reduction is obtained, the head is placed into neutral to slight extension and the weights are dropped to 10–20 lbs. Care should be taken not to hyperextend the neck to avoid causing a central cord syndrome. A final radiograph is obtained to confirm the reduction and the patient is sent to MRI and/or CT scan to complete the diagnostic imaging. If there is residual neurologic compression on the postreduction imaging, earlier surgical decompression and stabilization should be considered.

11.7 Conclusion

Closed reduction of unilateral and bilateral facet dislocations by cranial tong traction is a safe and effective procedure. Expedient reduction and decompression of neurologic structures enhances neurologic recovery. Recent studies support closed reduction prior to obtaining MRI in patients who are awake, alert, and cooperative. Timing of reduction with regard to obtaining MRI in patients with impaired cognition is controversial.

11.8 Pearls

Patience is important with closed reduction. Wait 5–10 min between each addition of weight.

- Careful evaluation of fluoro images with each addition of weight is important to avoid overdistraction.
- Manipulation is controversial but gentle flexion can unlock the facets to aid in reduction.
- Check the pin sites regularly, especially when adding heavier weights.
- Conscious sedation from trained staff can help tremendously to relax the patient and ease reduction.

11.9 Pitfalls

With heavier weights, pins can migrate – monitor them closely.

- Neurologic deterioration before or after reduction requires immediate attention. Be prepared for this possibility.
- Occult skull fractures may be present. Study prereduction CT scans carefully.
- Combative or inebriated patients can be difficult and may not be ideal candidates for closed reduction.
- Postreduction, the patient may still need surgical treatment.
- Fractured facet fragments can impinge nerve roots. Evaluate this if the patient has an isolated radiculopathy postreduction.

11.10 Complications

- Pin slippage
- Neurologic deterioration

11.11 Bailouts/Salvage

- Open ACDF
- Open posterior reduction

11.12 Post Procedure

- Rigid cervical collar such as Aspen or Miami-J.
- Anterior or posterior fusion may be necessary based on stability.

Further Reading

1. Anon (2002) Treatment of subaxial cervical spinal injuries. Neurosurgery 50(3 suppl):S156–S165, Review
2. Anon (2002) Initial closed reduction of cervical spine fracture-dislocation injuries. Neurosurgery 50(3 suppl):S44–S50, Review
3. Andreshak JL, Dekutoski MB (1997) Management of unilateral facet dislocations: a review of the literature. Orthopedics 20(10):917–926, Review
4. Moore KR, Frank EH (1995) Traumatic atlantoaxial rotatory subluxation and dislocation. Spine 20(17):1928–1930, Review
5. Shapiro SA (1993) Management of unilateral locked facet of the cervical spine. Neurosurgery 33(5):832–837; discussion 837, Review
6. Schwarz N, Sim E (1993) Treatment problems in unilateral locked facet syndrome of the cervical spine. Eur Spine J. 2(2):65–71, Review
7. Beyer CA, Cabanela ME (1992) Unilateral facet dislocations and fracture-dislocations of the cervical spine: a review. Orthopedics 1992;15(3):311–315, Review. Erratum in: Orthopedics 1992;15(5):545
8. Dailey AT, Shaffrey CI, Rampersaud R, Lee J, Brodke DS, Arnold P, Nassr A, Harrop JS, Grauer J, Bono CM, Dvorak M, Vaccaro A (2009) Utility of helical computed tomography in differentiating unilateral and bilateral facet dislocations. J Spinal Cord Med 32(1):43–48
9. Nassr A, Lee JY, Dvorak MF, Harrop JS, Dailey AT, Shaffrey CI, Arnold PM, Brodke DS, Rampersaud R, Grauer JN, Winegar C, Vaccaro AR (2008) Variations in surgical treatment of cervical facet dislocations. Spine 33(7):E188–E193
10. Dvorak MF, Fisher CG, Aarabi B, Harris MB, Hurbert RJ, Rampersaud YR, Vaccaro A, Harrop JS, Nockels RP, Madrazo IN, Schwartz D, Kwon BK, Zhao Y, Fehlings MG (2007) Clinical outcomes of 90 isolated unilateral facet fractures, subluxations, and dislocations treated surgically and nonoperatively. Spine 32(26):3007–3013
11. Spector LR, Kim DH, Affonso J, Albert TJ, Hilibrand AS, Vaccaro AR (2006) Use of computed tomography to predict failure of nonoperative treatment of unilateral facet fractures of the cervical spine. Spine 31(24):2827–2835
12. Vaccaro AR, Nachwalter RS (2002) Is magnetic resonance imaging indicated before reduction of a unilateral cervical facet dislocation? Spine 27(1):117–118
13. Ludwig SC, Vaccaro AR, Balderston RA, Cotler JM (1997) Immediate quadriparesis after manipulation for bilateral cervical facet subluxation. A case report J Bone Joint Surg Am 79(4):587–590

Cervical Open Posterior Reduction of Facet Dislocation

12

Eric Klineberg and Munish Gupta

12.1 Case Example

A 45-year-old woman, a restrained passenger, was involved in a rollover motor vehicle accident. She presented with a sensory level at C6 with 4/5 strength in biceps and deltoid and only a flicker of wrist extension on the right. There was no fundtional motor or sensory function below C6 in her bilateral upper or lower extremities. Initial CT scan, and model representation is shown in (Fig. 12.1).

CT scan demonstrates a fracture dislocation of C5/6 with significant displacement and neural compression. The patient was taken to the OR for open reduction and internal fixation.

12.2 Background

Facet dislocations are an uncommon injury in the subaxial cervical spine. The most common levels for injury are the C5/6 and C6/7 levels [9, 13], and the mechanism of injury is usually a motor vehicle or motorcycle accident [10]. The forces on the cervical spine are usually a hyperflexion and rotation moment that uncouples the posterior elements and results in disruption of the posterior ligamentous complex, facet capsule, and disk annulus. For a unilateral facet dislocation, section studies have demonstrated that disruption of the ipsilateral facet capsule, annulus fibrosis, and ligamentum flavum are sufficient to allow dislocation in a pure rotation moment [11]. A bilateral facet dislocation has traditionally thought to include facet disruption, posterior ligamentous complex disruption, as well as disruption of the posterior longitudinal ligament [12], although a recent MRI study found only a 40% rate of disruption of the PLL [2]. Facet fractures are also a common component of this constellation of injuries and occur in over 60% of these injuries. This has implications for how one considers reducing and stabilizing these fractures.

Neurologic injuries in these groups are common. For bilateral facet dislocations, severe neurologic injuries are common with 65% presenting with complete motor quadriplegia [9]. Unilateral facet dislocations have a much more benign clinical presentation and usually present either without neurologic injury or with a unilateral radiculopathy [10].

Conservative management of these complex injuries with a halo vest or cervicothoracic orthosis tends to lead to late subluxation or redislocation, and most authors recommend surgical stabilization [1, 10] (Fig. 12.2). Selection of a posterior approach for facet dislocations is predicated on several important factors. First, the most important consideration is the presence or absence of an anterior disk herniation that can be brought into the canal during the reduction and cause neurologic injury. Preoperative MRI can be useful in determining the presence of the herniation. Additionally, CT scans can be windowed to determine if there is intracanal pathology. There is still controversy regarding the timing of closed reduction and surgical approach [7]. But most authors

E. Klineberg (✉) and M. Gupta
Adult and Pediatric Spinal Surgery, Department
of Orthopaedics, University of California at Davis,
4860 Y Street, Suite 3800, Sacramento, CA 95817, USA
e-mail: eric.klineberg@ucdmc.ucdavis.edu

V.V. Patel et al. (eds.), *Spine Trauma*,
DOI: 10.1007/978-3-642-03694-1_12, © Springer-Verlag Berlin Heidelberg 2010

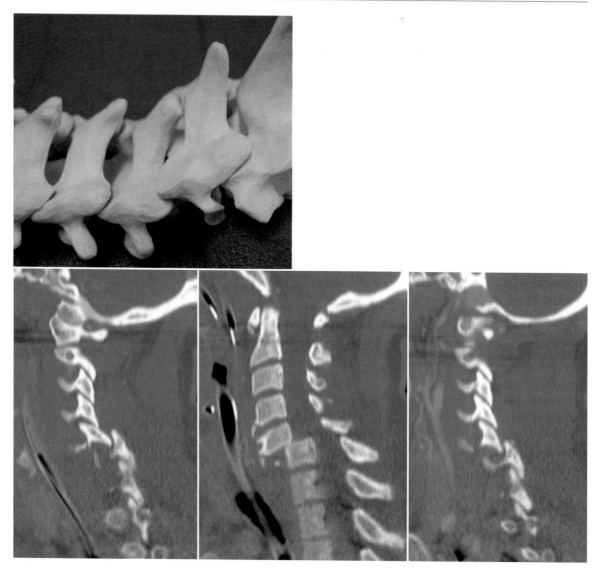

Fig. 12.1 Bilateral facet dislocation. CT scan and bone model representation

would advocate early reduction in awake patients who are cooperative with significant neurologic injuries. Even if there is disc pathology on the postreduction MRI, this rarely has implications for neurologic recovery [5]. If closed reduction is unsuccessful, open reduction is necessary to restore alignment and provide adequate neural decompression. Either an anterior or posterior reduction can accomplish the goals of reduction and the decision is based on surgeon preference, and the presence of a disc herniation on MRI imaging.

Facet fractures also have implications for using the posterior approach. If the facet is both fractured and dislocated then the fusion levels must extend beyond the fracture for adequate screw purchase. This often means including an additional level into the construct. With unilateral facet fractures and subluxation, the anterior approach has been successful in providing stability even without facet reduction [8]. However, control of this fractured facet through an anterior approach can be difficult and may require a staged approach is reduction is unsuccessful.

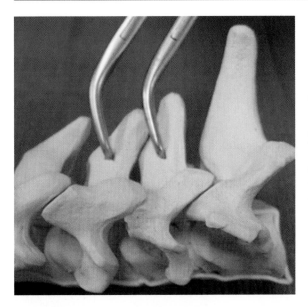

Fig. 12.2 Initial reduction with towel clamps

12.3 Indications and Advantages for Procedure

The posterior approach is advantageous to reduce facet dislocations for a variety of reasons. First, a posterior approach addresses the major ligamentous injury as well as the bony pathology directly. This can make the reduction easier and potentially safer. The anatomy is well known to spinal surgeons and can be approached and manipulated with relative ease.

Second, the posterior approach restores the major deforming force, which is the flexion moment and the restoration of the posterior tension band. For unilateral facet dislocations, biomechanical studies have shown that posterior fixation alone was superior to anterior fixation in decreasing motion at the injured segment [3]. Posterior fixation with reduction and bony fusion can still result in an 18% incidence of neck pain, although there was a 92% resolution of patients' radiculopathy [10]. Additionally, in a clinical study with facet dislocations or subluxations treated with anterior alone instrumentation, there is a 13% loss of postoperative alignment [6].

Third, the posterior approach allows for direct decompression of the spinal cord as well as the exiting spinal roots.

12.3.1 Contraindications and Disadvantages for Procedure

The most significant disadvantage of the posterior approach is the inability to address anterior pathology. If a preoperative MRI demonstrates a large disc herniation, the surgeon is obligated to first perform an anterior discectomy to prevent translation of the disc material into the canal with reduction. Additionally, if there are facet fractures, often the construct needs to be extended an additional level. The anterior approach, may be able to limit the levels fused.

12.4 Procedure

12.4.1 Equipment Needed

- OR table for prone positioning. (This surgeon's preference is for a slider table to allow movement into the fluoroscopy beam.)
- Mayfield tongs.
- Posterior cervical set.
- Posterior fixation system.
- 18-guage wire or cables for intraspinous wiring.
- Small lamina spreader.

12.4.2 Anesthetic and Neuromonitoring Considerations

- Fiberoptic or awake intubation due to neck instability.
- SSEP, MEP monitoring, preflip signals to determine baseline.

12.4.3 Patient Positioning and Room Setup

- Patient positioned prone on slider table in Mayfield tongs. This allows for safe and controlled head positioning.

12.4.4 Surgical Approach

- Posterior midline subperiosteal approach.
- Control any bony bleeding from fractures with bone wax and gelfoam.

12.4.5 Reduction Technique

- Reduction can then be obtained using two towel clamps placed in opposing positions that are secured through the lamia and spinous process of the affected vertebra (Fig. 12.2).
- A thin periosteal elevator can also be used within the facet joint to provide leverage and facilitate reduction.
- Once the facet joints have been reduced, they tend to sit in a subluxed position that can be verified using fluoroscopy (Fig. 12.3). To complete the reduction, the surgeon should reposition the head to provide additional lordosis. I find that this is usually inadequate to fully reduce the facet joints and I use an intraspinous single wire to complete the reduction and restore the appropriate lordosis (Fig. 12.4).

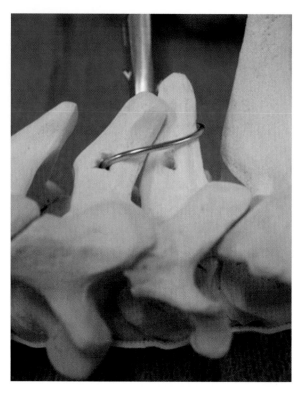

Fig. 12.4 Provisional reduction of facet joints with spinous process wiring

12.4.6 Fixation Technique

- Fixation is accomplished using rigid lateral mass screw rod constructs and/or figure of light spinous process wiring (Fig. 12.5).

12.4.7 Closure

- Tight fascial closure 1/8 in. hemovac drain
- Running 3–0 nylon suture

12.5 Technical Pearls and Pitfalls

12.5.1 Pearls

- After exposure, complete a midline decompression to remove any ligamentum flavum that could infold upon the spinal cord with reduction.

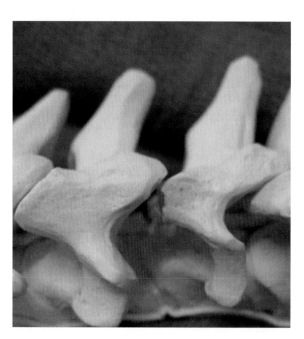

Fig. 12.3 Subluxed position of facet joints, despite adequate reduction

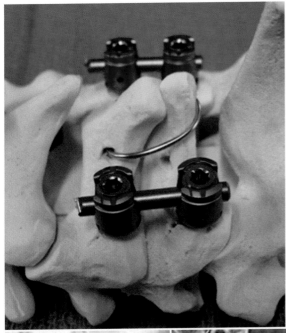

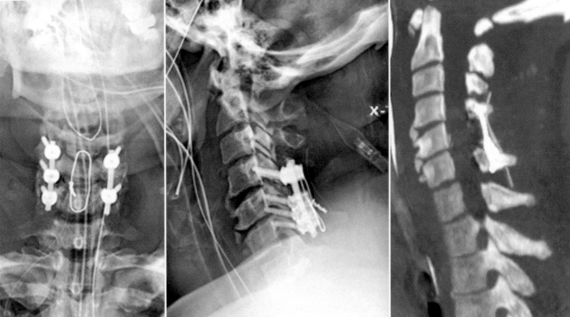

Fig. 12.5 Final stabilization with lateral mass construct. CT scan and bone model

- Denude the cartilage from the inferior facet joint as this will be exposed to you as the facet sits in the dislocated position.
- If the reduction cannot be obtained with gentle direct manipulation, then by using a Kerrison rongeur or high speed burr one can remove the most superior aspect of the superior facet joint and thus unlock the facets. Be careful in the amount of bone removed as this will have implications for stability after reduction (Fig. 12.6).
- Additionally, an interlaminar spreader can be used to provide the reduction force to allow for the distraction needed across the level [4] (Fig. 12.6).

Fig. 12.6 Pearls–Lamina spreader for longitudinal traction for facet reduction, and removal of the superior articular process with a kerrison rongeur for reduction of locked facets

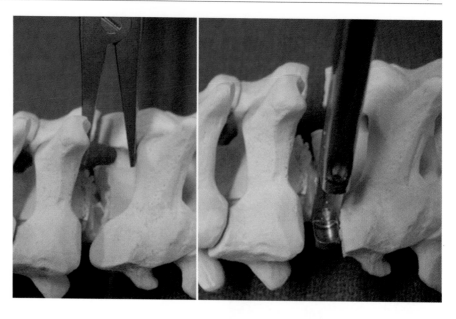

- Use a nerve hook to feel the foramen to assess for any residual compression after the reduction. If the nerve is compressed, a foraminotomy can be performed. Bony fragments may remain in the foramen after reduction and may need to be removed.

12.5.2 Potential Intraoperative Complications

- Dural tears from the fracture. This can induce surgeon angina, but can be managed successfully with either direct repair, if the tear is easily accessible and small, or with packing of the durotomy with gelform, with careful consideration to prevent cord compression. Head elevation postoperatively can reduce the incidence of pseuomeningocele.
- SSEP or MEP signal change during reduction. Stop reduction immediately, and make sure that additional compression has not occurred posteriorly through the ligamentum flavum. If this is not the case, then the likely cause is from the anterior disc. This obligates the surgeon to perform a discectomy prior to proceeding with the posterior reduction.
- Bleeding may also be an issue with bony fractures and the epidural plexus. Local control is usually effective in the form of bone wax or gelfoam. The surgeon should, however, be prepared and utilize cell saver and/or the patient should have blood available.

12.5.3 Bailout/Salvage for Procedure Failure

- If singe-level posterior fixation is inadequate due to facet fracture, extension of the fusion may be necessary to additional levels. Additionally, posterior fixation can later be augmented with anterior column decompression and support.

12.6 Postoperative Considerations

12.6.1 Bracing

- Three months in a Miami-J or Aspen collar.

12.6.2 Activity

- Mobilize as tolerated in collar.

12.6.3 Follow-Up

- Follow-up in 3 weeks for nylon suture removal and plain films to evaluate union and reduction.

12.6.4 Potential Complications

- Nonunion
- Malunion
- Continued neural compromise

12.6.5 Treatments/Rescue for Complications

- The rescue operations should focus on addressing the major problem. If stability is a question or there is a potential for nonunion, then an anterior approach can be performed and either a discectomy or corpectomy be completed depending upon the injury pattern. Similarly, if there is any residual compression, this will need to be addressed through an anterior approach or revision posterior foraminotomy.

References

1. Beyer CA, Cabanela ME, Berquist TH (1991) Unilateral facet dislocations and fracture-dislocations of the cervical spine. J Bone Joint Surg Br 73(6):977–981
2. Carrino JA, Manton GL, Morrison WB, Vaccaro AR, Schweitzer ME, Flanders AE (2006) Posterior longitudinal ligament status in cervical spine bilateral facet dislocations. Skeletal Radiol 35(7):510–514
3. Duggal N, Chamberlain RH, Park SC, Sonntag VK, Dickman CA, Crawford NR (2005) Unilateral cervical facet dislocation: biomechanics of fixation. Spine 30(7):E164–E168
4. Fazl M, Pirouzmand F (2001) Intraoperative reduction of locked facets in the cervical spine by use of a modified interlaminar spreader: technical note. Neurosurgery 48(2):444–445; discussion 445–446
5. Grant GA, Mirza SK, Chapman JR, Winn HR, Newell DW, Jones DT, Grady MS (1999) Risk of early closed reduction in cervical spine subluxation injuries. J Neurosurg 90 (1 suppl):13–18
6. Johnson MG, Fisher CG, Boyd M, Pitzen T, Oxland TR, Dvorak MF (2004) The radiographic failure of single segment anterior cervical plate fixation in traumatic cervical flexion distraction injuries. Spine 29(24):2815–2820
7. Nassr A, Lee JY, Dvorak MF, Harrop JS, Dailey AT, Shaffrey CI, Arnold PM, Brodke DS, Rampersaud R, Grauer JN, Winegar C, Vaccaro AR (2008) Variations in surgical treatment of cervical facet dislocations. Spine 33(7):E188–E193
8. Rabb CH, Lopez J, Beauchamp K, Witt P, Bolles G, Dwyer A (2007) Unilateral cervical facet fractures with subluxation: injury patterns and treatment. J Spinal Disord Tech 20(6):416–422
9. Shapiro SA (1993) Management of unilateral locked facet of the cervical spine. Neurosurgery 33(5):832–837; discussion 837
10. Shapiro S, Snyder W, Kaufman K, Abel T (1999) Outcome of 51 cases of unilateral locked cervical facets: interspinous braided cable for lateral mass plate fusion compared with interspinous wire and facet wiring with iliac crest. J Neurosurg 91(1 suppl):19–24
11. Sim E, Vaccaro AR, Berzlanovich A, Schwarz N, Sim B (2001) In vitro genesis of subaxial cervical unilateral facet dislocations through sequential soft tissue ablation. Spine 26(12):1317–1323
12. Vaccaro AR, Madigan L, Schweitzer ME, Flanders AE, Hilibrand AS, Albert TJ (2001) Magnetic resonance imaging analysis of soft tissue disruption after flexion-distraction injuries of the subaxial cervical spine. Spine 26(17):1866–1872
13. Wolf A, Levi L, Mirvis S, Ragheb J, Huhn S, Rigamonti D, Robinson L (1991) Operative management of bilateral facet dislocation. J Neurosurg 75(6):883–890

Open Anterior Reduction of Cervical Facet Dislocation

13

Anh X. Le

13.1 Introduction

Cervical spine injuries are observed in 2–5% of patients presenting with blunt trauma. The incidence of facet injuries is 6.7% of all cervical spine fractures [7]. Significant discussions have been generated over the years regarding diagnostic requirements (MRI before or after reduction), reduction maneuvers (open vs. closed, anesthetized vs. awake), and surgical approaches (posterior vs. anterior). Treatment algorithms have also been developed providing guidelines for the treatment of unilateral and bilateral facet dislocations [12] (Table 13.1).

At present, there is consensus for the need for MRI evaluation following both successful and failed closed reduction prior to an open surgical reduction; this is done to evaluate the amount of potential cord compression present, which may worsen during the surgical procedure.

Approximately 30–50% of patients with cervical dislocations have an associated acute disc herniation at the level of injury documented by magnetic resonance imaging [5, 8]. Closed reduction seems to increase the risks of disc herniation. Specifically, the incidence of cervical disc herniation is 18% before and 56% after closed reduction of cervical dislocations observed in a series of 11 patients [15]. Many centers have reported large series of patients successfully treated with awake, closed reduction without prereduction MRI with minor neurological consequences [14]. However, there are several case

reports documenting acute neurological deterioration after cervical reduction in patients with herniated discs. Although reduction in these reports was done under anesthesia rather than keeping patients awake, the devastating complications have prompted alteration in treatment protocols at many centers [6, 12]. Thus MRI vs. immediate awake reduction remains controversial, especially in patients with partial neurologic deficit. In either case, the surgeon must be prepared for immediate anterior discectomy with possible anterior reduction. Also, the statistics on MRI-documented disc herniation suggest that almost one third to one half of the patients with facet dislocations should undergo anterior reduction and fusion. Therefore, gaining familiarity with anterior reduction techniques can improve treatment outcomes of traumatic facet dislocations. Understanding the mechanism of injury that leads to facet dislocations is important in technique development and may improve the rate of successful reduction from an anterior approach.

13.2 Mechanism of Injury

13.2.1 Unilateral Facet Dislocations

During normal physiologic motion, cervical movements are coupled; lateral bending is coupled with axial rotation. During injury, these forces are exaggerated leading to disruption of normal tissues. Supraphysiologic combination of flexion, lateral bending, and axial rotation forces results in unilateral facet subluxation and dislocation. Rupture of facet capsules, attenuation of interspinous ligaments, partial disruption of the posterolateral corner of the disc, and uncinate process are observed in this type of injury [13]. Addition of shear or vertical compression to the existing deforming forces

A.X. Le
Alpine Orthopaedic Medical Group and Spine Center,
2488 North California Street, Stockton, CA 95204, USA and

Assistant Clinical Professor, Department of Orthopaedic
Surgery, University of California, Davis
e-mail: anhxlespine@yahoo.com

V.V. Patel et al. (eds.), *Spine Trauma*,
DOI: 10.1007/978-3-642-03694-1_13, © Springer-Verlag Berlin Heidelberg 2010

Table 13.1 Treatment guidelines for unilateral and bilateral facet dislocations

Injury	Type	Treatment
Unilateral facet dislocations	Reducible	Reduce and Halo vest for 3 months
	Not reducible	Open reduction and posterior fusion
	Associated with facet fractures	Open reduction and posterior fusion
	Associated with disc herniation	Anterior decompression, reduction, and fusion
Bilateral facet dislocations	Reducible without disc herniation	Closed reduction; then posterior fusion
	Not reducible, without disc herniation	Open posterior reduction and fusion
	Associated with disc herniation	Anterior decompression, reduction, and fusion

can lead to bony failures, such as unilateral facet, bilateral facet, and lateral mass fractures [10].

13.2.2 Bilateral Facet Dislocation

Bilateral facet subluxation, perched facet, and facet dislocation represent different stages of flexion distraction injury [9]. Severe tensile loading of the posterior elements causes significant posterior ligamentous disruption. In cases of bilateral facet dislocations, complete rupture of interspinous ligaments, facet capsules, and in 30–50% of the cases, traumatic disruptions of the posterior annulus have been documented [1, 5]. Unlike unilateral facet dislocations, the predominant deforming force in these cases is flexion and distraction without rotation. This difference represents an important consideration during the application of distraction pins for anterior reduction.

13.3 Surgical Technique

Attention to details during the perioperative period improves the chances of achieving successful anterior reduction of facet dislocations. I prefer using Gardner-

Wells tong to apply traction during surgery, though a Mayfield head holder can be used as long as traction can still be applied. The pins should be placed below the equator of the skull (1 cm superior to the pinna of the outer ear and approximately 2 cm posterior to the external auditory meatus) in order to apply a flexion moment on the cervical spine to dislodge overlapping articular processes (Fig. 13.1) [14]. A radiolucent Stryker frame or a Jackson frame is ideal for this procedure because the patient could be turned to a prone position without having to be moved from the surgical table in case of failed anterior reduction. C-arm imaging is helpful to prevent overdistraction. Prereduction image should be thoroughly scrutinized to understand the pathological landmarks prior to attempting reduction. Somatosensory and motor evoked potential should be routinely used to monitor neurological status prior to and after reduction. The injured patient is placed in a routine position for an anterior cervical discectomy and fusion. Shoulder taping and/or kerlix straps on the wrists are helpful in imaging the lower part of the subaxial spine. Shoulder rolls should be avoided as it hyperextends the cervical spine and blocks reduction. Intraoperative findings and reduction maneuvers are different between unilateral and bilateral facet dislocations.

13.4 Unilateral Facet Dislocation

The anterior approach as described by Smith and Robinson is utilized. The injury level has a unique appearance. The superior vertebra is rotated anteriorly relative to the inferior vertebra on the side of facet dislocation producing mild cervical scoliosis (Fig. 13.2). The injured disc typically exhibits asymmetrical collapse to the nondislocated side (Fig. 13.3). The anterior longitudinal ligament typically remains intact, and the posterior longitudinal ligament is partially disrupted. Standard discectomy with removal of the posterior longitudinal ligament and evacuation of herniated disc material is performed. Make sure the posterior aspect of the vertebral bodies is swept with a nerve hook or similar device to remove any sequestered disc fragments. After the canal is free of herniated disc material, a small towel roll is placed underneath the head to flex the neck and unlock the dislocated facets. Although Cloward intervertebral spreaders have been described in decompression and reduction, I prefer the Caspar pin distractors [3]. These pins should be

Fig. 13.1 Strategic applications of Gardner-Wells tong. (**a**) Posterior application of the pins produces a flexion moment of the head. (**b**) Normal placement of the pins generates neutral axial traction of the head

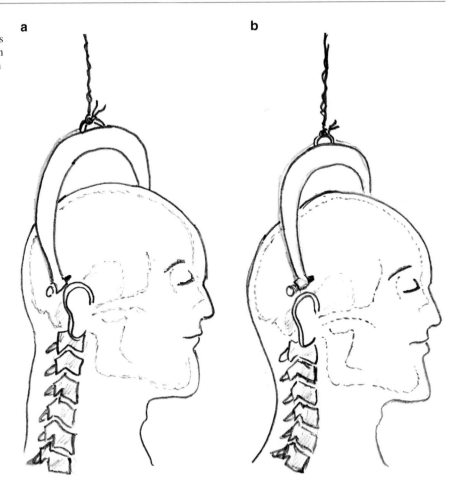

placed off the midline and more toward the dislocated side (Fig. 13.4). This asymmetrical pin placement effectively applies greatly distraction on the injured side while hinging on the normal side. Additional traction may be needed in the Gardner-Wells tongs or Mayfield at this time to assist reduction. Also, if needed, the Caspar distractor can be removed to allow manipulation of the pins to better effect the reduction. After the articular processes are perched and visible with the C-arm imaging, posterior force is applied to the superior pin reversing the deforming rotational force and reducing the injured facet joint. Distraction force is removed after C-arm imaging confirms successful reduction. At this point, the roll underneath the head should be removed, and if necessary, a roll should be placed between the shoulders to place the neck in extension for the purpose of fusion. Choice of graft and cervical plates is the preference of the surgeon; I have enjoyed success with cortical allograft spacers and fixed-angle cervical plates. Dynamic plates are not indicated in situations with posterior element instability.

13.4.1 Bilateral Facet Dislocation

In a bilateral facet dislocation, the entire superior vertebra protrudes anterior to the inferior vertebra. The injured disc exhibits symmetrical collapse. The anterior longitudinal ligament typically remains intact, but the posterior longitudinal ligament is partially or completely disrupted. After adequate decompression, the pins are placed in the middle of the vertebra, and the neck is then placed in slight flexion. I prefer using the Cloward intervertebral spreader to gain distraction to unlock the articular processes in these cases. Cotler et al. have described a technique where the head is rotated from side to side while under traction to achieve closed reduction [4]. Applying modified Cotler's technique to open reduction, the upper pin is rotated slowly, 30–40° beyond the midline, then toward the midline, and then 30–40° from the midline in the opposite direction reducing both facet joints. Distraction force is removed after C-arm imaging

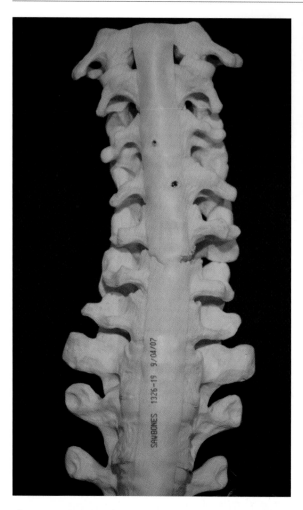

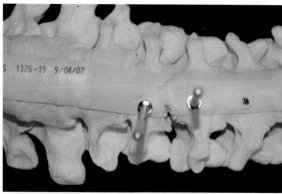

Fig. 13.4 Asymmetrical application of Caspar pins toward the dislocated side improves the chance of achieving reduction

confirms anatomic reduction, and neck extension is restored prior to fusion. Because of the extensive destruction of ligamentous structures in bilateral facet dislocation, one can overdistract the disc space during fusion. Thus it is important to measure the height of the adjacent uninjured disc on plain radiographs during graft selection. Also, monitoring the facets for excessive gap can also decrease overdistraction.

13.4.2 Irreducible Reduction

When anterior reduction efforts have failed, Howard An has described a technique where a graft is placed in the disc space, and the patient is then turned to a prone position for posterior reduction and fusion [2]. Occasionally, the graft is displaced during posterior reduction, and a return to the anterior position is necessary to reposition the graft, often referred to as a 540 degrees fusion [2]. A plate applied in the buttress fashion can help avoid such dislodgement. In a few cases, I have found that when placing a graft anteriorly, the segment stiffens making posterior reduction difficult. Currently, I prefer leaving the decompressed disc empty and proceeding to posterior reduction. After successful posterior reduction and fusion, anterior grafting is performed, and the anterior fusion is supplemented with a cervical plate.

Fig. 13.2 In unilateral facet dislocation, the superior vertebra is rotated anteriorly to the inferior vertebra on the side of facet dislocation producing mild cervical scoliosis

13.5 Postoperative Considerations

Postoperative bracing with hard cervical orthosis should be considered in these patients. I routinely brace my patients in a Miami J or an Aspen collar for

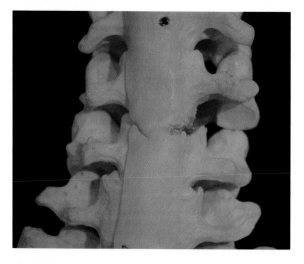

Fig. 13.3 In unilateral facet dislocation, the injured disc asymmetrically collapses to the non-dislocated side

3 months. Frequent office visits in the early follow-up period (the first 3 weeks after the operation) are necessary to detect potential loss of reduction. The patients are allowed to drive when surgical pain has subsided (typically 3 weeks after the operation). They are allowed to participate in nonlifting gym programs, and they may return to noncontact sports after 4 months. Participation in contact sports is resumed after successful radiographic fusion is ascertained. Although I have not experienced any loss of reduction, posterior cervical fusion with instrumentation is the procedure of choice for this complication.

13.5.1 Pitfalls

- Inadequate imaging, especially for lower cervicals. Use Kerlix on wrists for nurse to pull the arms.
- Positioning does not allow flexion and later extension of neck.
- Osteoporotic bone – may need to use two pins per level.

13.5.2 Pearls

- Use a combination of traction, pin manipulation, and intervertebral distraction to reduce in difficult cases.
- Add weight to the Mayfield or Gardner-Wells early in the case for ligamentous relaxation.
- Can add more weight at the time of reduction.

13.5.3 Complications

- Overdistraction.
- Insufficient facet overlap leading to insufficient resistance to shear force and subsequent listhesis.

13.5.5 Occult body fracture

- Be prepared to do corpectomy if needed.

References

1. Abitbol JJ, Kostuik JP (1998) Flexion injuries to the lower cervical spine. In: Clark CR (ed) The cervical spine, 3rd edn. Lippincott-Raven, Philadelphia
2. An H (1998) Cervical spine trauma. J Spine 23:2713–2729
3. Boyce RH, Hilibrand AS (2003) Operative techniques: anterior cervical decompression and fusion. In: Vaccaro AR (ed) Fractures of the cervical, thoracic and lumbar spine. Marcel Dekker, New York, pp 335–346
4. Cotler HB, Cotler JM, Davne SH et al (1987) Closed reduction of cervical dislocations. J Clin Orthoped 214:185–199
5. Doran SE, Ducker TB, Papadopoulos SM (1993) Magnetic resonance imaging documentation of coexistent traumatic locked facets of the cervical spine and disk herniation. J Neurosurg 79:341–345
6. Eismont FJ, Arena MJ, Green BA (1991) Extrusion of an intervertebral disc associated with traumatic subluxations or dislocation of the cervical facets; case report. J Bone Joint Surg (Am) 73:1555–1560
7. Hadley MN, Fitzpatrick BC, Sonntag VKH et al (1992) Facet fracture-dislocation injuries of the cervical spine. J Neurosurgery 30:661–666
8. Harrington JF, Likavec MJ, Smith AS (1991) Disc herniation in cervical fracture subluxations. J Neurosurgery 29:374–379
9. Le AX, Delamarter RB (2003) Classification of cervical spine trauma. In: Vaccaro AR (ed) Fractures of the cervical, thoracic and lumbar spine. Marcel Dekker, New York, pp 103–115
10. Levine AM (1992) Facet injuries in the cervical spine. In: Camins MB, O'Leary PF (eds) Disorders of the cervical spine. Williams & Wilkins, Baltimore, pp 289–302
11. Mahale YJ, Silver JR (1993) Neurological complications of the reduction of the cervical dislocations. J Bone Joint Surg (Br) 75:403–409
12. Pakzaban P (2008) Spinal instability and spinal fusion surgery. Emedicine, WebMD http://www.webmd.com
13. Savas PE (2003) Biomechanics of the injured cervical spine. In: Vaccaro AR (ed) Fractures of the cervical, thoracic and lumbar spine. Marcel Dekker, New York, pp 23–44
14. Spivak JM, Razi AE (2003) Cervical traction and reduction techniques. In: Vaccaro AR (ed) Fractures of the cervical, thoracic and lumbar spine. Marcel Dekker, New York, pp 263–277
15. Vaccaro AR, Flaatyn SP, Flanders AE et al (1999) Magnetic resonance evaluation of the intervertebral disc, spinal ligaments, and spinal cord before and after closed traction reduction of cervical spine dislocations. J Spine 24(12): 1210–1217

Anterior Cervical Discectomy and Fusion for Traumatic Disc Herniation

14

Ben B. Pradhan

14.1 Case Example

A 54-year-old right-hand dominant lady presented to the emergency room after being rear-ended in a motor vehicle accident. Her only complaints were in the neck and right arm. She had severe neck pain that radiated down the back of her right arm. She had dense numbness in the right C7 distribution and also had marked weakness in the right triceps. The biceps, triceps, and brachioradialis reflexes were all hyperactive on both sides. Hoffman's sign was positive in both hands. Her plain radiographs of the cervical spine, including best-effort flexion-extension views, revealed no fractures or instability. However, there was a degenerated disc space at C6–7 with bony osteophyte formation both anteriorly and posteriorly into the canal (Fig. 14.1). A computed tomography scan without contrast in the emergency room revealed the same, but with indications of a disc herniation into the canal as well. An MRI was ordered to get a better view of the spinal canal (Figs. 14.2 and 14.3). This showed a very large disc herniation at C6–7, right-sided, causing central canal stenosis in addition to foraminal stenosis.

She was placed on intravenous steroids for 24 h, but serial exams did not show any improvement in numbness or weakness. The pain remained quite severe as well, and the patient felt that she was not getting any better and, in fact, subjectively felt she may have been worsening. She was offered the surgical treatment of anterior cervical discectomy and fusion (ACDF), and after considering

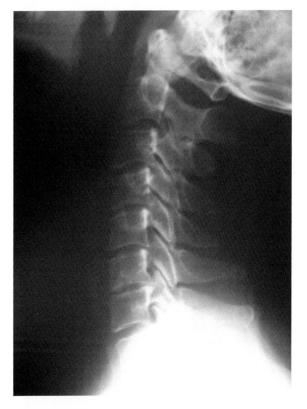

Fig. 14.1 Preoperative lateral radiograph demonstrating a small bony spur formation and disc height loss at C6–7

the risks and benefits or surgery vs. nonoperative management, she wished to proceed with the surgery.

A postoperative X-ray after C6–7 ACDF is shown in Fig. 14.4. The patient felt immediate relief of arm pain after the surgery. Her arm felt stronger and her sensation improved, but neither was completely normal when she was discharged from the hospital one day later. Over the next few months, however, her strength and sensation were effectively within normal limits.

B.B. Pradhan
Spine Surgeon, Director of Research, RISSER Orthopaedic Group, 2627 E Washington Boulevard,
Pasadena, CA 91107, USA
e-mail: benpradhan@yahoo.com

V.V. Patel et al. (eds.), *Spine Trauma*,
DOI: 10.1007/978-3-642-03694-1_14, © Springer-Verlag Berlin Heidelberg 2010

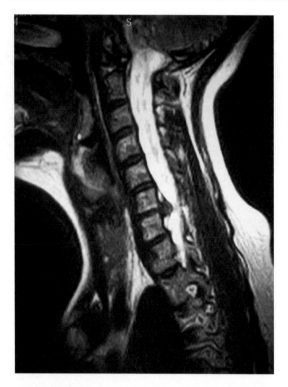

Fig. 14.2 Preoperative sagittal MRI showing C6–7 disc degeneration and a large herniation

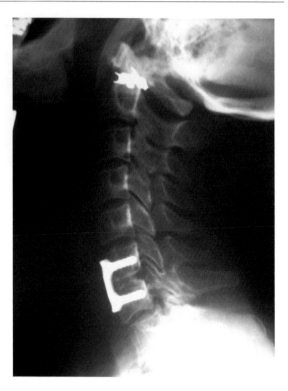

Fig. 14.4 Postoperative lateral radiograph showing C6 and C7 fusion with anterior cervical plate and screws

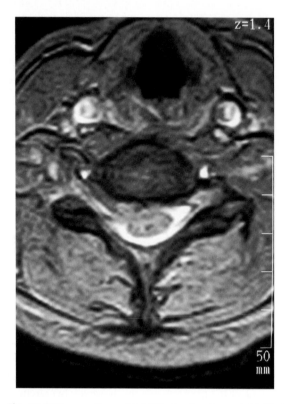

Fig. 14.3 Preoperative axial MRI showing large right-sided disc herniation at C6–7

14.2 Background

Unless there is a problem of the neural tissue itself (e.g., spinal cord or nerve tumor), spinal surgery really essentially means surgery on the tissues surrounding neural tissues. Rarely is surgery performed on the nerves. Rather, surgery involves the surrounding protective and structural tissues that have become damaged or dysfunctional. There are basically only two things that spinal surgery seeks to achieve: decompression and/or stabilization. All spinal surgeries have one or both of these purposes. Decompression means removing any tissue that is mechanically compressing the neural tissues, since, after all, the only tissues in the spine that are indispensable are the nerves themselves. Stabilization used to mean fusion only, but nowadays, a veritable plethora of nonfusion stabilizing options are available. For the purposes of this chapter, we will focus on decompression and stabilization with fusion for cervical spine traumatic injuries, using an anterior approach: specifically anterior cervical discectomy and fusion.

Cervical spine trauma is common in the adult population, in large part due to the high prevalence of pre-existing degenerative disc disease and neck stiffness, and has a number of different presentations. Cervical spine injury may present as purely axial neck pain, neck stiffness, or headaches. In cases of instability or compromise of the neural spaces, radicular symptoms in the upper extremities may be present. If the instability or spatial compromise is severe enough, myelopathy or upper motor neuron signs may be present.

14.3 Indications and Advantages

Spinal surgery may be indicated for patients with intractable or disabling pain, progressive neurologic deficits, dense neurologic deficits even if not progressive, myelopathy, instability that is likely not going to improve or may worsen, tumor or infection (especially if in the epidural space), and possibly lesser indications based on the patient's lifestyle and activity needs. ACDF in the trauma setting is indicated for disc herniations with neurologic compromise. Anterior cervical discectomy and fusion (ACDF) is a very effective and logical method of decompressing the spinal canal from any lesion that exists in front of the cervical spinal cord, as it is impossible to get to this from a posterior approach (the cervical spinal cord cannot be retracted safely). The lesion may be a herniated disc, a fracture fragment, tumor, infection, or hematoma. ACDF is also a very effective way of stabilizing the spine, since it stabilizes the anterior column, and most of the axial loading of the spine goes through this column (vertebra-disc-vertebra complex). Since a large intervertebral graft can be placed between the vertebrae, flexion stability is immediately achieved. Since a plate and screws can be placed in the front, extension stability is also imparted. So in fact, ACDF can be used to stabilize the spine for instability due to some posterior element dysfunction as well (e.g., some facet joint fractures or dislocations).

In addition to providing direct access to the anterior column, the ACDF technique has other advantages. Postoperative neck pain and rehabilitation in general are less after anterior surgery vs. posterior surgery because no muscle dissection is involved [1]. Sagittal alignment is easier to recreate and maintain through the customization of intervertebral graft height. Fusion is also biologically less challenging because of the large surface areas of contact between the graft and native bone. The graft remains in compression during the healing process, which is conducive for fusion.

14.4 Contraindications and Disadvantages

Pathology posterior to the spinal cord needs to be decompressed through a posterior approach since the cervical spinal cord cannot be retracted safely. So the approach is determined by where the lesion that needs to be decompressed lies in relation to the spinal cord.

Also locked, jumped facets that cannot be reduced (e.g., old fracture dislocations) may require a posterior or posterior and anterior approach. Cases of severe instability (e.g., complete fracture dislocation of bilateral facets) should also be considered for a combined approach due to the relative weakness of ACDF in resisting shear forces.

Other absolute and relative contraindications for an anterior approach would be the presence of other comorbidities, such as an active neck infection, a tracheostomy that is dirty and would be in the way, morbid obesity, etc. While there are no unique disadvantages specific to an ACDF procedure, there are several approach-related complications that will obviously be different from a posterior approach. These would involve breathing, swallowing, and vocal cord issues, which are discussed in the potential complications section further in this chapter.

14.5 Procedure

14.5.1 Equipment Needed

A basic cervical discectomy tray is required, along with the intervertebral graft and anterior spinal plate or fixation system of your choice. A fluoroscopy-compatible operating table for intraoperative X-rays is used as needed. Usually, reversing the head–foot orientation of a regular operating table is sufficient to allow a C-arm machine to take anteroposterior and lateral images. A head halter traction device with 10–20 lbs of weight for traction is used for holding the head looking straight ahead. For more controlled distraction during discectomy and graft placement, a Caspar pin distractor set is utilized. A microscope is a great advantage for

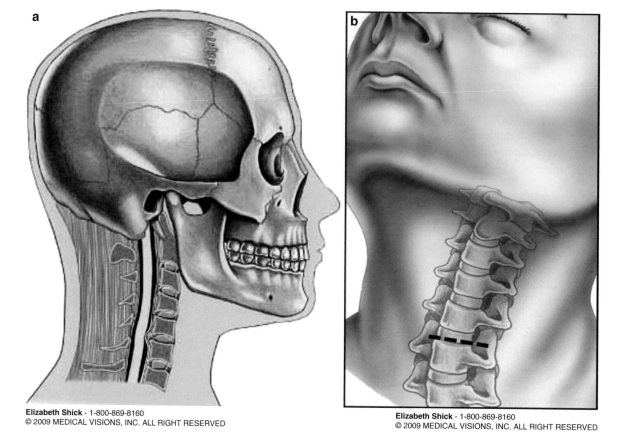

Fig. 14.5 (**a, b**) Schematics showing the positions of the discs with respect to the jaw, and how neck extension allows easier access to them. For 1–3 level discectomies, a transverse incision is sufficient. For more levels, an extensile vertical incision is better

visualization and detail work. In addition to curettes and Kerrison Rongeurs, a high-speed drill is used for uncovertebral bone removal, partial corpectomies, foraminotomies, and osteophyte decompression.

A small bump (can be a roll of linen) can be placed between the base of the neck and the scapulae to place the neck in some extension and to additionally stabilize the spine. The extension helps during the approach, disc excision, placement of the structural graft, and to recreate or maintain physiologic cervical lordosis, since a fusion is being performed and this position will be locked (Fig. 14.5a, b).

14.5.2 Anesthetic and Neuromonitoring Considerations

General anesthesia is necessary for this surgery. The details can be discussed between the patient and the anesthesiologist. Intraoperative neuromonitoring may be used for additional security. The neuromonitoring technologist, the surgeon, and the anesthesiologist should discuss the details of what is being monitored, and how the anesthesia should accommodate for that (e.g., whether full muscle relaxation is needed or not).

Because during intubation and surgery the neck will be placed in extension, it is important to have checked preoperatively how much extension is comfortable for the patient. It may also be valuable to run a baseline neuromonitoring scan before intubation and positioning, to ensure that there is no subsequent neurologic compromise. A fiberoptic intubation may be necessary if the patient cannot comfortably move the neck, or if there is risk of structural or neurologic compromise by moving the neck.

If the surgeon prefers, anesthesia can help apply variable amounts of traction during the surgery by pulling on a head halter traction device that can be applied

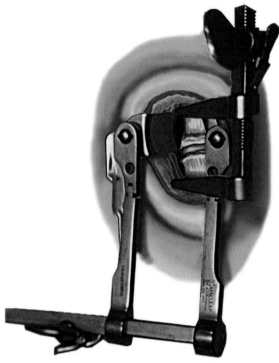

Fig. 14.6 Placement of retractors and distraction pins once the exposure is complete

to the patient preoperatively. I prefer to do this with Caspar pin distractors on the vertebrae inside the surgical field itself (Fig. 14.6). In addition, gentle skin traction is applied with wide tape on the shoulders pulling toward the foot of the bed. This makes it easier to view the inferior cervical vertebrae on intraoperative radiographs. Alternatively, some surgeons prefer assistants pull down on the arms of the patient during radiographs, in which case Kerlix rolls can be loosely attached to the wrists for traction from the foot end of the bed.

14.5.3 Surgical Approach, Pearls, and Pitfalls

Either a left or right-sided anterior approach to the cervical spine is performed. The recurrent laryngeal nerve is indirectly avoided with a left-sided approach, whereas with a right-sided approach, because it is visible, it can be isolated and consciously avoided. Otherwise, the approach is identical. If a previous anterior cervical

surgery has been performed, the other side can be used for an easier approach through virgin tissue planes, unless the recurrent laryngeal nerve was injured during the last approach, in which case the same side should be used to preserve the contralateral nerve and avoid complete vocal cord paralysis. Previous recurrent laryngeal nerve damage can be diagnosed by a history of increased hoarseness, or if any doubt, through a laryngoscopy.

The anterior neck is then prepped and draped with care taken not to restrict the surgical field. The level of the skin incision is determined by palpating the bony landmarks or, alternatively, by using a radio-opaque skin marker and a lateral radiograph. The inclination or angle of the disc space targeted should be taken into account when making the skin incision.

A transverse incision is then made through the skin (Fig. 14.5b) and subcutaneous fat and bleeding is controlled using electrocautery. The platysma muscle is carefully cut in line with the incision to avoid cutting the large superficial veins just beneath it. Beneath the platysma muscle, the deep cervical fascia is identified and divided laterally to the anterior of the sternocleidomastoid muscle where it is dissected inferiorly and superiorly off the muscle belly. A finger is then used for blunt dissection between the carotid sheath laterally and the trachea and esophagus medially down to the prevertebral fascia. A hand-held Cloward retractor is used to retract the midline structures allowing direct visualization of prevertebral fascia and underlying longus colli muscles and disc spaces. When a disc space is identified, a short needle is inserted into the disc space and a radiograph is obtained to confirm that the appropriate level has been approached.

When the appropriate level is confirmed, the longus colli muscles are dissected off the spine laterally and a self-retaining retractor is placed exposing the disc space to the uncovertebral joints. The operating microscope, sterilely draped, is then brought into the field. Under direct visualization using the microscope, the disc is incised with a scalpel and the anterior portion is removed using a pituitary forceps and an angled curette (Fig. 14.7). A high-speed drill may be used to complete the discectomy, along with partial removal of the vertebrae to expose bleeding subchondral bone (Fig. 14.8). This will help remove posterior osteophytes or fracture fragments that are overhanging into the canal and better expose the posterior longitudinal ligament (PLL).

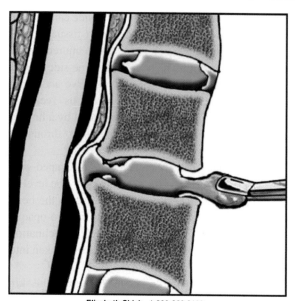

Fig. 14.7 Initial removal of disc fragments with a pituitary

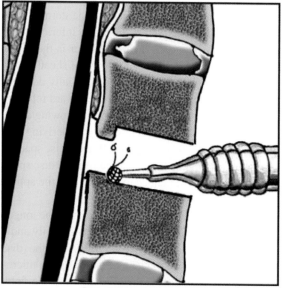

Fig. 14.8 Removal of end plate cartilage with a high-speed bur

After exposure, the PLL is elevated off of the posterior aspect of the vertebral bodies using a small 4–0 forward-angled curette and is then excised using 1 and 2 mm Kerrison Rongeurs. The PLL does not require routine removal if nuclear protrusion or extrusion through it is not present, but this has to be carefully

explored. If there is a dural leak along with a fracture, it may be necessary to remove the PLL as well to try and remove any bony fragments from the canal. The posterior aspect of the uncinate process can be excised using the 3–0 curette followed by the 1 and 2 mm Kerrison Rongeurs. The foramina can be probed with the 90° angled nerve hook to confirm adequate decompression or any remaining loose disc fragments. A high-speed burr can be used to remove osteophytes or other bony canal compromise, as well as for end plate preparation.

14.5.4 Reduction Technique

After the discectomy, removal of posterior uncinate process, and possible removal of the PLL, the segment should be mobile enough to reduce if necessary. Some additional traction, whether through a Caspar pin distractor, laminar spreader, or by head halter traction or tongs, may be needed, along with some flexion/extension maneuvering by moving the table at the hinge near the base of the neck. All these need to be done with careful neuromonitoring. Caspar pins can also be manipulated independent of the distractor as needed to facilitate reduction.

14.5.5 Fixation Technique

Single level cervical spine problems are most commonly treated with ACDF. For two or more adjacent levels, some surgeons choose to perform a corpectomy of the intervening vertebral bodies instead of multi-level ACDF. After the disc is removed, graft choices include harvested iliac crest bone graft or allograft, usually a fibular ring or strut. Synthetic interbody devices are also available, along with bone graft alternatives such as demineralized bone matrix. Currently, most surgeons will instrument with an anterior cervical plate fixed to the adjacent vertebral bodies to prevent graft displacement anteriorly and to provide stability while the fusion matures.

When the discectomy and foraminotomies are complete, the disc space is measured and an appropriately sized graft is chosen. Care should be taken to choose a graft that does not overdistract the disc space. The trials should have a similar height as the adjacent normal

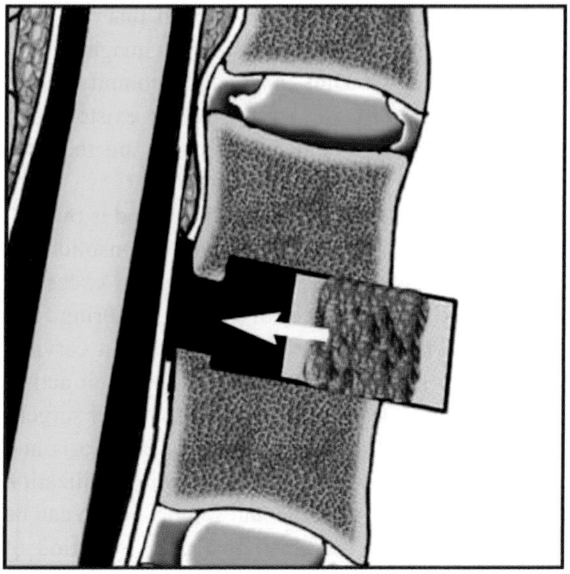

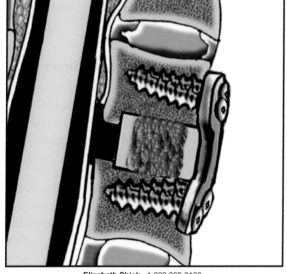

Fig. 14.9 Placement of interbody graft once discectomy and end plate removal are complete

Fig. 14.10 Completion of surgical construct with the placement of spanning anterior cervical plate and screws

disc spaces and the facet joints should be examined for continued apposition. Otherwise, overdistraction can reduce the shear resistance of the facet joints. For placement, increased traction is applied on the halter traction device or the Caspar pin distracters, and the graft is gently impacted into position (Fig. 14.9). When it is adequately positioned, all traction is removed. An appropriate-sized plate is then chosen and applied on the anterior aspect of the cervical spine. The plate should not be so long that it extends beyond the mid-vertebral point toward the adjacent disc space, as this increases the risk of adjacent segment breakdown, or as also known by, adjacent level ossification disease. Care is taken while drilling screw holes to choose a length that will be contained in the vertebral body. When the plate is in position, a lateral radiograph is obtained and graft and hardware positioning is checked (Fig. 14.10).

by performing blunt dissection down to the spine [2]. If any injury is detected to these structures, it is important to get an immediate otolaryngology or vascular surgery consultation in the operating room. During discectomy, injury to the vertebral arteries is largely avoided by not traveling beyond the uncovertebral joints laterally, and preoperative imaging should be carefully evaluated for an aberrant path into the disc space. If a vertebral artery is injured, it should be packed off and the other side should be left alone to preserve collateral flow. A vascular surgery consultation may be obtained.

If a dural tear occurs, a direct repair with sutures may be attempted though it can be very difficult. A watertight seal may be attained with a Duragen patch and fibrin glue. A fat graft or a fascial graft may also be used if the tear is amenable and the exposure is sufficient. If a dural tear occurs, the patient will have to be restricted to a head-elevated position for a day or two after surgery to avoid increased hydrostatic pressure at the tear site.

14.5.6 Potential Intraoperative Complications

Damage to nearby soft tissue structures such as the esophagus, trachea, and carotid sheath is largely avoided

14.6 Pearls

- Get prepositioning *baseline signals* on neuromonitoring.
- Do not overdistract the disc space.

- Use combinations of traction, Caspar distraction, laminar spreader, etc. for reduction as needed.

14.7 Postoperative Considerations

After instrumentation is complete, the wound is copiously irrigated and thoroughly checked for hemostasis. Often a drain is used even if the wound appears very dry because a postoperative hematoma may cause significant morbidity. The platysma muscle and subcutaneous tissue are then closed with interrupted absorbable sutures. This may be followed by a running layer of subcuticular suture, or steri-strips alone may be applied followed by a sterile dressing. The patient is then placed into a rigid cervical orthosis such as an Aspen collar prior to moving or extubation.

In the immediate postoperative period, the head of the patient's bed is maintained in an elevated position to decrease swelling in the neck. The patient should be able to walk, void, swallow liquids, and tolerate a diet before discharge. Most patients are discharged a day or two after surgery. Patients commonly complain of sore throat and pain with swallowing in the first few days after surgery. If these complaints seem more severe than usual, a single dose or short course of oral corticosteroids may be given in an attempt to minimize swelling.

Patients with radicular symptoms will often note immediate relief of symptoms after surgery. Most patients report a change in the quality of their axial neck pain to one more typical of postoperative pain. Generally, patients treated for radicular symptoms achieve greater than 90% satisfactory results, whereas those treated for axial neck pain generally achieve about 80% satisfactory results [3, 4]. Occasionally, the postoperative course may be complicated by a nerve root palsy (often the C5 nerve root). If this occurs, a short course of steroids may be tried. An imaging study may be needed to ensure no structural compromise of the root. If no structural compromise exists, often occupational therapy and rehabilitation are the only treatment options for such nerve palsies.

One concern in the postoperative period is overactivity before fusion is achieved. Stable consolidation of fusion often requires 6–12 weeks, so excessive motion and loading are discouraged during this period. Often patients are maintained in a cervical collar for 6–12 weeks in order to restrict their activities, but patients frequently recover from their surgery much sooner and desire to remove the orthosis and resume activities. Months of relative immobilization can result in significant deconditioning, which can be a challenge to the therapist. In the early period of return to activity and therapy, it is important to avoid injury due to overly strenuous exercises or an overzealous patient.

References

1. Carreon L, Glassman SD, Campbell MJ (2006) Treatment of anterior cervical pseudoarthrosis: posterior fusion versus anterior revision. Spine J 6(2):154–156
2. Fountas KN, Kapsalaki EZ, Nikolakakos LG et al (2007) Anterior cervical discectomy and fusion associated complications. Spine 32(21):2310–2317
3. Garvery TA, Transfeldt EE, Malcolm JR et al (2002) Outcome of anterior cervical disectomy and fusion as perceived by patients treated for dominant axial-mechanical cervical spine pain. Spine 27:1887–1894
4. Sidhu K, Herkowitz H (1999) Surgical management of cervical disc disease: surgical management of cervical radiculopathy. In: Herkowitz H et al (eds) The spine. W.B. Saunders, Philadelphia

Posterior Cervical Fusion for Trauma

15

F. Cumhur Oner

15.1 Case Example

This 70-year-old lady fell from stairs and presented with an incomplete SCI at the level of C6 with MRC 3 in upper and lower extremities. CT and MR images showed a fracture-subluxation at the level of C6–C7 with facet fracture on one side and dislocation on the other (Fig. 15.1). CT images showed that the low cervical and cervicothoracic junction were ankylotic. We decided to operate on this patient immediately because of her neurologic injury. No attempt was made to reduce the fracture by traction.

15.2 Background

In many types of traumatic subaxial spine injuries, there is substantial damage to the posterior elements such as the posterior ligamentous complex (PLC) and facet joints. Traditionally, most of these injuries have been stabilized by anterior surgical techniques largely due to the acquaintance of the surgeons with these procedures and lack of sufficient surgical techniques for rigid posterior fixation. Development of easy and reliable fixation techniques utilizing the lateral mass screws has largely changed the surgical care of these patients [1, 3, 7, 9].

15.3 Indications and Advantages of Technique

Posterior open reduction and fixation techniques allow the surgeon to directly reduce the facet joints, decompress the canal, and achieve rigid fixation. Mechanical studies have shown that posterior instrumentation with lateral mass screws is superior to anterior fixation alone especially if the PLC and facet joints are injured [2, 5]. Complications associated with these techniques are low [4, 8]. One prospective randomized study showed comparable results for anterior and posterior surgical stabilization in unilateral facet joint injuries in the subaxial spine [6].

15.4 Contraindications and Disadvantages

This procedure does not allow anterior decompression of the spinal canal of the disc or fracture fragments. Posterior reduction also has a chance of pulling the disc material into the canal.

Finally, fractured facets/lateral masses may not provide adequate screw purchase necessitating either cervical pedicle screws or additional levels of fixation.

15.5 Procedure

Careful attention must be paid to head position and neck alignment while positioning, as this will be the final position once fused. Check these both visually and on fluoroscopy to maintain cervical lordosis. The patient is

F.C. Oner
University Medical Center Utrecht,
HP G 05.228, 85500, 3508 GA Utrecht,
The Netherlands
e-mail: f.c.oner@umcutrecht.nl

V.V. Patel et al. (eds.), *Spine Trauma*,
DOI: 10.1007/978-3-642-03694-1_15, © Springer-Verlag Berlin Heidelberg 2010

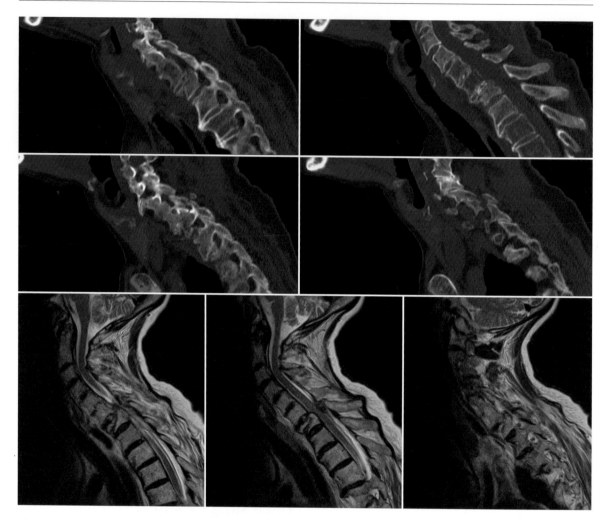

Fig. 15.1 Fracture-subluxation C6–C7. Note that the cervicothoracic junction is ankylotic. The facet joint is fractured on one side and the other side is dislocated and locked

positioned prone with her head attached to a Mayfield clamp (Fig. 15.2). Lateral fluoroscopy is used to determine the level. Pull on both arms to get a sufficient image of the lower C-spine. If this is not possible, the levels can also be determined on AP images based on the first rib.

Through a midline incision, the spine is exposed at the levels to be treated out to the lateral edge of the facet joints. Facet joint reduction can be performed as described in Chap. 9 (Fig. 15.3), and decompression can be performed as needed.

Lateral mass screws are strong and easy to insert at the levels of C3–C6. Once the lateral mass is fully exposed, it forms a square. The entry point for the screws has been described by various authors. We recommend

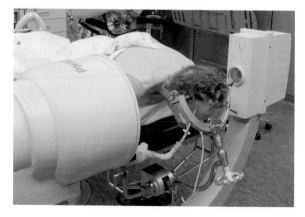

Fig. 15.2 Positioning of the patient with a Mayfield clamp

Fig. 15.3 To reduce a locked facet without distraction, remove the cranial part of the superior articular process of the caudal vertebra. This allows reduction by a simple translation force

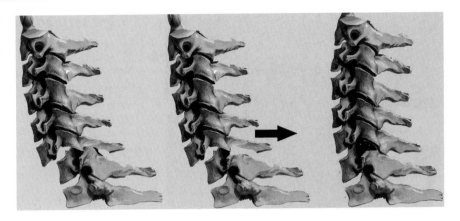

Fig. 15.4 Placement of lateral mass screws. The direction of the screw is parallel to the lamina on the transverse plane and parallel to the facet joints on the sagittal plane

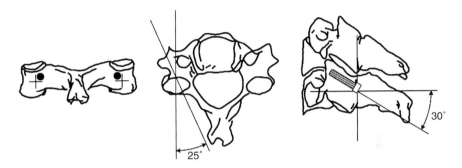

to start at about 2 mm. medial to the centre of the lateral mass and drill 30° cranial and 25° lateral; thus the drill shaft will typically touch the spinous process at the level below the one where the screw is to be placed. This actually means that the drill should be parallel to the lamina and the facet joint at the same time (Fig. 15.4). Screws with polyaxial heads can be used. The usual length is between 10 and 20 mm. In C7 the lateral mass may be thinner and shorter. In that case a pedicle screw can be inserted. When the lateral mass and pedicle screws are inserted at adjacent levels, the screw heads may lie too close to each other and jam. This should be anticipated. Choosing a slightly cranial entrance point for the lateral mass screw may be helpful. Otherwise, the anatomy may necessitate skipping a lateral mass screw at the level immediately above the level of pedicle screw insertion. In our case example, we chose to extend the construct to T1 because of the ankylosis of this area. The fractured lateral mass of C6 was skipped, and we were able to place lateral mass screws at C7 and pedicle screws at T1 (Fig. 15.5). After reduction, the screws are connected with the rods bent in the appropriate curvature. In this case with a partially ankylotic spine we used local bone from the laminectomy for fusion (Fig. 15.6). In younger

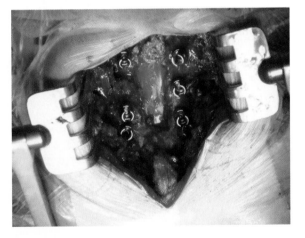

Fig. 15.5 Placement of the polyaxial screws. C5 and C7 bilateral lateral mass and T1 bilateral pedicle screws. The fractured left lateral mass of C6 was too weak to allow a screw. Here we used lateral mass screw on the other side. Note the proximity of the heads of the lateral mass C7 and pedicle T1 screws

patients we prefer iliac crest autograft to achieve reliable fusion. Post-op radiographs showed a good alignment of the spine (Fig. 15.7). Except for some paresthesia in her hands this patient recovered completely.

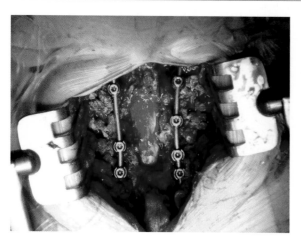

Fig. 15.6 Assembly of the rods and placement of bone graft lateral to the rods

15.5.1 Equipment needed

- Radiolucent bed with Mayfield attachment
- Traction device/method for reduction, if needed
- Lateral mass screw system
- Fluoroscopy
- Spinous process wiring system, if needed for backup
- Bone graft harvest tools or bone graft substitute
- High-speed drill for bone decortication/removal
- Neuromonitoring

15.5.2 Anesthetic considerations

- Neuromonitoring compatible anesthetic
- Fiberoptic intubation

15.5.3 Patient positioning

- Prone on Wilson frame or Jackson table
- Mayfield or other rigid head holder

15.5.4 Pearls

- Place a penfield or freer in the facet joint and use this to guide the drill trajectory parallel to the facet joint.
- Place the drill holes in lateral masses carefully as the vertebral artery can be injured.
- C7 lateral masses are typically small, check pre-op CT.
- If traumatic vertebral artery injury exists, do not attempt lateral mass screws in the contralateral side.

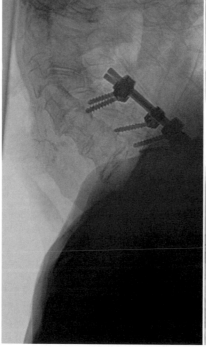
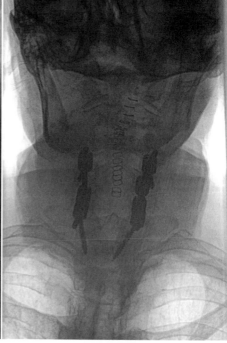

Fig. 15.7 Postoperative radiograms showing a good realignment of the spine

- Screw heads can impinge on each other, especially C7 and T1, space screw to avoid this.
- The spinous process of the lower adjacent level may need to be trimmed to allow the correct lateral angulation of the drill and screws.

15.5.5 Pitfalls

- Vertebral artery injury. In this case, place a screw quickly and do not place contralateral screws. Avoid vascular and IR involvement.
- Drill holes break out laterally. This is usually due to the drill "walking" when starting the hole at a steep angle. Avoid this by creating a starting a hole that is deep enough with a burr.
- Lateral mass fracture. May necessitate spinous process wires or adjacent level instrumentation.

15.5.6 Bailout

- Additional level fusion
- HALO

15.5.7 Bracing

- Cervical collar for 6 weeks

15.5.8 Complications

- Nonunion can be treated with revision posterior surgery or ACDF

References

1. Arnold PM, Bryniarski M, McMahon JK (2005) Posterior stabilization of subaxial cervical spine trauma: indications and techniques. Injury 36:S36–S43
2. Bozkus H, Ames CP, Chamberlain RH, Nottmeier EW, Sonntag VK, Papadopoulos SM, Crawford NR (2005) Biomechanical analysis of rigid stabilization techniques for three-column injury in the lower cervical spine. Spine 30(8):915–922
3. Deen HG, Birch BD, Wharen RE, Reimer R (2003) Lateral mass screw-rod fixation of the cervical spine: a prospective clinical series with 1-year follow-up. Spine J 3(6):489–495
4. Deen HG, Nottmeier EW, Reimer R (2006) Early complications of posterior rod-screw fixation of the cervical and upper thoracic spine. Neurosurgery 59(5):1062–1067
5. Duggal N, Chamberlain RH, Park SC, Sonntag VK, Dickman CA, Crawford NR (2005) Unilateral cervical facet dislocation: biomechanics of fixation. Spine 30(7):E164–E168
6. Kwon BK, Fisher CG, Boyd MC, Cobb J, Jebson H, Noonan V, Wing P, Dvorak MF (2007) A prospective randomized controlled trial of anterior compared with posterior stabilization for unilateral facet injuries of the cervical spine. J Neurosurg Spine 7(1):1–12
7. McCullen GM, Garfin SR (2000) Spine update: cervical spine internal fixation using screw and screw-plate constructs. Spine 25(5):643–652
8. Pateder DB, Carbone JJ (2006) Lateral mass screw fixation for cervical spine trauma: associated complications and efficacy in maintaining alignment. Spine J 6(1):40–43
9. Wu J, Huang W, Chen Y, Shih Y, Cheng H (2008) Stabilization of subaxial cervical spines by lateral mass screw fixation with modifived Magerl's technique. Surg Neurol 70(suppl 1)S1:25–33

Corpectomy for Burst Fracture

16

Harel Arzi and Paul M. Arnold

16.1 Case Example

While riding his motorcycle under the influence of alcohol and various narcotic drugs, a 45-year-old man ran into a fence without wearing a helmet. Upon arrival at the emergency room, he was hemodynamically stable. Complete assessment was compromised by the presence of alcohol in his system. He complained of cervical spine tenderness. He had multiple scalp and facial lacerations and abrasions. Further investigation revealed no intracranial, abdominal, or chest injury and no long bone fractures. The patient had decreased strength in the bilateral upper and lower extremities. He had 4/5 strength in the bilateral lower extremities, 4/5 strength in the right upper extremity, and 3/5 strength in his left upper extremity. The patient had decreased sensation in his bilateral lower extremities and decreased rectal tone.

CT of the cervical spine showed a compression fracture of C5 (Fig. 16.1). Compression fractures of T8–10 were diagnosed on chest CT. MRI of the cervical spine showed fracture of the vertebral body of C5 as well as significant injury to the posterior ligamentous complex and spinal cord compression (Fig. 16.2). The patient was subsequently taken to the operating room a day after admission, and underwent C5 vertebrectomy and fusion with autograft, metallic cage, and plate (Fig. 16.3). The patient tolerated the procedure well. He was mobilized while wearing a cervical collar and a TLSO and continued to be stable throughout the

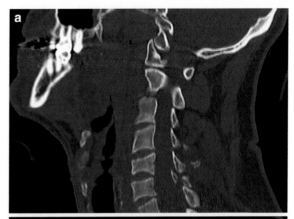

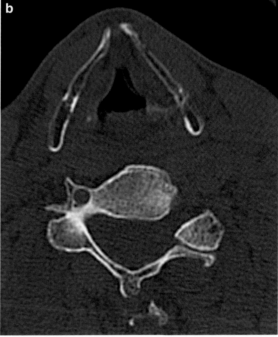

Fig. 16.1 (**a**, **b**) CT scan of the cervical spine showing compression fracture of the 5th cervical vertebral body with significant bony injury

P.M. Arnold (✉) and H. Arzi
Department of Neurosurgery, Mail Stop 3021,
3901 Rainbow Boulevard, Kansas City, KS 66160, USA
e-mail: parnold@kumc.edu

V.V. Patel et al. (eds.), *Spine Trauma*,
DOI: 10.1007/978-3-642-03694-1_16, © Springer-Verlag Berlin Heidelberg 2010

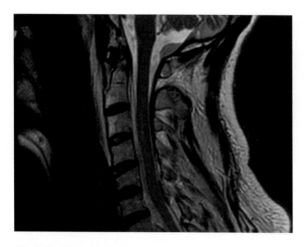

Fig. 16.2 T2-weighted MRI of the cervical spine showing burst fracture of the 5th cervical vertebra with significant posterior soft tissue injury

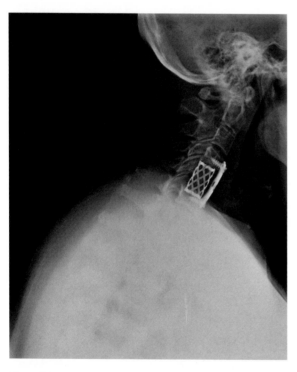

Fig. 16.3 Postoperative X-ray of the cervical spine showing reconstruction of C5 using metallic mesh cage and plate

remainder of his hospital stay. The patient regained near-normal motor activity in both upper and lower extremities as well as light touch and pain sensation, but was still complaining of some numbness around the affected extremities.

16.2 Background

Cervical burst fractures belong to the axial load and flexion-type spinal fractures, along with cervical tear drop fractures, as well as thoracic and lumbar burst and compression fractures. Burst fracture is a relatively common spinal injury, but the cervical spine is the least common site of injury [2]. The most frequent mechanism of injury is motor vehicle accident, followed by fall from height and sport-related injury, especially diving. The frequency of neurological injury in this type of fractures is greater than 50% [11]. As in other spine fractures, concomitant spinal injury at other levels as well as associated nonspinal injury should be thoroughly investigated and evaluated. According to White and Panjabi, burst fractures can meet the criteria for instability with either posterior injury or spinal cord injury [16]. Using the Magerl (AO) classification, burst fracture can be classified as type A or C depending on posterior element involvement [12]. It is important to distinguish between burst fractures and tear drop fractures. In the former, axial load causes fracture of both the anterior and posterior cortex of the vertebral body with the posterior bony fragment at risk for compromising the spinal canal, while in the latter, shearing forces cause fracture of only the anterior cortex and possible canal compromise as the result of retrolisthesis of the rest of the vertebral body [14].

16.3 Indications and Advantages for Procedure

Traditionally, cervical burst fractures were treated conservatively using traction or orthotics, but since the early 1960s, much knowledge about the surgical treatment of cervical spine fractures has accumulated [4]. The goals of surgical treatment for burst fracture are three-fold:

1. Decompression of the spinal cord.
2. Restoration of spinal stability and prevention of further cord injury.
3. Reconstruction of spinal alignment or prevention of future loss of alignment.

No consensus exists regarding the indications for surgical treatment of cervical burst fractures, but some points of agreement can be found. Anterior burst can be treated nonsurgically if there are no neurological deficits, no significant posterior injury, no significant local kyphosis, and no spinal canal compromise [6]. Nonsurgical treatment with a cervical collar or even traction can correct mild kyphosis and prevent further collapse. Posterior cervical spine fusion can restore spinal alignment and stabilize the spinal segment, and combined with laminectomy, can decompress the spinal canal, but does not allow for direct decompression of the anterior aspect of the spine from fractured bony fragments. Only anterior corpectomy can restore alignment, decompress the canal, and stabilize the segment all in one procedure. This can be achieved with favorable fusion rates and low morbidity [1, 5]. Some reports show that even patients with complete neurological injury can benefit from anterior decompression, with better chance for future neurological improvement [11].

16.4 Contraindications and Disadvantages for Procedure

There are no absolute contraindications to anterior cervical corpectomy. Some patients cannot be operated on because of other life-threatening injuries, head injuries, or hemodynamic instability. Relative contraindications include a stable fracture with no significant kyphosis, previous cervical surgery, previous recurrent laryngeal nerve (RLN) injury, and skin breakdown or infection at the anterior aspect of the neck. Disadvantages include a direct approach to the fracture site that can result in considerable bleeding and can turn a minimal, controlled traumatic dural tear into a major source of morbidity. Other disadvantages are the result of a surgical approach next to major vascular and neural structures of the neck. Injury of these structures is rare, but can lead to unfavorable results.

16.5 Procedure

16.5.1 Equipment Needed

A self-retaining blade retractor for anterior cervical approach is highly recommended. A high-speed burr is needed for the preparation of the disc spaces, removal of the fractured vertebra, and preparing drill holes for the plate screws. For reduction and maintenance of the

vertebral height throughout the procedure, Gardner-Wells tongs or an intraoperative device such as a Steinman pin-based distractor, Caspar distractor, or a laminar spreader can be used. Instruments for harvesting iliac crest bone graft such as osteotomes or chisels should be available if this option is to be used; otherwise, allograft or cages of adequate size range are required. Usually, there is enough bone available from the ventral decompression that harvesting of the iliac crest is not necessary. Anterior cervical plate as well as screws of different lengths and diameters should be accompanied by the drills and instruments needed for the internal fixation. Rigid rather than dynamic plates are indicated in these complex fractures with posterior element instability. X-ray or fluoroscopy is used to verify postreduction vertebral height and both coronal and sagittal axis, and later to verify proper placement of the bone graft and hardware.

16.5.2 Anesthetic and Neuromonitoring Considerations

Extension of the cervical spine should be avoided in all patients with unstable cervical spine injury. Despite the fact that burst fractures are flexion-type injuries, hyperextension can cause displacement of bony fragments, resulting in compression of the thecal sac [3]. A nonextension endotracheal intubation technique should be utilized, and fiber-optic intubation should be considered. Neuromonitoring can be useful in detecting spinal cord compromise as a result of positioning, reduction, or corpectomy, but meticulous technique during anesthesia, positioning, and surgery can lower the incidence of such complications.

16.5.3 Patient Positioning and Room Setup

The patient is positioned supine with the head resting on a soft round gel donut-type headrest or a horseshoe Mayfield headrest. If tongs are to be used, a proper traction device and weights should be readily available. Arms are tucked to the sides of the patient's body and secured with a sheet, a belt, wide adhesive tape, or all of the above. Mild extension can be achieved using a shoulder roll placed longitudinally under the thoracic spine and between the shoulder blades. Using an inflatable bag enables neck extension after removal of the bony fragments is completed. The patient's shoulders are pulled distally with tape to facilitate imaging of the caudal part of the cervical spine. Kerlix roll-type gauze can also be wrapped around the wrists for brief traction by the nurse during imaging as needed. Using long anesthesia tubing and wiring will allow the anesthesia unit to be taken further away from the patient's head and operative field and allow a wider workspace for the surgeon and assistant.

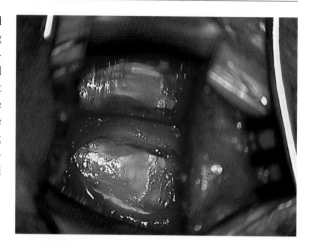

Fig. 16.5 Deep dissection showing the anterior aspect of the vertebral bodies covered by the anterior longitudinal ligament (ALL) and longus coli muscles

16.5.4 Surgical Approach

The anterior surgical approach to the cervical spine utilizes the plane between the sternocleidomastoid (SCM) muscle and the carotid sheath (CS) on the lateral side, and the strap muscles, trachea, and esophagus on the medial side. For a single level corpectomy, a transverse curved incision will permit sufficient exposure with the advantage of the possibility to follow a natural skin crease (Fig. 16.4). If a larger exposure is required, a longitudinal incision along the medial border of the SCM is selected. Radiography or fluoroscopy can be used to determine the location of the transverse skin incision. After undermining the subcutaneous tissue cranially and caudally, the platysma muscle is divided along its fibers. The plane between the SCM and the CS on the lateral side and the trachea and esophagus on the other side is identified and divided with palpation of the carotid pulse on the lateral side. This plane is

developed until the prevertebral fascia is encountered and dissected. At this point, the anterior aspect of the vertebra should be visible with the longus coli muscles on both sides and the anterior longitudinal ligament (ALL) to be used as an aid for marking of the midline (Fig. 16.5). The fractured vertebra should be easily identified and a radiograph or fluoroscopy can be used to confirm the correct level using a spinal needle inserted into the disc space. Once the level is verified, the coli muscles are stripped bilaterally so that the unco-vertebral joint can be identified. The retractor blades are secured beneath the coli muscle to prevent any excessive pressure on the esophagus or CS.

16.5.5 Reconstruction and Fixation Technique

Annulotomy and complete discectomy of the intervertebral discs on both sides of the affected vertebra is performed (Fig. 16.6). Special attention should be drawn towards the removal of all disc and cartilage from the end plates by careful curettage of the latter. To facilitate removal of disc material, axial traction can be applied using tongs. The discectomy and corpectomy should be limited laterally by the medial border of the unco-vertebral joint to prevent possible vertebral artery injury. Excision of the vertebral body is carried out first using a Lexell rongeur to obtain the bone graft to be used for fusion, followed by a high-speed burr for the removal of the posterior cortex. The

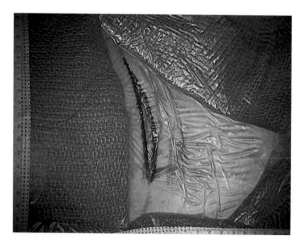

Fig. 16.4 Skin incision using a naturally occurring skin crease

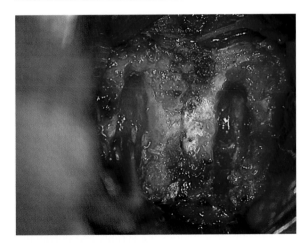

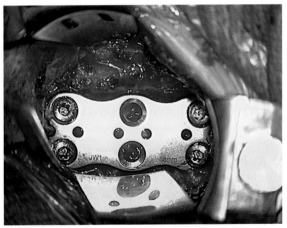

Fig. 16.6 Affected vertebral body after completion of cranial and caudal discectomies

Fig. 16.7 A metallic cage is inserted in the intervertebral space, and a metallic plate is used for fixation of the affected level

remainder of the cortex as well as the posterior longitudinal ligament (PLL) is removed using Kerrison rongeurs. Although complete removal of the PLL is not mandatory in this procedure, it serves to make sure that no bone or disc fragment is compressing the dura at this level. Once the corpectomy is completed, reconstruction of the spinal segment is performed. This can be done by using an iliac crest autograft, allograft, or a metallic cage packed with autograft taken from the excised vertebral body. An expandable cage can be used to assist in distraction in addition to providing anterior column support. Depth gage and a caliber can be used to determine the desired graft or cage diameter and length. The implant should be prepared to settle into the trough with gentle mallet tapping, allowing for solid setting of the implant against both end plates yet avoiding distraction injury to the cord or the nerve roots. When using the tongs, additional traction can be applied for the insertion of the implant. If using a Caspar distractor, this can also be adjusted as needed. X-rays should be taken at this point to ensure adequate alignment, especially lordosis. The anterior surface of the adjacent vertebra is prepared with the high-speed burr to accommodate the plate. A proper-sized plate is selected to allow for good screw purchase in the adjacent vertebral bodies, but with no protrusion into the next disc spaces (Fig. 16.7). X-ray is obtained to verify proper location of the implants as well as reduction and alignment (refer again to Fig. 16.3). Meticulous hemostasis is essential throughout the procedure as accumulation of hematomas can result in serious neurologic or airway compromise. The use of a vacuum drain is recommended for the same reason.

16.6 Technical Pearls and Pitfalls

16.6.1 Pearls

- Left- and right-sided approaches are both acceptable despite some reports of lower incidence of RLN injury when approaching from the left [9, 10].
- Application of tongs can cause local scalp bleeding, which is usually minor. Use of laminar disc space spreader can result in end plate fracture and Steinman pin distractor can damage adjacent vertebral body bone and interfere with the fixation of the anterior plate.
- For lower lesions (C5-T1) positioning in excessive lordosis should be avoided, and not using a shoulder roll should be considered.
- Crossing the midline and undermining the subcutaneous tissue enables wide exposure through a transverse incision.
- The surgeon should be aware of the higher bleeding tendency of the traumatized tissue and prepare hemostatic measures such as thrombin, gelfoam, and other commercially available products.
- Application of a self-retaining blade retractor can result in significant pressure across the tracheal wall. Deflation and reinflation of the endotracheal tube's cuff after application of the retractor can lower this pressure and decrease the rate of postoperative dysphagia.
- Sharp dissection of the plane between the carotid artery and esophagus is correlated with lower rates of esophageal injuries than is blunt dissection [7].

- Following the 16 mm rule for the width of the discectomy and corpectomy will allow for adequate decompression, fusion surface, and graft size while avoiding vascular and nerve root injury.
- Iliac crest bone graft can be associated with significant donor site morbidity [13].
- Infectious complications of properly treated allograft, including transmission of hepatitis and HIV, are extremely uncommon.
- All bone grafts should be carefully machined to fit into the trough; cage size selection should be based on end plate diameter as well as trough length and include the width of the cage end caps if in use.
- Posterior instrumentation should be considered in patients with posterior element disruption, especially if multilevel corpectomy is performed.
- Compared to titanium cages, PEEK cages cause smaller artifacts on postoperative MRI allowing for better evaluation of the spinal canal contents, but have smaller inner caliber for the insertion of bone graft.
- Creating a "posterior lip" at the adjacent end plates might prevent posterior slippage of the implant and possible nerve compression.
- Some bending of the anterior end plate can improve plate setting on the natural cervical lordosis.
- Application of traction during the procedure and extra traction during graft insertion can result in oversizing of the implant in cases with high degree of segmental instability. In such cases, the use of traction should be reconsidered for every step of the procedure. Monitor the facet joint gaps on fluoroscopy whenever possible to avoid this complication.
- Using fixed screws for plate fixation creates a rigid construct that might provide better short-term stability. Using variable angle screws enables load-sharing effect with possible better fusion rates.
- Screw trajectory should point 15–30° medial and parallel to the disc space or slightly divergent on the sagittal plane.

the bleeding, and prompt vascular surgery consultation obtained. Direct suture of the defect or endovascular catheterization and coil embolization of the artery are the two most common solutions to this potentially devastating complication.
- Vertebral artery: Minor lacerations may resolve with the application of local pressure and with the use of hemostatic agents or bone wax. Larger lacerations will necessitate packing and endovascular embolization, as direct repair is seldom feasible.
- Be aware that traumatic esophageal ruptures can be associated with these fractures.
- Esophageal injuries are serious and potentially lethal complications of this approach. Although rare, a high index of suspicion is the key to identification of such injury, and/or thoracic surgery. Consultation should be obtained prior to repair attempts.
- Dural tears: Dural tears can be a result of the primary trauma or can be iatrogenic, and are usually visualized when attempting to remove a compressing bone or disc fragment or dissecting the PLL. Small dural tears are best managed by direct suture, synthetic or muscle dural patch, a dura-sealing gel, or a combination of those options. Larger tears are usually traumatic and placement of a continuous lumbar CSF drain may be indicated.
- Poor screw purchase can result in the displacement of the plate creating unwanted pressure against adjacent structures. Drilling a new trajectory through the same plate hole can result in loss of cancellous bone beyond the size of the largest screw diameter. Other options are the use of larger diameter screws, longer screws if vertebral body dimensions permit, or non-self-drilling screws, which have more blunt and threaded tips with better purchase.

16.6.2 Potential Intraoperative Complications

- Damage to adjacent organs
  - Carotid artery: With significant carotid artery injury, direct pressure should be applied to stop

16.6.3 Bailout/Salvage for Procedure Failure

Bailout or salvage techniques may involve enlarging the procedure to add an adjacent level or performing a posterior fixation and fusion or posterior instrumentation.

16.7 Postoperative Considerations

16.7.1 Bracing

A rigid collar is recommended for a period of 4–12 weeks according to the level of instability and posterior injury. Removal of the collar is permitted for daily care and in the more stable cases while lying in bed.

16.7.2 Activity

Physical therapy for active and passive range of motion (ROM) of upper and lower extremities is recommended especially if neurological damage is present and the formation of joint contractures is to be prevented. Once removal of cervical collar is permitted, physical therapy should be targeted towards regaining passive and active ROM of the neck. Driving is prohibited until near-normal ROM is regained, otherwise automobile modification is necessary.

16.7.3 Follow-up

The first follow-up visit for the inspection of the surgical wound is within 2 weeks of discharge, followed by the first radiographic evaluation at 4 weeks. The next radiographic evaluations are at 3, 6, and 12 months. Early identification of nonunion or resultant deformity, usually kyphotic, enables early and possibly more simple and successful intervention.

16.7.4 Potential Postoperative Complications

16.7.4.1 Soft Tissue Hematoma

Soft tissue hematoma will usually manifest during the first hours after surgery and can present as progressive dysphagia or difficulty breathing, painful neck swelling, or neurological deterioration. Any case of rapidly evolving symptoms of the aforementioned type warrant emergent evacuation of the hematoma, which might even be done at the bedside in extreme conditions. Mild cases of painful swelling can be followed closely. Drain placement and meticulous hemostasis and preoperative identification of bleeding disorder or anticoagulant medication will help in preventing this devastating complication.

16.7.4.2 Dysphagia

Swallowing difficulties are one of the most common complaints after anterior cervical surgery. Symptoms include pain during swallowing, coughing, choking, regurgitation, or feeling of blocked throat. Most symptoms will resolve in a matter of days in the vast majority of patients. The minority of patients who have persistent dysphagia should be evaluated by a speech professional and put on an exercise and treatment plan. Rarely is a feeding tube necessary. Recovery rate approaches 100% with conservative treatment.

16.7.4.3 Recurrent Laryngeal Nerve (RLN) Injury

Prevalence of RLN injury is reported to be between 1.5–4%. Symptoms include new onset "wet" voice or hoarseness. Symptoms usually resolve within 12 weeks, but laryngoscopy is warranted for patients with prolonged symptoms of more than 2–4 weeks. Some patients will be asymptomatic despite unilateral RLN palsy. Patients with persisting preoperative hoarseness or previous cervical surgery should, whenever possible, have a documented ENT evaluation prior to surgery to avoid bilateral RLN injury and severe speech impairment; otherwise, it is best to use the same-sided surgical approach to avoid bilateral injury.

Arytenoid dislocation can be a cause of persistent hoarseness after trauma or crash intuition. This should be considered early in the postoperative period in patients with new vocal or swallowing difficulties.

16.7.4.4 Other Nerve Injuries

The superior laryngeal nerve and the 12th cranial nerve are at risk for injury, especially when approaching the upper cervical spine. Most of these injuries are traction injuries and will resolve with conservative treatment. Infrequent persistent paralysis might require exploration of nerve for possible repair. Horner's syndrome is a result of 10th cranial nerve traction in the CS and is usually transient. Malpositioning of the arms or over-traction upon the shoulder might cause brachial plexus injury. The best strategy of dealing with nerve injuries is prevention. Careful positioning of the patient, as well as handheld and self-retaining retractors will min-imize the occurrence of such injuries.

16.7.4.5 Continuous CSF Leak

This can be the result of an unrecognized dural tear or an unsuccessful attempt to repair a tear. Some cases will resolve with removal of the drain and suturing of the drain site opening. If the leak persists, lumbar CSF drain-age might be indicated. If the leak is persistent despite adequate lumbar drainage, surgical exploration and dural repair should be considered. Antibiotic treatment should be administered in order to prevent the develop-ment of possible wound infection or meningitis.

16.7.4.6 Hardware Failure and Nonunion

Among patients at risk for developing nonunion and failure of the hardware are smokers, diabetics, and those who are suffering from chronic renal failure. Unfortunately, there is a correlation between these comorbidities and the occurrence of burst fractures [15]. The consequences of this complication could be progressive segmental kyphosis, segmental instability, continuing neck pain, neurologic deterioration or dis-placement of the hardware, and compression of other neck structures. Strict postoperative follow-up protocol and extended cervical collar immobilization period for at-risk patients can assist in decreasing nonunion rates. Salvage procedures include revision of the anterior instrumentation (which is inevitable in cases of clini-cally significant hardware dislodgement), or perform-ing a posterior cervical instrumented fusion that will enable avoiding revision of the previous surgical site and related complications.

References

1. Aebi M, Zuber K, Marchesi D (1991) Treatment of cervical spine injuries with anterior plating. Indications, techniques, and results. Spine 16(3 Suppl):S38–S45

2. Bensch FV, Koivikko MP, Kiuru MJ, Koskinen SK (2006) The incidence and distribution of burst fractures. Emerg Radiol 12(3):124–129

3. Ching RP, Watson NA, Carter JW, Tencer AF (1997) The effect of post-injury spinal position on canal occlusion in a cervical spine burst fracture model. Spine 22(15): 1710–1715

4. Cloward RB (1961) Treatment of acute fractures and fracture-dislocations of the cervical spine by vertebral-body fusion. A report of eleven cases. J Neurosurg 18:201–209

5. Do Koh Y, Lim TH, Won You J, Eck J, An HS (2001) A biomechanical comparison of modern anterior and posterior plate fixation of the cervical spine. Spine 26(1):15–21

6. Dvorak MF, Fisher CG, Fehlings MG, Rampersaud YR, Oner FC, Aarabi B, Vaccaro AR (2007) The surgical approach to subaxial cervical spine injuries: an evidence-based algorithm based on the SLIC classification system. Spine 32(23):2620–2629

7. Fountas KN, Kapsalaki EZ, Nikolakakos LG, Smisson HF, Johnston KW, Grigorian AA, Lee GP, Robinson JS Jr (2007) Anterior cervical discectomy and fusion associated compli-cations. Spine 32(21):2310–2317

8. Gaudinez RF, English GM, Gebhard JS, Brugman JL, Donaldson DH, Brown CW (2000) Esophageal perforations after anterior cervical surgery. J Spinal Disord 13(1): 77–84

9. Jung A, Schramm J, Lehnerdt K, Herberhold C (2005) Recurrent laryngeal nerve palsy during anterior cervical spine surgery: a prospective study. J Neurosurg Spine 2:123–127

10. Kilburg C, Sullivan HG, Mathiason MA (2006) Effect of approach side during anterior cervical discectomy and fusion on the incidence of recurrent laryngeal nerve injury. J Neurosurg Spine 4(4):273–277

11. Koivikko MP, Myllynen P, Karjalainen M, Vornanen M, Santavirta S (2000) Conservative and operative treatment in cervical burst fractures. Arch Orthop Trauma Surg 120(7-8): 448–451

12. Magerl F, Aebi M, Gertzbein SD, Harms J, Nazarian S (1994) A comprehensive classification of thoracic and lum-bar injuries. Eur Spine J 3(4):184–201

13. Pollock R, Alcelik I, Bhatia C, Chuter G, Lingutla K, Budithi C, Krishna M (2008) Donor site morbidity follow-ing iliac crest bone harvesting for cervical fusion: a compari-son between minimally invasive and open techniques. Eur Spine J 17(6):845–852

14. Toh E, Nomura T, Watanabe M, Mochida J (2006) Surgical treatment for injuries of the middle and lower cervical spine. Int Orthop 30(1):54–58

15. van der Klift M, de Laet CE, McCloskey EV, Johnell O, Kanis JA, Hofman A, Pols HA (2004) Risk factors for inci-dent vertebral fractures in men and women: the Rotterdam Study. J Bone Miner Res 19(7):1172–1180

16. White AA, Panjabi MM (1990) Physical properties and functional biomechanics of the spine. In: White A, Panjabi M (eds) Clinical biomechanics of the spine, 2nd edn. Lippincott Williams & Wilkins, Philadelphia

Posterior Pedicle Screw Fixation

17

Yasutsugu Yukawa

17.1 Case Example

A 38-year-old man sustained a C5–7 fracture dislocation (CE stage 5, Allen classification [3]) with ASIA A
neurological deficit in a traffic accident. Lateral X-ray,
sagittal and axial CT images showed C5–7 laminae
fractures, left C5 and right C6 pedicle fractures, and
C7 vertebral body fracture (Fig. 17.1 a–c). Posterior
open reduction, halo vest fixation, and tracheotomy
due to respiratory failure were conducted in the primary care hospital near the trauma site. After transfer
to our hospital, CT scan demonstrated good alignment
and a tracheal tube anterior to the cervical spine. We
performed C5–7 pedicle screw fixation (Fig. 17.1 d, e).
The patient started his rehabilitation one day following
the surgery without external fixation. Postoperative CT
scan showed good placement of the pedicle screws
within the pedicle cortex (Fig. 17.1 f, g).

17.2 Background

Pedicle screw fixation emerged as a safe and effective
means of posterior spinal instrumentation for spinal
arthrodesis in the lumbar spine. Abumi et al. introduced the concept of pedicle screw fixation in cervical
spine surgery, and have applied pedicle screws to the
mid and lower cervical spine since 1994 [1]. They, and
others, have reported good clinical results and relatively low rates of complications from this procedure

[1, 2, 16, 17]. Pedicle screw fixation can provide the
best initial stability among the various internal fixation
systems available for the cervical spine. Kotani and his
colleagues showed the biomechanical advantages of
pedicle screw fixation [10]. However, because it has
the potential to seriously injure the spinal cord, nerve
roots, or vertebral arteries, pedicle screw fixation has
generally been considered a very risky surgery. Therefore,
if the safety of the procedure can be ensured, cervical
pedicle screw fixation becomes an effective procedure
for reconstructing the cervical spine.

This chapter introduces pedicle screw fixation in the
treatment of unstable cervical injuries, and describes
its indication, procedural steps, intraoperative imaging
technique, technical pitfalls, and postoperative course
in detail.

17.3 Indications and Advantages for Procedure

Pedicle screw fixation technique can be applied to any
type of unstable cervical injury; subluxations, dislocations, burst fractures, and fracture dislocations. This
fixation is applicable to all levels between C2 and C7.
Connection with the occipital bone or the thoracic spine
is easily possible. Supplementary anterior decompression
and strut graft is sometimes needed in limited cases;
however, the majority of unstable cervical injuries can
be treated by pedicle screw fixation alone. The best indications are the cases in which posterior wiring or lateral
mass plating cannot be applied, due to the damage to the
posterior elements or poor bone quality. Transpedicular
screw fixation may provide optimal stabilization for
such unstable motion segments, if the pedicles are intact
[5, 10, 11]. Short segment fixation, usually 1 above and

Y. Yukawa
Department of Orthopaedic Surgery, Chubu Rosai Hospital,
1-10-6 Komei, Minato-ku, Nagoya, 455-0019, Japan

V.V. Patel et al. (eds.), *Spine Trauma*,
DOI: 10.1007/978-3-642-03694-1_17, © Springer-Verlag Berlin Heidelberg 2010

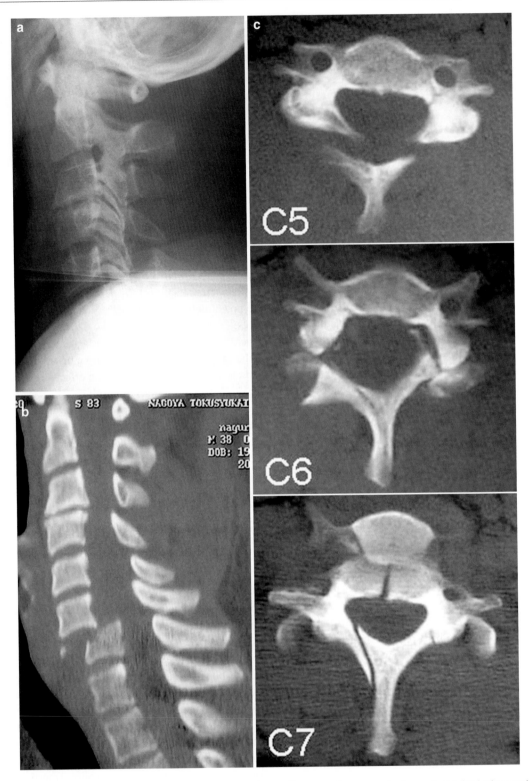

Fig. 17.1 Imaging studies of an illustrative case. Preoperative lateral X-ray showing C5 lamina fracture and vertebral body widening (**a**). Preoperative sagittal and axial CT images show C6/7 dislocation, C5-7 laminae – vertebral body separation and left C5 and right C6 pedicle fracture without displacement (**b**, **c**). Good alignment after open reduction and a tracheal tube anterior to the cervical spine are seen on another sagittal and axial images (**d**, **e**). Postoperative AP and lateral radiograph shows good alignment with C5-7 pedicle screw fixation (**f**). Postoperative CT scans show good placement of the pedicle screws at C5-7 levels (**g**)

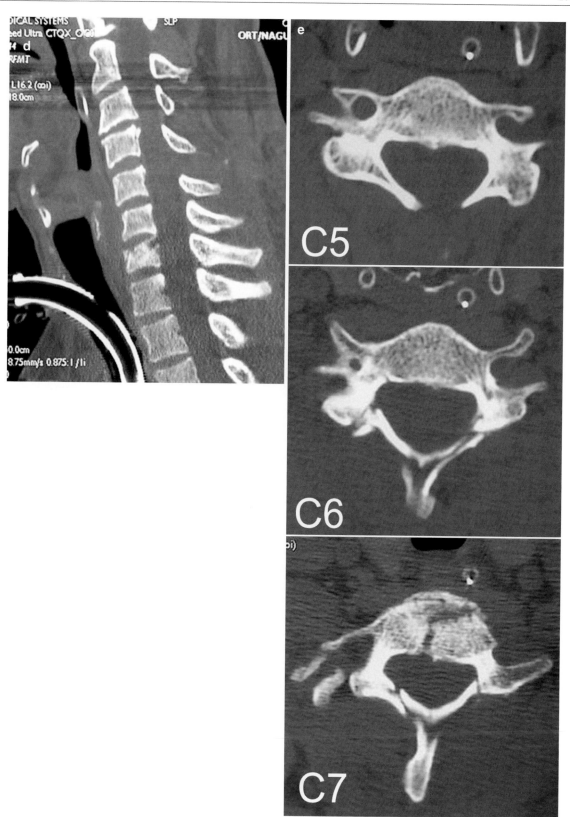

Fig. 17.1 (continued)

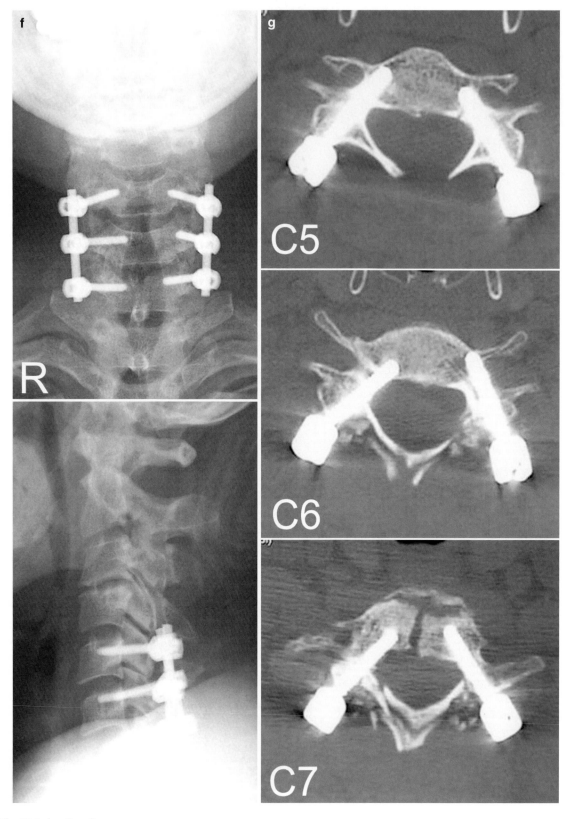

Fig. 17.1 (continued)

1 below the lesion, is possible. This method provides strong fixation even in patients with osteoporosis.

Pre- and postoperative tracheotomy is often required in patients with severe spinal cord injuries due to respiratory insufficiency. This technique can provide three-column fixation by posterior surgery alone and omits the need for postoperative external fixation. The tracheotomies could be easily performed in these patients without hesitation, in contrast to the patients who would undergo anterior or combined surgery.

In cases of the lower cervical spine where good lateral views cannot be obtained due to the overlying shoulders, the pedicle axis view technique by fluoroscopy shows the pedicle entry point matched with the trajectory angle [16].

17.4 Contraindications and Disadvantages for Procedure

Pedicle screw insertion at levels with pedicle fracture or narrow pedicles <4 mm is a contraindication for this procedure. In such cases, it is recommended to lengthen the fixation one more level without screw insertion at the level of the pedicle fracture. It is preferable not to insert pedicle screws in the side of the remaining vertebral artery (VA), if occlusion of contralateral VA is seen on preoperative MR or CT angiography.

17.5 Preoperative Imaging Study

Plain X-ray (AP, lateral, and two oblique views), computed tomography (CT), and magnetic resonance imaging (MRI) should be obtained preoperatively in all patients. It is of paramount importance for the surgeon to review all the preoperative radiographic studies to ensure that no destruction of the pedicle exists which would preclude the placement of pedicle screws. Pedicle morphology and medial inclination of the pedicle axis are fully visualized and noticed preoperatively.

CT angiography and/or MR angiography are necessary to observe the presence of VA anomaly or disruption preoperatively. The course and patency of the VA must be clearly delineated to avoid injury to that structure.

17.6 Timing of Surgery

An issue that is clearly controversial is the timing of surgical intervention in patients with neurological deficits. An indication for emergent surgical intervention in cases of cervical trauma includes a progressive neurologic deficit in unstable fracture/dislocation patterns with significant spinal cord compression. However, previous studies have reported that even a delayed decompression of persistent spinal cord compression can be beneficial in terms of improved neurologic status [8]. Finally, the timing should be decided, taking into consideration the availability of a trained spine team and the general/neurological conditions of the patient. Please see Chap. 4 for further discussion.

17.7 Procedure

17.7.1 Equipment Needed

Screw and rod systems used for lateral mass screws can also be used as pedicle screws. Curved probes are better than straight ones. In midcervical spine, the diameter of the pedicle screws used is usually 3.5 mm and the length is 20 or 22 mm. Occasionally, 4.0 mm diameter screws are used in cases with wider pedicles or osteoporosis, and screws longer than 22 mm are used at C2 and C7.

Fluoroscopy is absolutely necessary to visualize the screw insertion during surgery. If computer-aided navigation system is available, it could provide better identification of the insertion point and trajectory angle of pedicles.

The angle gauge indicates the trajectory angle and is very helpful, if it is available.

17.7.2 Anesthetic and Neuromonitoring Considerations

Excessive extension during intubation may induce additional neurological injury in patients with unstable cervical spines. Awake intubation using fiberscope is usually used for such patients to avoid neurological deterioration.

Patients with spinal cord lesions, or potentials for cord deficits, need to maintain adequate blood flow to the spinal cord throughout the surgery. This requires careful monitoring by the anesthesiologist, as well as clear communication from the surgeon informing his expectations, anticipated blood loss, and the time of surgery.

Neurological deterioration is the most feared complication of the surgery. Neurological injury is not simply a by-product of the surgery itself. It can occur preoperatively during transfer of the patient to the operating table, neck extension during intubation, or patient positioning. From a surgical prospective, appropriate preoperative preparation, careful surgical planning, surgical execution, and constant surgical vigilance can minimize the risk of neurological complications. An additional mean of injury prevention is continuous neurophysiological monitoring of the spinal cord and spinal nerve root function. Therefore, intraoperative neurophysiological monitoring of spinal cord and spinal nerve root function is gaining importance to reduce the incidence of new or additional neurological deficits during surgery. Technological advances in neurophysiological instrumentation permit the neurophysiologist to monitor somatosensory evoked potentials, transcranial motor-evoked potentials, and both spontaneous and stimulated electromyography in a single test protocol, all displayed simultaneously. Intraoperative neurophysiological monitoring should be considered an integral adjunct to the surgical management of the spine-injured patient [15].

17.7.3 Patient Positioning and Room Setup

Patients are placed on a Jackson table Relton–Hall frame or comparable frame with their skull fixed in a Mayfield three-point fixator and the cervical spine is positioned parallel to the floor. Shoulder girdles are pulled caudally and fixed by taping. (Fig. 17.2)

A multiplanar fluoroscope is set on the right side of the patient in prone position. It is checked preoperatively to obtain a true lateral view of the cervical spine and pedicle axis view which demonstrates the approximately circular portion of the pedicle cortex wall in the inclination of the pedicle axis.

17.7.4 Surgical Approach

Midline posterior approach is used. There are few vital structures between the skin and the spine, and a longitudinal midline exposure through the ligamentum nuchae is performed. This exposure is usually bloodless and truly internervous, preventing denervation of the musculature. Strict subperiosteal dissection creates a bloodless

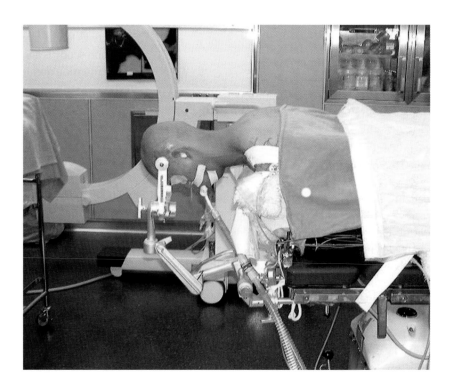

Fig. 17.2 Patient positioning on a Relton–Hall frame with his skull fixed in a Mayfield three-point fixator

field. Adequate exposure of the lateral mass is crucial for accurate screw placement (Fig. 17.3). If adequate exposure of the surgical field cannot be obtained, an additional small incision can be considered (Fig. 17.4).

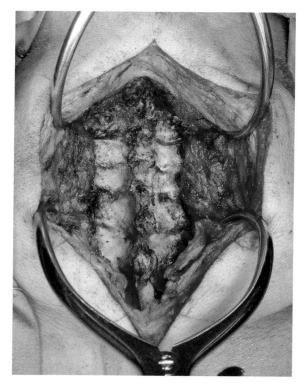

Fig. 17.3 Adequate exposure of the lateral mass during surgery

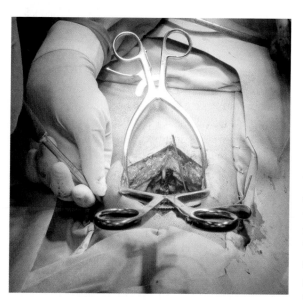

Fig. 17.4 Supplemental incision

17.7.5 Reduction Technique

Subluxation is usually reduced by neutral position setting in the Mayfield fixator. Unilateral or bilateral facet dislocation is reduced in about half of the cases by gentle longitudinal traction following general anesthesia. In the remaining cases, the reduction is obtained by partial resection of the superior articular process and application of longitudinal traction with bone holding forceps. Vertebral fractures with or without dislocations are partially reduced by the surgical position setting. Protrusion of the posterior wall into the spinal canal is almost totally reduced by pedicle screw and rod techniques. If significant canal compromise remains postoperatively, supplemental anterior decompression and strut bone graft should be considered.

17.7.6 Fixation Technique

Accurate screw placement needs precise identification of the screw entry point matched with the trajectory angle. For that purpose, several techniques are employed; the original technique described by Abumi et al. [1], the pedicle axis view technique by fluoroscopy [16], the laminoforaminotomy technique [12, 13], and the computer-assisted navigation technique [4, 9].

In this chapter, we introduce our pedicle axis view technique by fluoroscopy in C3–7 pedicle screw placement. During the placement of the C2 pedicle screw, direct visualization and palpation of the medial and superior walls of the C2 pedicles is recommended, as the overlapping teeth and mandible often prevent appropriate visualization of the pedicle axis view.

Fluoroscopy is set to obtain a true lateral view of the cervical spine. Then the fluoroscope is rotated so that an approximately circular portion of the pedicle cortex wall can be visualized in the transverse plane of the vertebral body; thus the axis of rotation is set to the cervical pedicle longitudinal axis (Fig. 17.5). This is the pedicle axis view and the screw insertion point is located at the center of the circle on the cervical lateral mass (Fig. 17.6). This point is close to the inferior margin of the inferior articular facet of the cephalad segment. The inclined axis of the fluoroscopy shows that the pedicle axis matches with the insertion point. Usually, the axis inclines from 30 to 55° from the midsagittal plane (C2–7) [6, 12, 14]

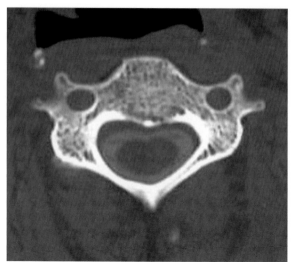

Fig. 17.7 Axial CT scan of C5

(Fig. 17.7). Because a larger inclination of the screw trajectory would require further surgical exposure, we employed a trajectory angle of 30–35° from the sagittal plane at the C3–7 levels. An entry hole is created with an awl, and a fine pedicle probe with a blunt tip is inserted through the entry hole into the pedicle cavity, the craniocaudal direction being parallel to the upper vertebral body endplate. Guide wires are inserted into the pedicle holes, and the accuracy of the trajectory angle is confirmed on lateral and pedicle axis views using the fluoroscope. The guide wires are reinserted into the pedicle if they are not correct. Tapping is performed before inserting the pedicle screws. For the mid- and lower cervical spine, we used 3.5 mm (diameter)×20–22 mm (length) screws. Anatomic lordosis is created by bending the rods. Decortication of the facets, laminae, and lateral masses is performed with a burr, and local bone chips from the spinous processes are grafted into the facets and onto the laminae and lateral masses. All the steps are done manually to acquire tactile feedback. No power drill is used to avoid injury to the neurovascular structures.

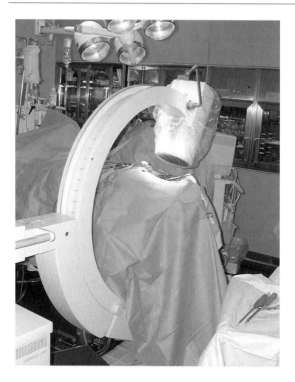

Fig. 17.5 Setting of the fluoroscopy to obtain the left pedicle axis view

17.8 Technical Pearls and Pitfalls

17.8.1 Pearls

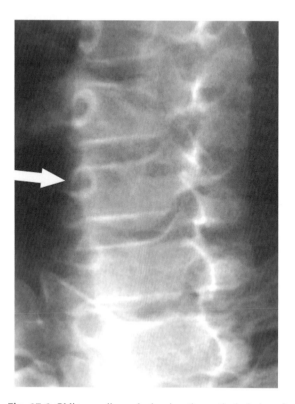

Fig. 17.6 Oblique radiograph showing the cortical circles of left C4–T1 pedicles. Left C6 pedicle is seen as a round circle just below the upper endplate; this is the pedicle axis view (*arrow*)

A good combination of the insertion point and the trajectory angle is crucial to insert the screws accurately. If either of those is not accurate, the screw placement

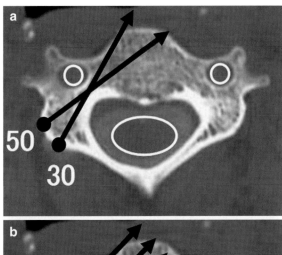

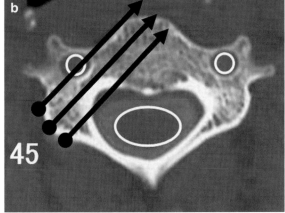

Fig. 17.8 Pedicle screw insertion point and trajectory angle. Insertion points change with the trajectory angles (**a**). Even if the trajectory angle is ideal, the screws may be aimed incorrectly according to the insertion points (**b**)

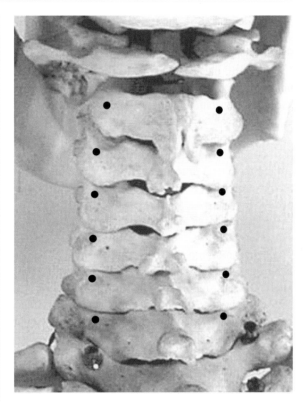

Fig. 17.9 Ideal insertion points for C2-7 pedicle screw. Even if the insertion points are correct, screw malpositioning can occur with unmatched trajectory angles

will fail (Fig. 17.8 a, b). Sometimes ideal insertion points are demonstrated as in Fig. 17.9. Those insertion points are usually matched with the anatomical axis of the pedicles. Those axes are inclined by about 45°. If the trajectory angle is less than 45°, the screws will aim too lateral or towards the VA.

The fluoroscopy-assisted pedicle axis view technique helps to determine the appropriate entry point that coincides with the correct trajectory angle for each cervical vertebra in both sagittal and transverse planes. Sometimes, in lateral images, the pedicles in the lower cervical spine are difficult to visualize due to the overlying shoulders, but such a problem is avoided in locating the correct entry points using the pedicle axis view technique. This technique can reduce the rate of pedicle perforation, as compared to the reports of the conventional technique (3.9 vs. 6.7%) [7, 16].

The all-manual procedure without using a power drill which the authors employed resulted in only few neurovascular complications and clinically innocent violations of the pedicle wall, when such violations are occasionally detected [7].

17.8.2 Pitfalls

Fluoroscopic lateral imaging is recommended in a study describing the conventional technique, but this method provides information regarding the vertical plane only and not the horizontal plane. Sometimes in the lateral images, the pedicles in the lower cervical spine are difficult to visualize due to the overlying shoulders.

If the patient is positioned with the cervical spine near the operative table, the handling of the fluoroscopy may be disturbed and the visualization of the pedicle axis view may be difficult.

Although cadaver studies have described detailed surface landmarks for posterior cervical pedicle entry points [17], the cervical lateral masses have small bony undulations that differ from that of thoracic or lumbar spine. In fact, during surgery, there are fewer morphometric landmarks than in cadaver demonstrations. Furthermore, the location of the pedicle entrance is unique to each level of the cervical vertebra and large variations are found among different individuals even at the same vertebral level.

Cortical wall is thicker in medially than laterally [6, 14]. Inadequate dissection might cause the screws aiming too lateral or towards the VA. Therefore screw malposition is likely to occur on the lateral side of the pedicle [17].

Violation of the upper facet capsules sometimes causes instability.

Cervical roots run just above the pedicles, unlike that in lumbar spine. Cephalad malposition of screws is more likely to cause root injury than caudal malposition.

Some studies recommend direct visualization and palpation of the superior, medial, and inferior pedicle walls using a small nerve retractor through a laminoforaminotomy. However, this technique may increase the risk of spinal cord and root injury by manipulation errors during the instrumentation.

17.8.3 Potential Intraoperative Complications

Intraoperative complications include problems related to the particular surgical approach, patient positioning, and neurological deterioration.

Iatrogenic neurological deterioration is the most serious complication that must be avoided. It might occur not only during surgery, but also during patient intubation or positioning.

Pedicle screw fixation has the potential to injure the spinal cord, nerve roots, or VA, and this technique between the C3 and C6 levels has generally been considered too risky. Complications related to cervical pedicle screw malposition depend on the direction of the cortical breech. Lateral perforation can injure the VA. Since the VA does not occupy the whole of the foramen transversarium, minimal violations of the foramen transversarium may not be as risky as expected. Medial breech may cause epidural venous bleeding. However, spinal cord injury is very rare, as the space between the medial wall of the pedicle and the spinal cord is relatively wide (Fig. 17.7 and 17.8). Superior perforation can injure the exiting nerve root, which

lies in the inferior portion of the foramen. Inferior perforation has the least incidence. Superior and inferior breech usually do not happen under accurate lateral imaging by fluoroscopy. Surgical manipulation itself might induce secondary neurological injury in an unstable spine.

17.8.4 Bailout/Salvage for Procedure Failure

During surgery, reduction is the first-line treatment to decrease the risk of possible subsequent neurological deterioration. If the cervical spine is unstable despite proper reduction, all manual procedures should be performed while holding the manipulated vertebra by grasping forceps.

If violation of the VA occurs, prompt packing with bone wax can stop the bleeding. Pedicle screw insertion should be aborted in the contralateral side. Other kinds of fixation in this level or single level extension of fixation should be considered.

Postoperative CT scan shows malpositioning of the screw in some cases. It is still controversial if such screws should be removed or not, when neurovascular symptoms related to the malpositioned screw are not seen.

If neurological deterioration related to traumatic disc herniation is seen postoperatively and is established in the imaging studies, anterior decompression and reconstruction should be considered promptly.

17.9 Postoperative Considerations

17.9.1 Bracing

A rigid cervical collar is worn for approximately 4 weeks postoperatively; however, no external fixation is applied to patients with ASIA A or B neurological deficit.

17.9.2 Activity

The patients are allowed to ambulate after removal of the postoperative drain and start postoperative rehabilitation on the same day or a few days later.

17.9.3 Follow-Up

Patients with paralysis are transferred to the rehabilitation unit several days after surgery. For them, prevention of secondary disease, optimization of function, and reintegration into the community are paramount.

Usually, patients are instructed to visit the clinic and take follow-up X-rays at 1, 3, 6, 12, and 24 months after surgery, when properly done.

17.9.4 Potential Complications

Postoperative complications fall into four broad categories, including general medical complications, problems associated with the specific surgical approach and positioning, postoperative infection, and instrument failure following pseudoarthrosis.

When the patient complains of headache, dizziness, vertigo, tinnitus, unsteady gait, dysarthria, diplopia, visual field defect, blurry vision, ptosis, drowsiness, syncope, altered level of consciousness, nystagmus, and dysphasia postoperatively, vertebrobasilar ischemia should be suspected. Late-onset vertebrobasilar ischemia might occur due to vascular occlusion by thrombus formation after incomplete VA injury. MR or CT angiography should be done promptly.

Delayed neurological deterioration is very rare. In such cases, imaging studies are necessary to exclude postoperative redislocation.

17.9.5 Treatments/Rescue for Complications

Dissolution of thrombus should be considered when VA occlusion is diagnosed by the imaging studies.

Early ambulation of patients with paralysis or multisystem trauma is important to prevent pulmonary complications, skin breakdown, deep vein thrombosis, and pulmonary embolism.

Diagnosis of a postoperative infection requires a high index of suspicion. Infections after posterior surgical approaches are generally more common than after anterior approaches. Wound drainage and unexplained fever are usually the earliest signs of infection. CT scan imaging may demonstrate the presence of an abscess at the operative site. Early irrigation, debridement, and appropriate antibiotic usage are the hallmarks of successful treatment of this complication.

Once loss of fixation is noted on postoperative radiographs, the surgeon should take immediate steps to prevent further implant displacement or spinal malalignment. This may include reoperation at the same site with revision of the instrumentation and/or stabilizing the spine from an alternative surgical approach.

Other methods of fixation or extending levels of fixation could provide better results.

The patients with spinal cord injury are often given high-dose steroids (NASCIS II protocol) and require prophylaxis against gastric ulcers, and vigilance for other side effects.

References

1. Abumi K, Itoh H, Taneichi H, Kaneda K (1994) Transpedicular screw fixation for traumatic lesions of the middle and lower cervical spine: description of the techniques and preliminary report. J Spinal Disord 7(1):19–28
2. Abumi K, Shono Y, Ito M, Taneichi H, Kotani Y, Kaneda K (2000) Complications of pedicle screw fixation in reconstructive surgery of the cervical spine. Spine 25(8):962–9
3. Allen BL Jr, Ferguson RL, Lehmann TR, O'Brien RP (1982) A mechanistic classification of closed, indirect fractures and dislocations of the lower cervical spine. Spine 7(1):1–27
4. Assaker R, Reyns N, Vinchon M, Demondion X, Louis E (2001) Transpedicular screw placement: image-guided versus lateral-view fluoroscopy: in vitro simulation. Spine 26(19):2160–4
5. Jones EL, Heller JG, Silcox DH, Hutton WC (1997) Cervical pedicle screws versus lateral mass screws. Anatomic feasibility and biomechanical comparison. Spine 22(9):977–82
6. Karaikovic EE, Daubs MD, Madsen RW, Gaines RW Jr (1997) Morphologic characteristics of human cervical pedicles. Spine 22(5):493–500
7. Karaikovic EE, Kunakornsawat S, Daubs MD, Madsen TW, Gaines RW Jr (2000) Surgical anatomy of the cervical pedicles: landmarks for posterior cervical pedicle entrance localization. J Spinal Disord 13(1):63–72
8. Kostuik JP (1988) Anterior fixation for burst fractures of the thoracic and lumbar spine with or without neurological involvement. Spine 13(3):286–93
9. Kotani Y, Abumi K, Ito M, Minami A (2003) Improved accuracy of computer-assisted cervical pedicle screw insertion. J Neurosurg Spine 99(3):257–63
10. Kotani Y, Cunningham BW, Abumi K, McAfee PC (1994) Biomechanical analysis of cervical stabilization systems. An assessment of transpedicular screw fixation in the cervical spine. Spine 19(22):2529–39
11. Kothe R, Ruther W, Schneider E, Linke B (2004) Biomechanical analysis of transpedicular screw fixation in the subaxial cervical spine. Spine 29(17):1869–75

12. Ludwig SC, Kramer DL, Vaccaro AR, Albert TJ (1999) Transpedicle screw fixation of the cervical spine. Clin Orthop Relat Res 359:77–88 (review)

13. Miller RM, Ebraheim NA, Xu R, Yeasting RA (1996) Anatomic consideration of transpedicular screw placement in the cervical spine. An analysis of two approaches. Spine 21(20):2317–22

14. Panjabi MM, Shin EK, Chen NC, Wang JL (2000) Internal morphology of human cervical pedicles. Spine 25(10):1197–205

15. Schwartz DM (2003) Intraoperative neurophysiological monitoring during post-traumatic spine surgery. In: Vaccaro AR (ed) Fractures of the cervical, thoracic and lumbar spine. Marcel Dekker, New York, pp 373–383

16. Yukawa Y, Kato F, Yoshihara H, Yanase M, Ito K (2006) Cervical pedicle screw fixation for 100 cases of unstable cervical injuries using pedicle axis views by fluoroscopy. J Neurosurg Spine 5(6):488–93

17. Yukawa Y, Kato F, Ito K et al. Placement and complications of cervical pedicle screws in 144 cervical trauma patients using pedicle axis view techniques by fluoroscope. Eur Spine J. 2009 Sep;18(9):1293-9. Epub 2009 Jun 2.

Thoracic Spinal Stability: Decision Making

18

Jeremy Smith and Nitin N. Bhatia

18.1 Introduction

The unique anatomic and biomechanical characteristics of the thoracic spine (T2–T10) require special attention when evaluating patients with spinal fractures. Careful attention to these characteristics during the clinical and radiographic assessment aids in the successful management of these patients. Although controversy exists regarding the radiographic interpretation of instability, identifying the potential for further instability and resultant neurologic decompensation is pivotal to preventing suboptimal outcomes.

18.2 Anatomic and Biomechanical Considerations

The thoracic spine is the longest segment of the spine, and its anatomic and biomechanical features make its response to mechanical stress and potential for instability different than other more mobile spinal segments.

The distinguishing characteristics of the thoracic spine are the presence of the ribs and their articulations (Fig. 18.1). The rib cage restricts motion and adds stiffness to the spine. As a result, the thoracic spine is more resistant to bending and axial rotational forces than the cervical or lumbar spine. In addition to the increased stability provided by the rib head articulations, the facet joints are oriented in the coronal plane,

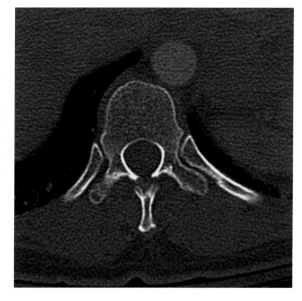

Fig. 18.1 Axial CT scan of a normal thoracic vertebra showing the bilateral articulations between the rib and the vertebral body

which helps to limit the anterior translation of the thoracic vertebrae during flexion loading. With the addition of the rib cage, two to three times the amount of compressive load can be tolerated before instability develops relative to other spinal segments. As a result of these differences, very high mechanical forces are required to cause thoracic vertebral injuries, making concomitant injuries to the chest, cervical spine, and head very common [4, 25, 38].

Kyphosis of the thoracic spine is caused by a 2–3 mm discrepancy in the height in the anterior vertebral body relative to the posterior height. Relative to the cervical and lumbar spine, the intervertebral disks are smaller in height, but have a thickened annulus fibrosis. This has been shown to increase the rotational stability in the thoracic spine [34, 44]. Although, because of this stability,

N.N. Bhatia (✉) and J. Smith
Department of Orthopaedic Surgery, UC Irvine Medical Center, 101 The City Drive South, Orange, CA 92868, USA
e-mail: bhatian@uci.edu

V.V. Patel et al. (eds.), *Spine Trauma*,
DOI: 10.1007/978-3-642-03694-1_18, © Springer-Verlag Berlin Heidelberg 2010

disk herniations in the thoracic spine are relatively rare, they can be devastating as they have a propensity to compromise the narrow spinal canal and spinal cord [4]. Given the limitations of rotatory motion placed on the thoracic spine by rib articulations, facets, and intervertebral disks, most injuries to the vertebral column occur in flexion and axial loading [4].

Another important anatomic feature of the thoracic spine differentiating it from the lumbar spine is the presence of the spinal cord. The spinal canal is relatively narrow in the thoracic spine, making the interval distance between the bony osseous ring and the cord significantly smaller. Thus injury to the upper thoracic spine that results in canal compromise or segmental translation has a high likelihood of resulting in some degree of neural injury. The blood supply to the central thoracic spinal cord is relatively sparse, increasing this segment's susceptibility to ischemia with lesser degrees of compression [44] Damage to intercostal nerve roots at the thoracic levels does not have as great of a functional consequence as do similar injuries to nerve roots in the lumbar and sacral levels due to the relative lack of motor function associated with the thoracic nerve roots.

18.3 Evaluation and Imaging

The initial goal while evaluating any trauma patient is to assess for life-threatening injuries and to provide necessary resuscitation efforts. Spinal injuries are common in the multiple-system trauma patients, but unfortunately they are frequently unrecognized. Anderson et al. described a 24% incidence of missed thoracolumbar fractures on initial evaluation [2]. Spinal fractures are more likely to be overlooked in the obtunded trauma patients who are unable to localize pain.

During the initial comprehensive evaluation of the trauma patient, a thorough examination of the spine is critical. Direct examination by visual inspection and especially palpation of all spinal segments is necessary. A step-off or soft spot between spinous processes can sometimes be the only indication of instability. Soft tissue trauma including laceration, swelling, or ecchymosis might indicate underlining spinal instability. Localized tenderness should be noted at every palpated segment. Soft tissue trauma to the chest and/or abdomen might suggest a seat-belt type injury that can be

associated with a flexion-distraction injury. A thorough neurologic examination is also very important in every trauma patient. Motor strength, sensory function, and reflexes should be documented. In the patient with suspected spinal cord injury, serial examinations need to be performed to assess for changes in neurologic status. The American Spinal Injury Association Impairment Scale provides a validated and reproducible method for documenting and following the level and severity of the spinal cord injury. In the obtunded or uncooperative patient, a repeat examination should be performed if the initial evaluation is inadequate. In those patients suspected of having spinal trauma or spinal cord injury, perianal sensation, rectal tone, and bulbocavernosus reflex should be documented, and the patients are maintained on spinal precautions until spinal trauma can be ruled out by radiographic and clinical evaluations.

Any abnormal finding or suspicion of spinal trauma during the initial examination warrants radiographic evaluation. Initial imaging should include plain radiographs or computed tomography (CT), but keep in mind that it is often difficult to visualize the thoracic spine on a lateral plain radiograph. In addition, paraspinous hemorrhage can cause mediastinal widening, giving the appearance of a ruptured thoracic aorta [4].

In cases where there is a high suspicion of spinal trauma or there are subtle findings on plain radiography, CT scan can provide a more detailed description of the injured segment. With modern CT scanners available, the morphology of the spinal fractures can be viewed rapidly in detail. CT images can reveal the degree of canal stenosis in burst fractures, aid in defining unstable rotational injuries, and indirectly assess ligamentous and intervertebral disk injury by displaying subtle differences in the alignment of adjacent spinal segments. Key examples include the "naked facet sign," found in cases of facet dislocation, and posterior interspinous widening in which injury to the posterior interspinous ligamentous complex results in increased distance between spinous processes, which is often seen in distraction type injuries. CT scans are also extremely useful in assessing hardware placement and adequacy of reduction in the postoperative period.

Magnetic resonance imaging (MRI) is the study of choice to evaluate the integrity of soft tissue structures and compression of the neural elements. In the setting of thoracic trauma, evaluation of the intervertebral disks, spinal cord, and posterior ligamentous complex is crucial in defining instability, identifying the amount of spinal cord compression, and deciding to treat patients conservatively or with surgery. In patients with neurologic deficit, MRI can define the extent of ongoing spinal cord compression and associated edema or hemorrhage that may help the prognosis for neurologic recovery.

18.4 Spinal Cord Injury

Because the thoracic spine is naturally kyphotic, has a narrowed spinal canal, and has a rather limited spinal cord blood supply relative to other areas, there is an increased risk of neurologic damage in the face of instability. Although most traumatic spinal cord injuries occur in the cervical and thoracolumbar junction, a high percentage of patients with thoracic spine fractures will have a spinal cord injury. Additionally, up to 80% of the spinal cord injuries in the thoracic spine may be complete injuries [5].

Despite continuous efforts with numerous laboratory studies and clinical trials, there remains no cure for spinal cord injury. Although we have seen improvement in both the survival rate and long-term outcome of spinal cord injury patients with advances in clinical management over the past fifteen years, there is still no clinically relevant therapeutic intervention. Both initial medical management and the timing of surgery remain controversial topics.

Although methylprednisolone can be administered for the spinal cord-injured patient, its efficacy continues to be questioned. The National Acute Spinal Cord Injury Study (NASCIS) has tested the effectiveness of methylprednisolone in three independent trials, NASCIS I, II, and III [6–16]. The NASCIS trials suggested that methylprednisolone may be beneficial for a selected group of SCI patients with nonpenetrating trauma, when administered within the first eight hours postinjury. Results from the NASCIS trials were initially viewed as promising and the administration of methylpredisolone was often considered the standard of care in the acute SCI setting. However, more recent studies have been highly critical of the interpretation of these trials, particularly the statistical analysis [28]. Currently, many spine trauma surgeons do not use methylprednisilone for patients with SCI or use it selectively in patients who are incomplete or have low risk-factor profile for steroids.

Decompression of the spinal cord is the hallmark of operative intervention for acute traumatic spinal cord injury. The timing of decompression remains controversial and a number of experimental and clinical studies have explored this issue. It is generally accepted that urgent surgical decompression is indicated in patients with progressive neurologic deficit in the presence of persistent spinal cord compression. It should be noted that decompression does not involve laminectomy, but more important stable realignment of the spine. The timing of surgical intervention in neurologically stable patients is less certain, and in general, they should be optimized medically prior to surgical intervention.

18.5 Classification of Thoracic Spine Injuries

Classification systems for defining thoracic and lumbar spinal trauma have a 70-year history with multiple variations on a few common themes. Using pathoanatomy and mechanism of injury as a premise for defining fracture patterns has enabled modern radiographic techniques to use static images to define more complex dynamic instability patterns. Ideally, a classification system can identify a mechanism, associate it with a musculoskeletal component, and aid in formulating a treatment strategy. Although such a classification system does not exist as a standard for defining thoracic spinal trauma, a few systems are commonplace. Still, there is no consensus as to which is most clinically relevant. A few of these classifications are outlined below.

Although the Denis' three-column concept [18] has traditionally been the most commonly utilized system for classifying thoracolumbar injuries, there remains controversy regarding its nomenclature, particularly when used in the thoracic spine. The original classification system is applied to regions extending from T1 to L5, which is ambiguously termed the thoracolumbar spine. The marked difference in intrinsic regional stability and sagittal alignment between the upper thoracic, thoracolumbar, and lower lumbar spine makes the incidence of fracture types in these three areas quite different. Nevertheless, the basic principles of this classification system are applied to other classification systems and warrant mentioning.

In his theory, Denis proposed that the spine was mechanically defined by three columns. The middle column, composed of the posterior longitudinal ligament, the posterior annulus, and the posterior aspect of the vertebral body, was hypothesized to be the most critical segment. The anterior column is composed of the anterior longitudinal ligament, the anterior annulus, and the anterior aspect of the vertebral body. The posterior column includes the neural arch, facet joints, ligamentum flavum, and interspinous ligament complex. This classification system mechanistically defines patterns of injury and categorizes the degree of instability based on the number of columns disrupted. The fracture pattern relates to the force applied to the spinal column, and the degree of instability is defined by the number of columns disrupted. Failure of two of the three columns is required for an unstable pattern of injury. Spinal injuries are classified into four different categories: compression fractures, burst fractures, seat-belt type injuries, and fracture-dislocations. The classification also includes 16 subgroups that help further define the morphology and mechanism of injury.

A more comprehensive classification was proposed by Magerl et al. in 1994 and is based on progressive pathomorphology and the mechanism of injury [24]. These types are subdivided into three groups that are defined by the fracture pattern and column involved [24, 33]. This system takes into account injury to the soft tissue and helps to differentiate unstable fracture patterns along with predicting the likelihood of an associated neurologic deficit.

In 2005, Vaccaro et al. [41, 42] proposed an injury classification system that is based on the morphologic/mechanistic model and factors in injury severity. Using this method of classification, it is thought that a single composite injury severity score will more accurately reflect the management of these injuries. This more clinically relevant system may aid in the decision making process in treating thoracic and lumbar spine trauma, although further data are required to confirm the validity and usefulness of this classification scheme (Table 18.1).

Table 18.1 AO classification system for spinal injuries. Refer to Figs. 18.2–18.21

A. Compression injury
A1: Impaction fracture
A1.1 Endplate impaction
A1.2 Wedge impaction
A1.3 Vertebral body collapse
A2: Split fracture
A2.1 Sagittal split fracture
A2.2 Coronal split fracture
A2.3 Pincer fracture
A3: Burst fracture
A3.1 Incomplete burst fracture
A3.2 Burst-split fracture
A3.3 Complete burst fracture
B. Distraction injury
B1: Posterior ligamentary lesion
B1.1 With disk rupture
B1.2 With type A fracture
B2: Posterior osseous lesion
B2.1 Transverse bicolumn
B2.2 With disk rupture
B2.3 With type A fracture
B3: Anterior disk rupture
B3.1 With subluxation
B3.2 With spondylolysis
B3.3 With posterior dislocation
C. Rotation injury
C1: Type A with rotation
C1.1 Rotational wedge fracture
C1.2 Rotational split fracture
C1.3 Rotational burst fracture
C2: Type B with rotation
C2.1 B1 Lesion with rotation
C2.2 B2 Lesion with rotation
C2.3 B3 Lesion with rotation

18.6 Fracture Types

Flexion and axial loading account for the majority of the fractures in the thoracic spine. Because of the

unique mechanical stability imparted by the rib cage, incidence and fracture pattern differ somewhat

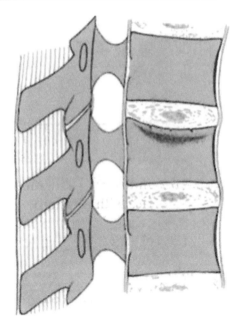

Fig. 18.2 End plate impaction (A1.1)

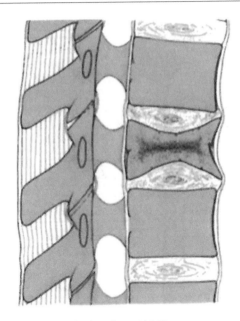

Fig. 18.4 Vertebral body collapse (A1.3)

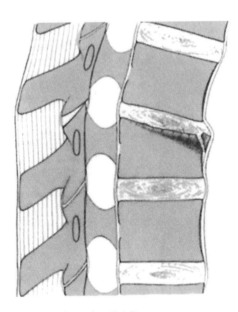

Fig. 18.3 Wedge impaction (A1.2)

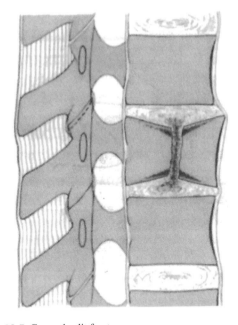

Fig. 18.5 Coronal split fracture

from those occurring in the thoracolumbar junction. Here we review the basic morphologic/mechanistic models as originally proposed by Denis and the unique characteristics of these injuries in the thoracic spine.

18.6.1 Compression Fractures

Although a considerable amount of force is required to produce a compression injury in the upper thoracic spine, compression wedge fractures remain the most

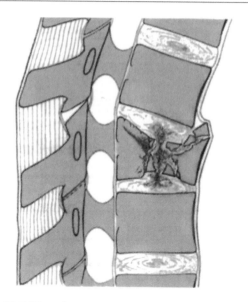

Fig. 18.6 Pincer fracture

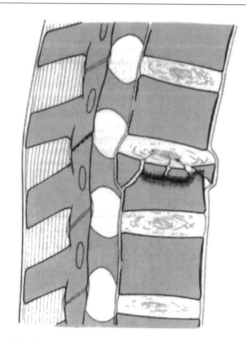

Fig. 18.7 Incomplete burst fracture

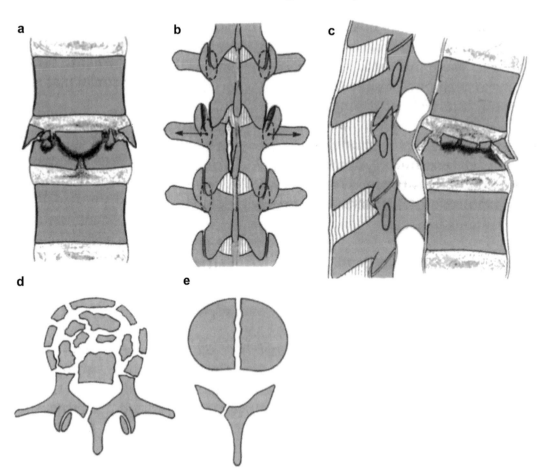

Fig. 18.8 (**a–c**) Appearance on standard radiographs, note the increased interpedicular distance (**b** *arrows*). (**d, e**) CT scan of the upper and lower part of the vertebral body

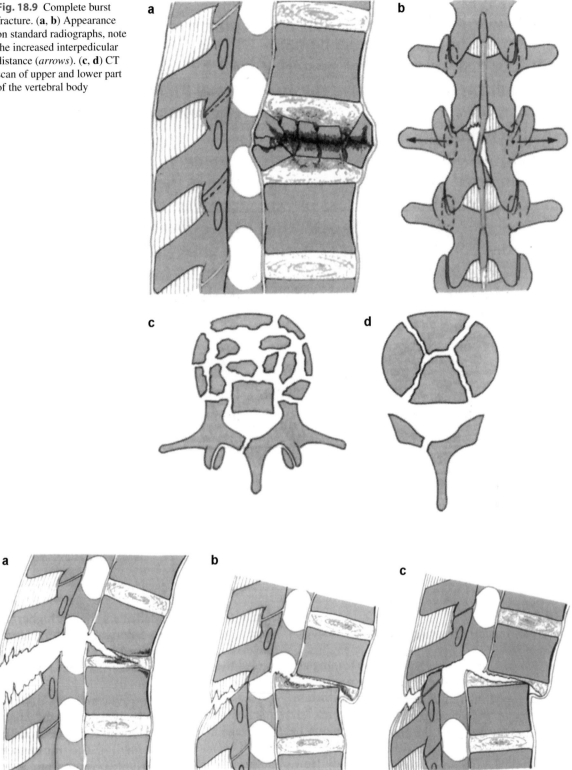

Fig. 18.9 Complete burst fracture. (**a**, **b**) Appearance on standard radiographs, note the increased interpedicular distance (*arrows*). (**c**, **d**) CT scan of upper and lower part of the vertebral body

Fig. 18.10 Examples of posterior disruption associated with an anterior lesion through the disk. (**a**) Flexion subluxation (B1.1.1) (**b**) Anterior dislocation (B1.1.2). (**c**) Anterior dislocation with fracture of the articular processes (B1.1.3)

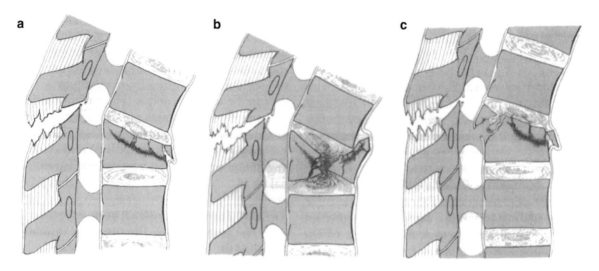

Fig. 18.11 Examples of posterior disruption predominantly ligamentous with subluxation of the facet joints associated with a type A fracture of the vertebral body (B1.2.1) (**a**) Flexion subluxation associated with a superior wedge fracture (B1.2.1+A1.2.1).

(**b**) Flexion subluxation associated with a pincer fracture (B1.2.1+A2.3). (**c**) Flexion subluxation associated with an incomplete superior burst fracture (B1.2.1+A3.1.1)

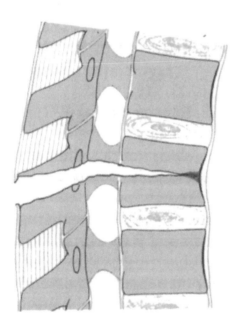

Fig. 18.12 Transverse bicolumn fracture (B2.1)

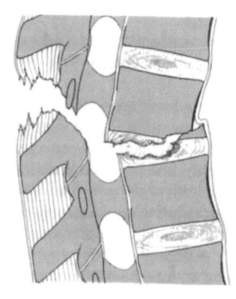

Fig. 18.13 Posterior disruption predominantly osseous associated with an anterior lesion through the disk: flexion-spondylolysis (B2.2.2)

common fracture type in this region [17, 47]. A combination of axial compression loading and forward flexion is responsible for producing the characteristic wedge-shaped deformity. In young and middle-aged patients, motor vehicle accidents and significant falls result in these types of injuries [19, 20, 23, 38]. In the

elderly population, osteoporosis makes the vertebral bodies more susceptible to compression injuries from even low-energy trauma [26, 45].

Compression fractures as defined by the Denis classification involve only the anterior column and are differentiated and subtyped according to the end plate

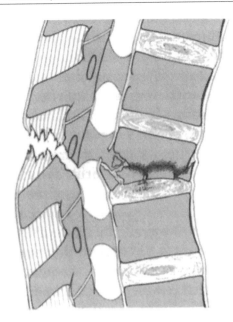

Fig. 18.14 Posterior disruption predominantly osseious associated with a type A fracture of the vertebral body: flexion-spondylolysis associated with an inferior incomplete burst fracture (B2.3.2+A3.1.3)

that fails [18]. The most common type (type B) results from a failure of the superior end plate. In a pure flexion-compression injury the less compressible intervertebral disk transmits load to the contiguous bone, resulting in end plate failure and subsequent collapse of the subcortical cancellous bone. The middle column does not fail in these injuries and acts as a fulcrum for anterior compression.

Radiographic evaluation by lateral radiograph or CT shows the severity of the compression fracture and can be calculated as a percentage of vertebral body collapse and the resulting kyphotic deformity. By dividing the height of the anterior wall of the injured segment by the average vertebral body height of the adjacent uninjured vertebral bodies, the percentage collapse can be calculated. To assess the degree of kyphotic deformity, the sagittal Cobb angle is measured between the injured segment and the first adjacent intact end plate.

Although the stability of compression fractures in the upper thoracic spine differs somewhat from injuries to the thoracolumbar junction, assessment of mechanically unstable fracture patterns in both regions has been traditionally approached in a similar manner. Stable fracture patterns are able to resist anterior compression, posterior tensile, and rotational forces, which may result in the progression of deformity or in neurologic compromise [46]. With more severe compressive

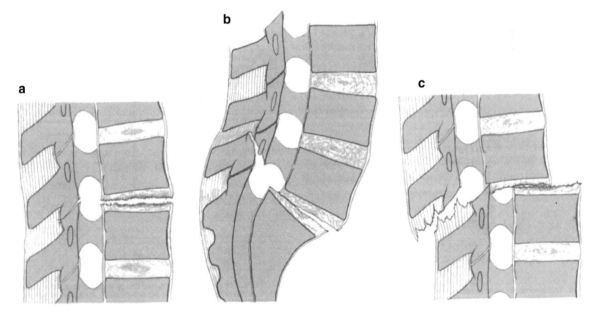

Fig. 18.15 Examples of anterior disruption through the disk (hyperextension-shear injuries). (**a**) Hyperextension-subluxation without fracture of posterior vertebral elements (B3.1.1). (**b**) Hyperextension-spondylolysis (B3.2) in the lower lumbar spine. (**c**) Posterior dislocation (3.3)

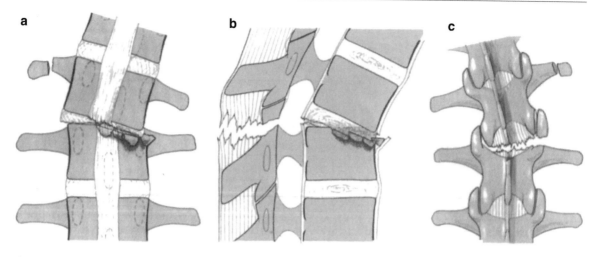

Fig. 18.16 Example of a type A fracture with rotation: rotational wedge fracture (C1.1)

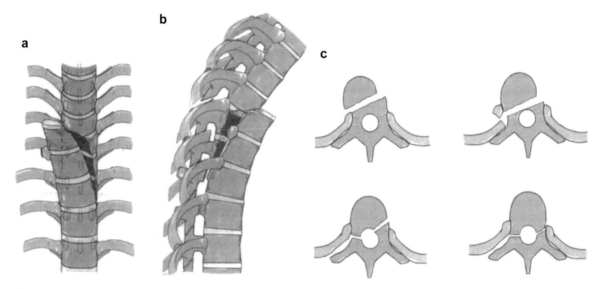

Fig. 18.17 Vertebral body separation (C1.2.4). (**a, b**) Appearance on standard radiographs. (**c**) CT scans of the fractured vertebrae

and forward flexion forces exerted on the vertebral segment, the posterior ligamentous complex resists further distraction until loaded to failure. With complete ligamentous disruption, the spine bends around an intact middle column and greater forces on the anterior column cause further wedging and collapse. As wedging and kyphotic deformation progress, a larger moment arm is created resulting in a greater tendency toward further progression [4, 40].

As a result of this proposed mechanism of instability and tendency toward progression, biomechanical theories of how the degree of anterior wedging correlates with the likelihood of posterior ligamentous disruption have been studied. One figure proposed by White and Panjabi (*Clinical Biomechanics of the Spine*) has been widely accepted and cited extensively in the literature [1, 21, 22, 29, 30, 43]. They suggested that greater than 50% anterior vertebral body wedging correlates with a greater likelihood of posterior ligamentous failure and a risk of progression. This cut-off for acceptable wedging is widely used as a guide for the treatment of these fractures. Considerations must be made in regard to the amount of force that is required to cause a thoracic compression fracture. In addition, the normal kyphosis of the upper thoracic spine predisposes to further progression. Bohlman

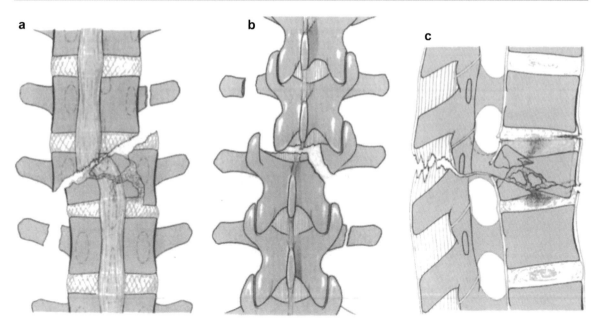

Fig. 18.18 Example of a type A fracture with rotation: complete burst fracture with rotation (C1.3.3). (**a**) Vertebral body. (**b**) Posterior elements. (**c**) Lateral view

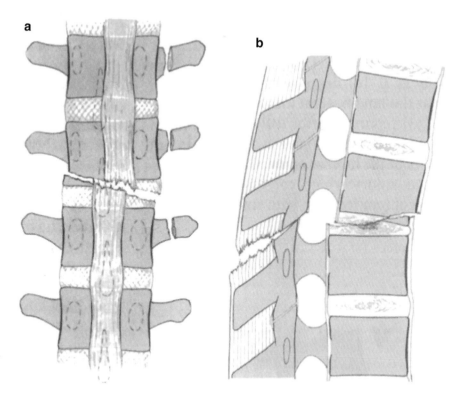

Fig. 18.19 Example of a type B injury with rotation: rotational flexion subluxation (c2.1.1). (**a**) Lateral view. (**b**) Posterior elements

suggests treatment for those injuries that display greater than 40° of kyphosis. Some authors advocate surgical stabilization only in those cases with progressive angulation or neurologic deficit [36]. Nevertheless, most authors agree that compression fractures with less than 40% of compression are stable and can be treated conservatively in the neurologically intact patient. Nonsurgical treatment generally involves

Fig. 18.20 Example of a type B injury with rotation: unilateral dislocation (C2.1.3). (**a**) Lateral view. (**b**) Posterior elements

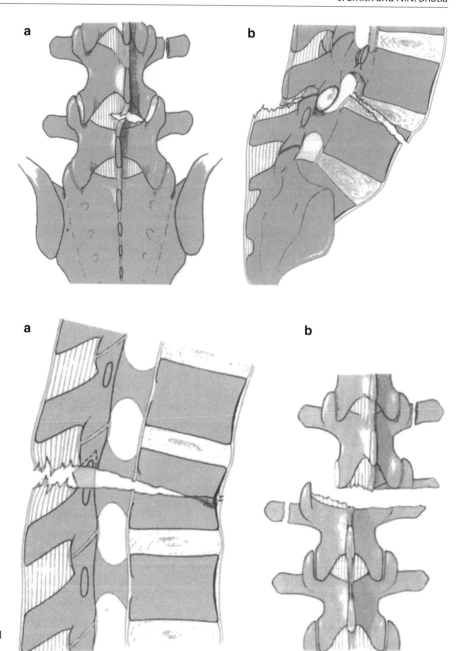

Fig. 18.21 Example of a type B injury with rotation: transverse bicolumn fracture with rotation (C2.2.1) (**a**). Anterior elements. (**b**) Lateral view

treatment with a rigid orthosis when the patient is in the upright position for approximately 3 months [4, 29]. The treatment of vertebral compression fractures with 40–50% of collapse is not as clearly defined in the literature. Some authors advocate surgical stabilization in those with greater than 40% compression [4], although there is poor agreement in the literature with regard to surgical treatment indications and options.

18.6.2 Burst Fractures

Burst fractures are extensions of the compression fracture with involvement of the posterior vertebral body, or middle column. The increased stability provided by the rib cage and sternum makes burst fractures a less common injury pattern in the thoracic spine vs. the thoracolumbar junction. The rib cage aids in dissipating axial loads and increases resistance to frontal and sagittal bending [3]. This, along with the relative stability imparted by the orientation of the thoracic facets, makes burst fractures relatively rare cephalad to the thoracolumbar junction. Nevertheless, when they do occur in this region, they can have a devastating impact on neurologic function. Careful attention must be paid to the patient's neurologic examination when there is even subtle radiographic evidence of spinal canal compromise. The same basic principles of the evaluation and management of thoracolumbar burst fractures apply to thoracic burst fractures and are covered in more detail in the other section of this book.

18.6.3 Fracture Dislocation

Facet fractures and dislocations are much less common in the upper thoracic spine relative to the thoracolumbar junction. The coronal plane orientation of the facet joints, combined with the significant amount of force required to overcome the stability imparted by the rib cage, decreases the likelihood of a facet dislocation [4, 27, 35]. Given the narrow spinal canal in this region, however, the likelihood of a catastrophic neurologic injury in the face of a traumatic dislocation is significant. The predominant mechanism of injury in this fracture pattern is flexion and distraction requiring failure of the posterior ligamentous complex, the facet capsules, and posterior annulus. Complete dislocation requires failure of both the posterior and anterior ligaments, as well as the intervertebral disk. Radiographically, patients have interspinous widening and variable degrees of sagittal plane vertebral body translation. Unilateral facet dislocations generally have translation less than 20%, while bilateral facet dislocations have translation of at least 30% of the width of the vertebral body.

Levine et al. reported nine cases of bilateral facet dislocations with an associated 89% incidence of complete spinal cord injury [31]. Similarly, Gellad et al. reported nine cases of bilateral locked facets in the thoracic spine associated with 100% complete paraplegia. Unilateral facet dislocations are reported in much smaller numbers [32]. This is likely due to the necessity of a rotary force strong enough to disrupt the rib cage along with flexion and distraction. Patients with these types of injuries are more likely to have an intact neurologic examination or an incomplete spinal cord injury pattern. Surgical stabilization is recommended for both types of these injuries.

18.6.4 Flexion-Distraction Injuries

Initially described by Chance in 1948, flexion-distraction injuries of the thoracic spine result from high-energy forces that result in forward flexion and distraction. The most common mode of injury is motor vehicle accidents, and they may be associated with high-riding lap seat-belts. Although flexion-distraction injuries in the thoracolumbar spine are described much more extensively in the literature, they do occur in the thoracic spine. As with other injuries to the thoracic spine, an extensive amount of force is required to overcome the stability provided by the rib cage. Based on Denis' three-column theory, flexion-distraction injuries result from failure of the middle and posterior columns under tension and possible failure of the anterior column with compression forces associated with flexion (Fig. 18.22). Flexion-distraction injuries can result in various fracture patterns in the vertebrae: they can be purely osseous, osteoligamentous, or purely ligamentous injuries. These injuries are distinguished from fracture-dislocations by the absence of translation (Table 18.2).

As with other injury patterns in the thoracic spine, these injuries have a high propensity to result in neurologic compromise. In addition, as a result of the high degree of flexion and resultant compression on the abdominal cavity, visceral injuries are common. The abdominal injury may be discovered prior to the injury to the spinal column. Because of the high incidence of neurologic injury and significant instability, these injuries are usually treated surgically.

18.7 Summary

The thoracic spine possesses unique anatomic characteristics, which influence the evaluation and decision making process of injuries to this area. The relative inherent stability imparted upon the thoracic spine by the rib cage and facet joint orientation decreases the risk of injury in this region; although when fractures or dislocations occur, they are frequently accompanied by significant spinal cord injuries. Appropriate clinical and radiographic evaluation is necessary to identify the nature of the injury and the appropriate treatment mechanism for both the structural instability and any accompanying spinal cord injury.

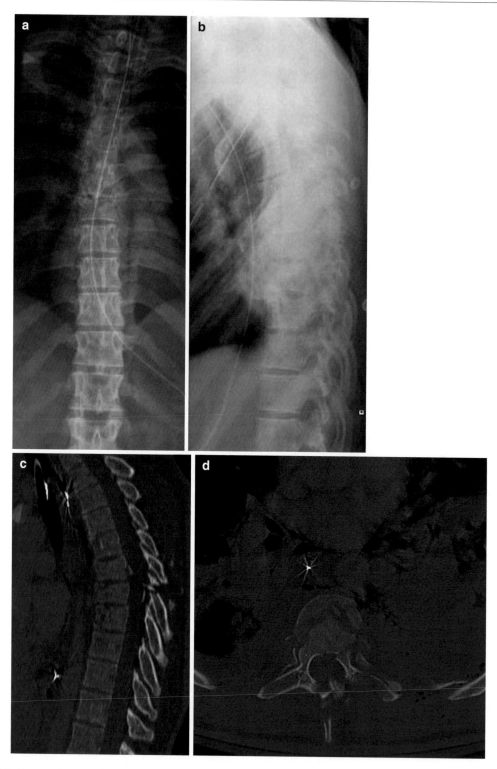

Fig. 18.22 Flexion-distraction injury in the thoracic spine. (**a**) AP radiograph showing malignment in the upper thoracic spine; (**b**) lateral radiograph demonstrating the difficulty in viewing upper thoracic injuries with plain radiographs; (**c**) sag- ittal CT scan with anterior vertebral body compression and spinous process distraction compatible with a flexion-distrac- tion type injury; (**d**) axial CT scan indicating severe three col- umn involvement

Table 18.2 Subaxial injury classification and severity scale

Morphology	Points
No abnormality	0
Compression	1
Burst	+1 = 2
Distraction (e.g., facet perch, hyperextension)	3
Rotation/translation (e.g., facet dislocation, unstable teardrop, or advanced staged flexion-compression injury)	4
Discoligomentous complex	
Intact	0
Indeterminate (e.g., isolated interspinous widening, MRI signal change only)	1
Disrupted (e.g., widening of anterior disk space, facet perch or dislocation, kyphotic deformity)	2
Neurological status	
Intact	0
Root injury	1
Complete cord injury	2
Incomplete cord injury	3
Ongoing cord compression (in setting of a neurologic deficit)	+1
Treatment	Total score
Nonoperative (rigid orthoses, halo-vest, etc.)	<4
Operative (surgical decompression/ stabilization)	>4

The AO system is very detailed and specific describing the anatomical fractures. However, it is a difficult system to quantify in the middle of the night when an emergency room physician is calling over the phone. Therefore, Dr. Paul Anderson has developed what he describes as a more practical anatomical approach, "Cervical Spine Injury Severity Score." It quantifies stability using a four-column analog analysis. The spine is divided into four columns, the anterior column, the posterior column, and then both left and right pillars, which include the pedicle and the lateral mass. The analog point scoring relates to the amount of comminution and displacement of the bone fragments in that particular column and ranges from 0 to 5. The four columns are then totaled with a maximum score being 20. If the total is above 7, then surgery is usually indicated; if below 7, nonoperative care is most appropriate. Dr. Anderson's severity score has been validated, as you can see in the slides, correlating to both treatment and neurological status.

References

1. AB BDS, Winter RB et al (1977) Surgical stabilization of fracture and fracture-dislocations of the thoracic spine. Spine 2:185–196
2. Anderson S, Biros MH, Reardon RF (1996) Delayed diagnosis of thoracolumbar fractures in multiple-trauma patients. Acad Emerg Med 3(9):832–839
3. Andriacchi T, Schultz A, Belytschko T, Galante J (1974) A model for studies of mechanical interactions between the human spine and rib cage. J Biomech 7(6):497–507
4. Bohlman HH (1985) Treatment of fractures and dislocations of the thoracic and lumbar spine. J Bone Joint Surg Am 67(1):165–169
5. Bohlman H, Freehafer A, Dejak J (1985) The results of treatment of acute injuries of the upper thoracic spine with paralysis. J Bone Joint Surg Am 67(3):360–369
6. Bracken M (1991) Treatment of acute spinal cord injury with methylprednisolone: results of a multicenter, randomized clinical trial. J Neurotrauma 8(suppl 1):S47–S50; discussion S51–S42
7. Bracken M (1993) Pharmacological treatment of acute spinal cord injury: current status and future projects. J Emerg Med 11(suppl 1):43–48
8. Bracken M (2000) Methylprednisolone and spinal cord injury. J Neurosurg 93(1 Suppl):175–179
9. Bracken M (2001) High dose methylprednisolone must be given for 24 or 48 hours after acute spinal cord injury. BMJ 322(7290):862–863
10. Bracken M (2001) Methylprednisolone and acute spinal cord injury: an update of the randomized evidence. Spine 26(24 suppl):S47–S54
11. Bracken M (2002) Methylprednisolone and spinal cord injury. J Neurosurg 96(1 suppl):140–141; author reply 142
12. Bracken M, Collins W, Freeman D et al (1984) Efficacy of methylprednisolone in acute spinal cord injury. JAMA 251(1):45–52
13. Bracken M, Shepard M, Collins W et al (1990) A randomized, controlled trial of methylprednisolone or naloxone in the treatment of acute spinal-cord injury. Results of the Second National Acute Spinal Cord Injury Study. N Engl J Med 322(20):1405–1411
14. Bracken M, Shepard M, Collins WJ et al (1992) Methylprednisolone or naloxone treatment after acute spinal cord injury: 1-year follow-up data. Results of the second National Acute Spinal Cord Injury Study. J Neurosurg 76(1):23–31
15. Bracken M, Shepard M, Hellenbrand K et al (1985) Methylprednisolone and neurological function 1 year after spinal cord injury. Results of the National Acute Spinal Cord Injury Study. J Neurosurg 63(5):704–713
16. Bracken M, Shepard M, Holford T et al (1998) Methylprednisolone or tirilazad mesylate administration after acute spinal cord injury: 1-year follow up. Results of the third National Acute Spinal Cord Injury randomized controlled trial. J Neurosurg 89(5):699–706
17. Day B, Kokan P (1977) Compression fractures of the thoracic and lumbar spine from compensable injuries. Clin Orthop Relat Res 124:173–176

18. Denis F (1984) Spinal instability as defined by the three-column spine concept in acute spinal trauma. Clin Orthop Relat Res 189:65–76

19. Dickson JH, Harrington PR, Erwin WD (1978) Results of reduction and stabilization of the severely fractured thoracic and lumbar spine. J Bone Joint Surg Am 60(6):799–805

20. Edwards CC, Levine AM (1986) Early rod-sleeve stabilization of the injured thoracic and lumbar spine. Orthop Clin North Am 17(1):121–145

21. Esses SI (1988) The placement and treatment of thoracolumbar spine fractures. An algorithmic approach. Orthop Rev 17(6):571–584

22. Ferguson RL, Allen BL Jr (1984) A mechanistic classification of thoracolumbar spine fractures. Clin Orthop Relat Res 189:77–88

23. Flesch JR, Leider LL, Erickson DL, Chou SN, Bradford DS (1977) Harrington instrumentation and spine fusion for unstable fractures and fracture-dislocations of the thoracic and lumbar spine. J Bone Joint Surg Am 59(2): 143–153

24. Gertzbein SD, Court-Brown CM (1989) Rationale for the management of flexion-distraction injuries of the thoracolumbar spine based on a new classification. J Spinal Disord 2(3):176–183

25. Harkonen M, Kataja M, Lepisto P, Paakkala T, Patiala H, Rokkanen P (1979) Fractures of the thoracic spine. Clinical and radiological results in 98 patients. Arch Orthop Trauma Surg 94(3):179–184

26. Harma M, Heliovaara M, Aromaa A, Knekt P (1986) Thoracic spine compression fractures in Finland. Clin Orthop Relat Res 205:188–194

27. Holdsworth F (1970) Fractures, dislocations, and fracture-dislocations of the spine. J Bone Joint Surg Am 52(8): 1534–1551

28. Hurlbert R (2000) Methylprednisolone for acute spinal cord injury: an inappropriate standard of care. J Neurosurg 93 (1 Suppl):1–7

29. Jacobs RR, Asher MA, Snider RK (1980) Thoracolumbar spinal injuries. A comparative study of recumbent and operative treatment in 100 patients. Spine 5(5):463–477

30. Jacobs RR, Casey MP (1984) Surgical management of thoracolumbar spinal injuries. General principles and controversial considerations. Clin Orthop Relat Res 189:22–35

31. Levine A, Bosse M, Edwards C (1988) Bilateral facet dislocations in the thoracolumbar spine. Spine 13(6):630–640

32. Lucas M, Berg E (1997) Unilateral thoracic facet dislocation. Clin Orthop Relat Res 335:162–165

33. Magerl F, Aebi M, Gertzbein SD, Harms J, Nazarian S (1994) A comprehensive classification of thoracic and lumbar injuries. Eur Spine J 3(4):184–201

34. Maiman DJ, Pintar FA (1992) Anatomy and clinical biomechanics of the thoracic spine. Clin Neurosurg 38:296–324

35. Maiman D, Pintar F (1992) Anatomy and clinical biomechanics of the thoracic spine. Clin Neurosurg 38:296–324

36. McAfee PC, Yuan HA, Fredrickson BE, Lubicky JP (1983) The value of computed tomography in thoracolumbar fractures. An analysis of one hundred consecutive cases and a new classification. J Bone Joint Surg Am 65(4):461–473

37. McCormack T, Karaikovic E, Gaines R (1994) The load sharing classification of spine fractures. Spine 19(15):1741–1744

38. Meyer PR Jr (1986) Posterior stabilization of thoracic, lumbar, and sacral injuries. Instr Course Lect 35:401–419

39. Scher AT (1983) Associated sternal and spinal fractures. Case reports. S Afr Med J 64(3):98–100

40. Sutherland CJ, Miller F, Wang GJ (1983) Early progressive kyphosis following compression fractures. Two case reports from a series of "stable" thoracolumbar compression fractures. Clin Orthop Relat Res 173:216–220

41. Vaccaro A, Lehman RJ, Hurlbert R et al (2005) A new classification of thoracolumbar injuries: the importance of injury morphology, the integrity of the posterior ligamentous complex, and neurologic status. Spine 30(20): 2325–2333

42. Vaccaro A, Zeiller S, Hulbert R et al (2005) The thoracolumbar injury severity score: a proposed treatment algorithm. J Spinal Disord Tech 18(3):209–215

43. Weitzman G (1971) Treatment of stable thoracolumbar spine compression fractures by early ambulation. Clin Orthop Relat Res 76:116–122

44. White AA 3rd, Panjabi MM, Posner I, Edwards WT, Hayes WC (1981) Spinal stability: evaluation and treatment. Instr Course Lect 30:457–483

45. White AA III, Panjabi MM, Thomas CL (1977) The clinical biomechanics of kyphotic deformities. Clin Orthop Relat Res 128:8–17

46. Whitesides TE Jr (1977) Traumatic kyphosis of the thoracolumbar spine. Clin Orthop Relat Res 128:78–92

47. Young MH (1973) Long-term consequences of stable fractures of the thoracic and lumbar vertebral bodies. J Bone Joint Surg Br 55(2):295–300

Anterior Corpectomy with Fixation, Thoracic

19

Peter G. Whang, Jonathan N. Grauer,
and Alexander R. Vaccaro

19.1 Case Example

A 56-year-old female was involved in a motor vehicle collision at which time she sustained an injury to her spine. The patient presented to the emergency department where she complained of axial pain in her lower thoracic region as well as bilateral leg pain and paresthesias. The patient's initial physical examination revealed focal tenderness to palpation over her distal thoracic spine with no palpable step-off as well as decreased sensation and subjective weakness in both lower extremities. Anteroposterior (AP) and lateral radiographs demonstrated a burst fracture involving the T12 vertebral body, which was associated with approximately 50% height loss and 50% canal compromise as evident on sagittal and axial CT images, respectively (Fig. 19.1a–c); however, a subsequent magnetic resonance imaging (MRI) study did not exhibit any findings consistent with frank disruption of the posterior ligaments (Fig. 19.1d, e). Given the inherent instability of the spinal column and the risk of neurologic decline secondary to ongoing compression of the thecal sac, the decision was made to proceed with a T12 corpectomy and anterior thoracic fusion from T11 to L1 with a stand-alone construct consisting of a titanium expandable cage and anterior instrumentation (Fig. 19.1f, g).

P.G. Whang (✉) and J.N. Grauer
Department of Orthopaedics and Rehabilitation,
Yale University School of Medicine,
208071, New Haven, CT 06520-8071, USA
e-mail: peter.whang@yale.edu

A.R. Vaccaro
Departments of Orthopaedic Surgery and Neurological Surgery,
Thomas Jefferson University and The Rothman Institute,
925 Chestnut Street, 5th Floor, Philadelphia, PA 19107, USA

19.2 Background

It has been estimated that nearly 90% of all spinal fractures involve the thoracic or lumbar regions of the vertebral column [6]. Because the motion segments between T11 and L2 that comprise the thoracolumbar junction represent the transitional zone between the rigid, kyphotic thoracic spine and the more flexible, lordotic lumbar vertebrae, these levels are subjected to greater biomechanical forces during a traumatic event and are therefore more susceptible to injury. Despite the additional stability afforded by the rib cage and the coronal orientation of the zygoapophyseal joints, fractures affecting the thoracic spine regularly give rise to catastrophic neurologic injuries as a result of the smaller canal to cord ratio as well as the vascular watershed that exists in this area.

The accurate diagnosis and successful management of thoracic spinal injuries are contingent upon the results of a comprehensive neurologic assessment and pertinent imaging studies, which may be utilized to evaluate the integrity of the various bony and soft tissue structures that serve to maintain spinal stability. Although the majority of thoracic fractures that are not associated with any neurologic compromise or instability are often effectively treated with immobilization and early ambulation, any patients with radiographic evidence of progressive deformity, disruption of the posterior ligaments, or symptomatic impingement of the spinal cord or nerve roots may benefit from operative intervention [10]. Surgery is frequently performed to impart immediate stability to the spinal column, correct any posttraumatic deformities, and facilitate neurologic recovery by addressing any ongoing compression of the neural elements. While the indications for the operative management of thoracic fractures remain somewhat controversial, multiple reports

V.V. Patel et al. (eds.), *Spine Trauma*,
DOI: 10.1007/978-3-642-03694-1_19, © Springer-Verlag Berlin Heidelberg 2010

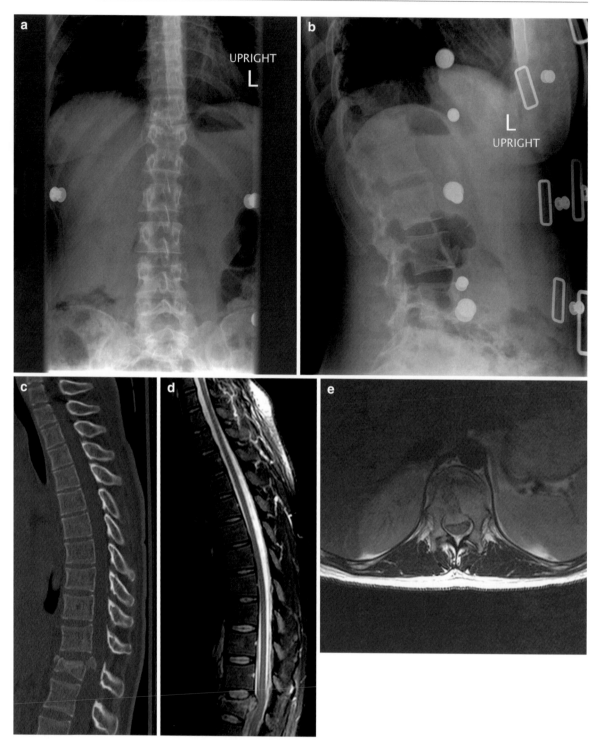

Fig. 19.1 AP (**a**) and lateral (**b**) x-rays demonstrate a compression-type injury of the T12 vertebral body. Sagittal (**c**) CT image reveals a T12 burst fracture with significant height loss and retropulsion of the posterior cortex into the canal but there is no clear evidence of posterior ligamentous disruption present on a subsequent MRI study (**d**, **e**). AP (**f**) and lateral (**g**) radiographs were obtained postoperatively after the patient underwent a T12 corpectomy and arthrodesis procedure with the placement of an expandable titanium implant and anterior instrumentation

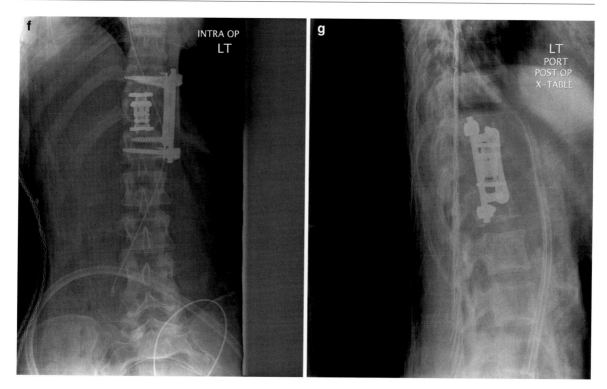

Fig. 19.1 (continued)

have suggested that in many instances these procedures may bring about superior clinical outcomes by allowing for more rapid rehabilitation and avoiding many of the complications inherent to nonoperative care [1, 14]. In particular, individuals with incomplete spinal cord injuries arising from thoracolumbar fractures are more likely to experience more timely improvements in their neurologic deficits following surgery than those who are treated conservatively [8, 10].

At this time, a number of surgical techniques have been described for the decompression and fixation of fractures localizing to the thoracic spine including those that incorporate either anterior, posterior, or circumferential approaches. The ideal operative strategy for a given injury may not always be readily apparent, largely because of the absence of a standardized therapeutic protocol and the paucity of Class I data confirming the superiority of one method over the others. Nevertheless, the process of determining which procedure is most appropriate is typically influenced by several different biomechanical and clinical factors such as the specific fracture pattern, the degree of focal kyphosis, the amount of canal stenosis, and the condition of the posterior ligamentous complex as noted on imaging

studies; the neurologic status of the patient; and the presence of other signs or symptoms of frank instability. Furthermore, the surgical plan may also be dictated by any significant medical comorbidities or concomitant traumatic injuries. Regardless of which approach is selected, the goals of operative intervention are ultimately the same: stabilization of the spinal column, restoration of physiologic alignment in the sagittal and coronal planes, optimization of neurologic function, relief of axial pain, and expedited rehabilitation.

19.3 Indications and Advantages

In most patients with thoracic spine fractures, encroachment of the spinal cord is usually attributed to retropulsed fragments of bone and soft tissue that have been displaced posteriorly into the spinal canal. Consequently, an anterior procedure may be beneficial for cases where there is critical stenosis (i.e., a decrease in total cross-sectional area of least 67%) resulting in an incomplete neurologic deficit because this strategy provides an unimpeded view of the spinal canal for the purpose of decompressing the contents of the thecal sac [7]. Anterior reconstructive techniques that entail the placement of interbody grafts or load-sharing instrumentation are also indispensable for fractures exhibiting substantial comminution or kyphosis greater than 30°, both of which are known risk factors for pseudarthrosis and worsening deformity [9, 13]. While certain burst injuries may be amenable to indirect reduction using posterior distraction and ligamentotaxis, this maneuver is less successful when performed more than 4 days after the injury has occurred [5]; thus, if surgical treatment is not initiated promptly for these fractures, an anterior operation may be more expedient for addressing any residual impingement of the neural elements. In these situations, anterior decompression and arthrodesis have been shown to be effective methods for alleviating chronic pain and enhancing neurologic outcomes even when these operations are delayed for as long as several years after the original traumatic event [2]. Fractures of multiple bony fixation points, undersized pedicles, or any other circumstances that do not permit the safe insertion of posterior instrumentation may also dictate that a thoracic injury should be managed anteriorly. Finally, the removal of any extruded disk material may be best achieved though a thoracotomy. Additionally, the combination of anterior lumbar support with a cage and anterior fixation allows for shorter segment fusion that may then be necessary if posterior fixation alone is used.

19.4 Contraindications and Disadvantages

Stand-alone anterior reconstructions normally do not confer sufficient stability to thoracic fractures that involve the posterior ligamentous complex because this tension band limits the distractive forces across the injured segment, which may otherwise lead to the development of a nonunion. For example, the introduction of an intervertebral device alone may not be suitable for many chance injuries or fracture–dislocations, which often require a posterior-based procedure in order to acquire a stable reduction and subsequent arthrodesis of the spinal column. Anterior techniques should be employed judiciously in patients with osteoporosis who may be predisposed to graft settling and hardware loosening secondary to a mismatch between the modulus of elasticity of the vertebral body and

that of the more rigid implant. Since the posterior epidural space is not accessible from an anterior exposure of the thoracic spine, it is generally not feasible to evacuate compressive hematomas, repair symptomatic durotomies, or extract trapped nerve roots with this approach. Aside from its propensity for prolonging surgical times and increasing blood loss, a thoracotomy may be too hazardous to attempt in the setting of preexisting pulmonary disease or other concurrent traumatic injuries to the chest where opening the thoracic cavity may prove to be life-threatening.

19.5 Procedure

19.5.1 Equipment Needed

- Preoperative imaging studies – X-rays, CT, and MRI
- Intraoperative imaging modality – plain radiography vs. fluoroscopy, surgical navigation (if available)
- Electrophysiologic neuromonitoring system
- Thoracotomy retractor
- Basic spinal instruments – Penfield dissector, Kerrison/Leksell/pituitary rongeurs, periosteal elevator, osteotomes, curettes, and lamina spreader
- High-speed burr
- Bipolar electrocautery and thrombostatic agents
- Interbody implant – autograft, allograft, and metal/synthetic devices
- Anterior instrumentation
- Thoracostomy tube
- Vascular repair set (back up)
- Posterior spinal instrumentation/fusion equipment as needed.

19.5.2 Anesthetic and Neuromonitoring Considerations

Since many thoracic fractures are observed in conjunction with other serious traumatic injuries to the chest, abdomen, and extremities, it is essential that the medical and general surgical services are consulted to clear these individuals for an anterior spinal operation. In preparation for the administration of general anesthesia, the patient is intubated while lying supine on a radiolucent operating room table. For injuries requiring a thoraco-tomy approach, the placement of a double-lumen endo-tracheal tube is recommended so that the ipsilateral lung may be selectively deflated to broaden the exposure of the vertebral column. Intraoperative recordings of soma-tosensory and transcranial electric motor-evoked poten-tials provide real-time electrophysiologic data that is useful for assessing the status of neurologic structures such that any documented deterioration in these signals may be indicative of an acute insult to the spinal cord. Although we believe that these modalities are manda-tory for any individual with either a normal neurologic examination or an incomplete deficit, it may even be worthwhile to monitor upper extremities signals in those with a complete spinal cord injury in an effort to reduce the incidence of an intraoperative neuropraxia.

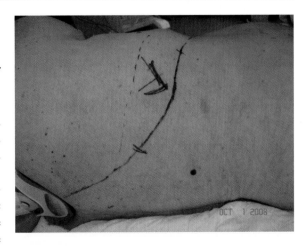

Fig. 19.2 Preoperative photograph of a patient secured in the left lateral position with the intended skin incision required for a thoracotomy exposure

19.5.3 Patient Positioning and Room Setup

Strict compliance with spinal precautions must be adhered to during all transfers as a preventative measure against any iatrogenic neurologic injuries, especially when handling an individual with a grossly unstable fracture. Depending upon the side from which the tho-racic spine will be approached, the patient is carefully logrolled into the right or left lateral decubitus position and secured with an inflatable beanbag or multiple exter-nal bolsters (Fig. 19.2). By centering the injured seg-ment over the break in the table, a flexion moment may be applied to the apex of the deformity, which not only improves the exposure by enlarging the intercostal spaces but also distracts the fracture site prior to the implantation of an intervertebral graft. An axillary cush-ion is situated beneath the chest wall to safeguard the neurovascular structures of the dependent shoulder while the upper extremity ipsilateral to the thoracotomy incision is supported on a Mayo stand. The hips and knees should be maintained in slight flexion and all bony prominences should be adequately padded to minimize any compression of peripheral nerves and avoid exces-sive pressure on the skin. Before proceeding any further, it may be prudent to acquire a series of preliminary fluo-roscopic images to localize the fracture and ensure that unobscured views of the vertebral column may be obtained in both the AP and lateral planes. Because of the considerable amount of bleeding that may be

encountered with these types of injuries, many surgeons may also elect to utilize a cell saver device when address-ing thoracic fractures through an anterior approach.

19.5.4 Surgical Approach

While the majority of thoracic injuries may be approached through either side of the chest cavity, it may be advantageous to perform a left-sided thoraco-tomy for fractures involving the thoracolumbar junction (i.e., between T11 and L4) in order to bypass the liver as well as the inferior vena cava, which is more difficult to dissect away from the spinal column than the adjacent aorta. The entire flank region is sterilely prepped and draped, making sure to include the iliac crest if a struc-tural autograft is to be implanted. An oblique incision extending from the anterior chest to the posterior ele-ments is developed through the skin and subcutaneous tissues in line with a rib that is typically one or two lev-els cephalad to the fractured vertebra (Fig. 19.3). The intercostal musculature is gently mobilized from the rib in a subperiosteal fashion without violating the travers-ing nerve and blood vessels within the subcostal groove. Even though it is frequently possible to achieve a satis-factory exposure of the injured segment by simply opening the intercostal space, the visualization of the thoracic spine may be improved even further if the intervening rib is excised in which case it must be dislo-cated from both the sternum and the transverse process

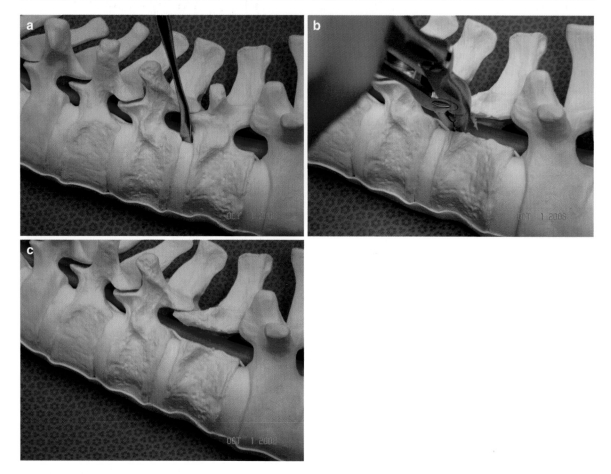

Fig. 19.3 In this model, a Penfield dissector has been placed in the neuroforamen (**a**) to facilitate the excision of the transverse process and pedicle with a Kerrison rongeur (**b**) so that the contents of the spinal canal may be clearly visualized (**c**)

before it is removed. After a self-retaining retractor has been placed between the ribs to expand the thoracotomy incision, the ipsilateral lung is deflated for the remainder of the procedure. For fractures of the lower thoracic spine or thoracolumbar junction, which may require the diaphragm to be detached from the chest wall, a circumferential rim of tissue measuring at least 1 cm in length should be maintained and tagged with stay sutures to facilitate a meticulous repair of this critical structure.

Through a thoracotomy approach, a surgeon should have access to several convex disks and concave vertebral bodies (i.e., "hills" and "valleys," respectively) of the thoracic spine. The bony fragments of the fracture ordinarily give rise to a palpable step-off, but in situations where there is any uncertainty regarding the location of the injured segment the various levels of the spine may be accurately identified by placing a needle within one of the disk spaces and verifying its position

with an intraoperative imaging study. The iliopsoas muscle is subsequently elevated and retracted posteriorly away from the fracture site. As a final step, the layer of parietal pleura overlying the spinal column is divided and the segmental vessels situated over the midportion of each vertebra are carefully ligated to reduce the risk of excessive bleeding during the ensuing portions of the operation. Excessive ligation of the segments should also be avoided to maintain spinal cord perfusion.

19.5.5 Thoracic Corpectomy and Decompression of Neural Structures

The transverse process and pedicle of the disrupted vertebra are identified by separating the remnants of the rib head from the costotransverse articulation. The borders of the pedicle are palpated by inserting a Penfield dissector into the neuroforamen; using the Penfield as a soft tissue retractor, the entire pedicle is eradicated with a high-speed burr and a Kerrison rongeur all the way to its junction with the posterior aspect of the vertebral body so that the anterior and lateral margins of the spinal canal may be fully visualized (Fig. 19.4). Diskectomies are completed adjacent to the fractured segment by incising the anulus fibrosis with a scalpel and removing the nucleus pulposus with a rongeur (Fig. 19.5). Once this tissue has been cleared from the disk space, the cartilage from the end plates

may be stripped with a curette or periosteal elevator to reveal the underlying bony surfaces.

As the initial step of the corpectomy, the more sizable pieces of bone are extracted from the fracture site with an osteotome, rongeur, or burr so that they may be set aside for later use as autogenous graft for the subsequent arthrodesis (Fig. 19.6). With an angled curette, any retropulsed fragments within the spinal canal may be mobilized away from the thecal sac and swept anteriorly into the space created by the corpectomy. Whenever possible, the anterior cortex of the body with its associated ligamentous attachments should be maintained in order to increase the stability of the spinal column and prevent

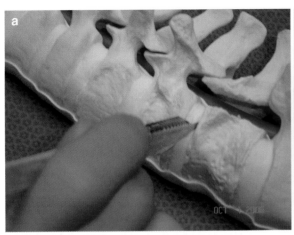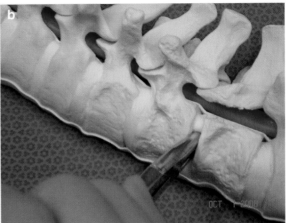

Fig. 19.4 Diskectomies are performed adjacent to the fractured segment by incising the anulus fibrosis at each level (**a**) and extracting the nucleus pulposus tissue with a rongeur (**b**)

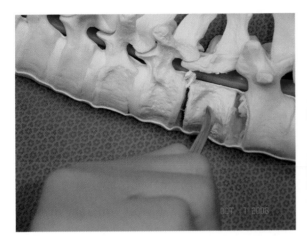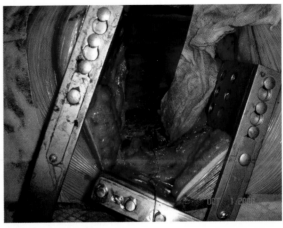

Fig. 19.5 The fractured vertebra is split with an osteotome so that the bony fragments may be safely removed in order to decompress the neural elements

Fig. 19.6 Intraoperative photograph demonstrating the defect that exists between the vertebral bodies following the completion of the corpectomy

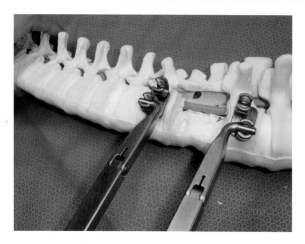

Fig. 19.7 Any deformity in the sagittal plane may be addressed by using anterior instrumentation to apply distractive forces across the injured segment

graft dislodgement. The vertebrectomy is continued laterally to the level of the contralateral pedicle to confirm that the spinal cord and nerve roots are thoroughly decompressed with no residual impingement of the dural tube (Fig. 19.7).

19.5.6 Reduction Technique

The normal sagittal alignment of the spinal column may be restored by performing a variety of reduction maneuvers. For instance, manual pressure on the posterior spine at the level of the fracture may diminish any focal kyphosis that may be present. Additional deformity correction may also be accomplished by placing a lamina

spreader within the corpectomy defect. In patients with supplemental anterior instrumentation spanning the injured segment, a reduction may be effected by applying distraction directly across the construct (Fig. 19.8). Also remember, if a bump was placed or the table was extended to laterally flex the patient and facilitate exposure, these should be corrected and the spine aligned in the coronal and sagittal planes prior to fixation.

19.5.7 Placement of Interbody Graft

Autogenous bone is still largely the "gold standard" for anterior thoracic reconstructions because a tricortical piece procured from the iliac crest is currently the only substance that delivers all of the elements that are obligatory for an intervertebral fusion, that is, stem cells with osteoblastic potential, osteoinductive growth factors, and an osteoconductive scaffold that promotes cellular adhesion and neovascularization. Since the morbidity associated with the harvesting of structural autograft is not insignificant, a number of alternative techniques have been advocated including allogeneic bone, expandable metal cages, and other devices consisting of synthetic materials such as carbon fiber or polyetheretherketone (i.e., PEEK). Even though all of these implants are generally able to withstand the substantial biomechanical forces that exist within the spinal column, none of these options provide any type of meaningful osteogenic signal when inserted alone; not surprisingly, these interbody spacers are virtually always filled with bony fragments from the corpectomy, demineralized bone matrices,

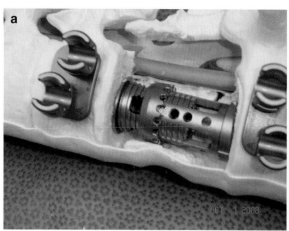

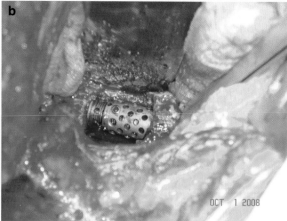

Fig. 19.8 Insertion of a metal expandable cage within the corpectomy defect as seen in a model (**a**) and an intraoperative photograph (**b**)

recombinant human bone morphogenetic proteins, or other commercially available products designed to augment the fusion response. However, the relative safety and efficacy of each of these methods have not yet been established by any randomized, controlled clinical studies so the ideal bone-grafting strategy for the treatment of thoracic injuries remains a matter of some debate.

At this point it is important to confirm once again that the cartilaginous end plates have been abraded to generate bleeding surfaces that may serve as a vascular supply to stimulate graft incorporation. While the implant may be seated within slots that have been fashioned in each vertebral body, the supporting layers of subchondral bone must be left intact to limit progressive settling of the construct. Once the intervertebral space has been prepared, an appropriately sized strut graft containing cancellous bone is inserted into the corpectomy defect under direct visualization so that the neural elements and the neighboring vascular structures are free of any compression (Fig. 19.9). The spinal column may be provisionally stabilized by loosening any intersegmental distraction and removing the break in the operating room table.

19.5.8 Fixation Technique

In recent years, more surgeons have elected to employ adjunctive internal fixation in the anterior thoracic spine in an attempt to enhance fusion rates and decrease the incidence of adverse events such as graft displacement or subsidence. By increasing the rigidity of the reconstructed levels, the implementation of these instrumentation techniques often precludes the need to perform a concomitant posterior arthrodesis such that it may be feasible to address various thoracic fractures through an anterior approach alone.

The "safe zone" for this hardware is restricted to the posterolateral aspect of the vertebral bodies so that they do not encroach upon the more anteriorly located aorta and vena cava. Any osteophytes or end plate abnormalities should be removed with a pituitary rongeur or high-speed burr to minimize the profile of the construct. The holes for the transverse screws or bolts are developed by passing an awl or drill across the contiguous vertebral bodies without penetrating the uninvolved disk spaces. Biomechanical studies have suggested that

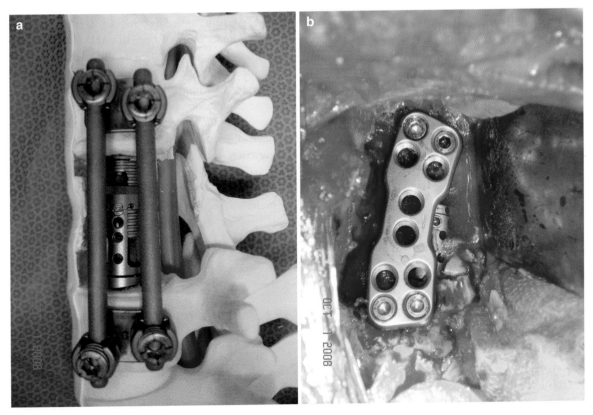

Fig. 19.9 Anterior instrumented constructs depicted in a model (**a**) and an intraoperative photograph (**b**) using dual rods and a plate, respectively

bicortical implants demonstrate significantly greater resistance to failure than those that only engage the near cortex [4]; nevertheless, the tips of these implants must not extend more than a few millimeters into the chest cavity to avoid any injury to the great vessels. Although an accurate estimate of the approximate screw lengths necessary to attain bicortical purchase may be derived from preoperative axial images of the thoracic vertebrae, the positioning of the internal fixation should be assessed with intraoperative X-rays or multiplanar fluoroscopy to verify that the hardware is not too long and does not violate either of the adjoining intervertebral disks. The screws or bolts are connected with a plate or rods, which may be used to administer additional compression across the strut graft prior to final tightening of the instrumentation with a single rod, it may be advisable to consider performing an adjunctive posterior fusion to support this construct.

19.5.9 Closure

At the completion of the procedure, the entire surgical site is copiously irrigated and any significant bleeding from the bone or surrounding soft tissues may be managed with bipolar electrocautery and hemostatic agents such as thrombin-soaked gelfoam or other vascular sealants. The parietal pleura lining is reapproximated and any defects in the diaphragm are addressed with an anatomic repair. A chest tube is normally utilized postoperatively and is immediately placed on suction to eliminate any collections of fluid or air within the thoracic cavity. The collapsed lung is reinflated by the anesthesiologist and the rib retractor is withdrawn from the intercostal space. The remaining layers of the wound are securely closed to establish a tight seal over the thoracotomy incision.

19.6 Technical Pearls and Pitfalls

19.6.1 Pearls: Decompression

- The use of a microscope or loupe magnification is strongly recommended for anterior thoracic procedures because adequate lighting and magnification

may facilitate a safe and thorough decompression of the thecal sac.
- One method of enhancing the visualization of the spinal column is to change the orientation of the operating room table as needed during the various steps of the corpectomy and arthrodesis. However, when inserting anterior instrumentation it may be helpful to return the patient to the true lateral decubitus position to reestablish a proper frame of reference for the surgeon and reduce the incidence of misdirected implants.
- It may be easier to address fractures of the thoracolumbar junction through a left-sided exposure because this approach avoids the liver and entails less manipulation of the inferior vena cava, which is more susceptible to injury than the aorta.
- With most thoracic fractures, the greatest amount of spinal cord compression characteristically occurs adjacent to the pedicles; thus, in these situations it may be preferable to excise the inferior portions of the vertebral body first since the interval between the bony fragments and the dura is larger at this level.
- Whenever possible, the posterior cortex of the disrupted vertebra should be preserved to protect the neural elements from inadvertent injury as the fracture fragments are being removed. Similarly, retaining an intact layer of cortical bone anteriorly will not only increase the stability of the reconstructed segment but also prohibit any gross displacement of the interbody implant.
- In addition to incorporating both intervertebral disks, the corpectomy must span the entire width of the interpedicular space to ensure that there is no residual encroachment upon the spinal cord or nerve roots.
- The posterior longitudinal ligament will usually protrude evenly into the vertebrectomy site once the underlying dural tube is free of any compression and if this is not the case, this structure should be incised so that any extruded bone or disk resulting in residual stenosis may be extracted from the spinal canal.

19.6.2 Pearls: Interbody Fusion

- The integrity of the vertebral bodies must be maintained when scraping the cartilaginous end plates or creating grooves to accommodate the graft because any violation of the subchondral bone may lead to progressive subsidence of the construct.

- Increasing the size of the interbody implant that is introduced into the corpectomy defect allows for improved load sharing, which augments the stability of the spinal segment and minimizes the incidence of graft complications such as pseudarthrosis and migration. Likewise, securing the graft more anteriorly between the vertebrae may also yield greater deformity correction in the sagittal plane.
- Structural autograft or allograft struts may be more appropriate for patients with osteoporosis because cages or spacers comprised of metal, carbon fiber, or PEEK may exhibit an unacceptable degree of settling when these types of synthetic devices are utilized in osteopenic bone as a result of the considerable disparity that exists between their moduli of elasticity.

19.6.3 Pearls: Anterior Instrumentation

- Stand-alone anterior reconstructions may be suitable for certain fractures of the thoracic spine but individuals with radiographic signs of posterior instability (e.g., translation in the coronal or sagittal planes, loss of vertebral body height >50%, focal kyphosis >30°, or evidence of significant posterior ligamentous injury on MR images) who undergo an anterior decompression and instrumented arthrodesis may require posterior fixation as well in an effort to reestablish the normal tension band of the spine.
- Anterior instrumentation is ordinarily positioned along the posterolateral aspect of the spinal column to lower the risk of injury to the great vessels; for this reason, it is important to detach any degenerative osteophytes or bony prominences from these vertebral bodies so that these implants may lie flush again this surface.
- Intraoperative imaging modalities such as plain radiography or fluoroscopy may be useful for guiding the placement of screws so that they do not perforate the intact disk spaces that are cephalad and caudal to the intended arthrodesis.
- A bicortical technique is often advocated for these constructs because it provides greater fixation within the vertebrae; however, it is imperative that the screws do not project more than a few threads past the second cortex because of the potential for acute or delayed vascular complications.

- While a single anterior rod connection may be sufficient when included as part of a circumferential fusion, a dual rod or plate system is preferable for stand-alone constructs that may benefit from the added stability.

19.6.4 Potential Intraoperative Complications

Aside from the morbidity related to a thoracotomy exposure (e.g., pulmonary dysfunction) and the inherent hazards to visceral and vascular structures associated with this approach, anterior thoracic procedures may give rise to a number of serious intraoperative complications. Even though an anterior corpectomy affords greater visualization of the contents of the spinal canal compared to posterior interventions, iatrogenic neurologic injuries or durotomies may still occur during the decompression of these fractures. Any insults to the spinal cord that are suspected either clinically or detected as a result of changes in electrophysiologic signals may warrant the initiation of vasopressor therapy to elevate the mean arterial blood pressure and improve tissue perfusion, reversal of any reduction maneuvers that may have been performed, and the administration of corticosteroids according to the National Acute Spinal Cord Injury Study III protocol if indicated [3]. The customary treatment for dural tears is primary repair, but if a watertight seal is unable to be attained, then these defects should also be augmented with fibrin glue and some type of patch material; postoperatively, persistent cerebrospinal fluid leaks may even require that an indwelling subarachnoid catheter be passed into the lumbar spine to diminish the pressure within the thecal sac so that a secure closure may be achieved. Profuse bleeding from the bony fragments or the epidural space may also be encountered throughout the course of the operation and should be addressed with bipolar cautery, hemostatic agents such as bone wax or thrombin-soaked gelfoam, and prompt resuscitation with intravenous fluids and blood products. Depending upon its location, malpositioned anterior thoracic instrumentation may also have grave consequences if it penetrates any of the various neurologic, vascular, or visceral structures in close proximity to the spinal column.

19.6.5 Bailout/Salvage for Failed Procedures

If a satisfactory decompression of the neural elements cannot be obtained through an anterior approach or the disrupted spinal column is not able to be adequately stabilized with a stand-alone interbody construct, it may be necessary to perform a subsequent posterior laminectomy or instrumented fusion as well in order to successfully accomplish these goals.

19.7 Postoperative Considerations

19.7.1 Bracing

Although a thoracic orthosis would be expected to restrict segmental motion at the levels of interest, there are still no randomized, controlled studies confirming that postoperative immobilization translates into meaningful improvements in either arthrodesis rates or clinical outcomes. Despite the lack of compelling data corroborating the utility of bracing regimens, many surgeons may elect to employ an external appliance for several weeks or even months after the procedure based on multiple factors including the severity of the original fracture, the use of internal fixation, and the presence of any patient comorbidities that may have detrimental effects on bone formation (e.g., osteoporosis and ongoing consumption of tobacco products).

19.7.2 Activity

Taking into account any concomitant traumatic injuries, individuals undergoing anterior thoracic interventions should be evaluated and treated by the physical therapy staff as quickly as possible to expedite their gait training because early ambulation may prevent many of the adverse events associated with protracted bed rest such as pneumonia, deep venous thrombosis (DVT), and decubitus ulcers.

19.7.3 Follow-Up

In addition to regular clinical examinations, standing AP and lateral X-rays of the thoracic spine should be acquired prior to hospital discharge, throughout the immediate postoperative time period, and for at least 1 year after surgery to monitor these patients for coronal or sagittal plane malalignment, graft settling, hardware failure, or any other radiographic signs of pseudarthrosis.

19.7.4 Potential Postoperative Complications

Regardless of whether their spinal injuries are treated conservatively in a rigid orthosis or addressed surgically, individuals with thoracic fractures are at risk for a myriad of medical sequelae such as pulmonary disorders, gastrointestinal ailments (e.g., constipation, ileus, or reflux disease), skin breakdown, and thromboembolic phenomena. In one series of thoracolumbar fractures, the rate of postoperative wound infections following anterior instrumented fusion procedures was reported to be approximately 14% [12]. If the biological or biomechanical conditions present at the host bone–implant interface are not conducive to bony healing, the reconstructed portion of the spinal column may demonstrate progressive collapse or worsening deformity, loss of fixation, or other deleterious effects of an established nonunion.

19.7.5 Treatment of Postoperative Complications

Any concurrent medical issues should be attended to in an expedient manner to eschew the significant morbidities that these patients may experience postoperatively; in particular, the recruitment of a multidisciplinary team may be essential for the proper care of those who have sustained spinal cord injuries as a result of their fractures. According to one investigation, symptomatic DVT or pulmonary embolism is observed in at least 2% in this population, which clearly justifies the implementation of prophylactic measures including the application of lower extremity sequential compression device sleeves, the deployment of a vascular filter in the inferior vena cava, or even the administration of anticoagulable agents (e.g., warfarin and low-molecular weight heparin) [11]. While an initial course of oral or intravenous antibiotics may be an efficacious therapeutic strategy for benign infections, the isolation of more virulent organisms or any involvement of the deeper structures frequently necessitates a formal irrigation and debridement of the skin incision and the entire thoracotomy site. Finally, most patients with stand-alone anterior constructs who display clinical or radiographic findings consistent with a pseudarthrosis are likely to be reasonable candidates for a supplementary posterior thoracic stabilization procedure, which may ultimately promote the formation of a solid arthrodesis across the injured segment.

References

1. Bohlman HH, Freehafer A, Dejak J (1985) The results of treatment of acute injuries of the upper thoracic spine with paralysis. J Bone Joint Surg Am 67:360–369
2. Bohlman HH, Kirkpatrick JS, Delamarter RB et al (1994) Anterior decompression for late pain and paralysis after fractures of the thoracolumbar spine. Clin Orthop Relat Res 300:24–29
3. Bracken MB, Shepard MJ, Horford TR et al (1997) Administration of methylprednisolone for 24-48 hours or tirilized mesylate for 48 hours in the treatment of acute spinal cord injury. Results of the Third National Acute Spinal Cord Injury Randomized Controlled Trial. JAMA 277:1597–1604
4. Breeze SW, Doherty BJ, Noble PS et al (1998) A biomechanical study of anterior thoracolumbar screw fixation. Spine 23:1829–1831
5. Crutcher JP, Anderson PA, King HA et al (1991) Burst fractures of the thoracic and lumbar spine. Clin Orthop Relat Res 3:39–48
6. DeWald RL (1984) Burst fractures of the thoracic and lumbar spine. Clin Orthop Relat Res 189:150–161
7. Esses SI, Botsford DJ, Kostuik JP (1990) Evaluation of surgical treatment for burst fractures. Spine 15:667–673
8. Jacobs RR, Asher MA, Snider RK (1980) Thoracolumbar spinal injuries. A comparative study of recumbent and operative treatment in 100 patients. Spine 5:463–477
9. McCullen G, Vaccaro AR, Garfin SR (1998) Thoracic and lumbar trauma: rationale for selecting the appropriate fusion technique. Orthop Clin North Am 29:813–828
10. McEvoy RD, Bradford DS (1985) The management of burst fractures of the thoracic and lumbar spine. Experience in 53 patients. Spine 10:631–637
11. Platzer P, Thalhammer G, Jaindl M et al (2006) Thromboembolic complications after spinal surgery in trauma patients. Acta Orthop 77:755–760
12. Rechtine GR, Bono PL, Cahill D et al (2001) Postoperative wound infection after instrumentation of thoracic and lumbar fractures. J Orthop Trauma 15:566–569
13. Schnee CL, Ansell LV (1997) Selection criteria and outcome of operative approaches for thoracolumbar burst fractures with and without neurologic deficit. J Neurosurg 86:48–55
14. Wilmot CB, Hall KM (1986) Evaluation of acute surgical intervention in traumatic paraplegia. Paraplegia 24: 71–76

Kyphoplasty, Osteoporotic and Traumatic 20

Yu-Po Lee and Robert A. Keller

20.1 Case Example

A 78-year-old female with a history of osteoporosis presents for evaluation of sudden mid back pain. She was in her usual state of good health when she tripped and fell 6 weeks ago. The fall caused sudden pain and she has since been in a Jewett brace. While her pain is improved slightly, she is still restricted and has pain with activities. The pain is described as a sharp pain in her mid back. The pain is provoked with activity or any changing of positions. Her pain is worsened with prolonged standing and is improved by lying down. Narcotic analgesics help, but she has constipation from taking the medications. Radiographs (Fig. 20.1a, b) and magnetic resonance imaging (MRI) (Fig. 20.2) show a compression fracture at L2.

20.2 Background

Kyphoplasty is a relatively new surgical technique that is used to treat patients with vertebral compression fractures (VCFs). VCFs are the most common type of osteoporotic fracture. They occur when axial and/or bending loads on the vertebral column are larger than the stability and stiffness of the vertebral bodies. The National Osteoporosis Foundation estimates the annual incidence of VCFs from osteoporosis is 700,000 in the USA alone [9]. VCFs are also the most common skeletal complication of metastatic cancer [1]. In addition, 90% of all traumatic fractures occur in the thoracolumbar region, with 66% of these fractures being VCFs [6].

Kyphoplasty is a percutaneous bone cement augmentation technique that is performed with the aim to decrease pain and correct the local kyphosis and height loss caused by the VCFs. This approach is a modification of the vertebroplasty technique, which was first developed in the 1980s. Vertebroplasty and kyphoplasty both employ the use of a transpedicular or extrapedicular needle approach to reach the vertebral body. Where the two approaches differ is that vertebroplasty is a direct percutaneous injection of bone cement (commonly PMMA) into the vertebral body, while kyphoplasty employs an inflatable balloon tamp (IBT) that expands the trabeculae of the vertebral body [2]. This process functions to restore vertebral body height, correct spinal deformities, and create a low-pressure space to inject the bone cement. The entire procedure utilizes fluoroscopic imaging. Kyphoplasty is now used in the treatment of VCFs due to osteoporosis, cancer metastasis, and trauma [10].

20.3 Indications and Advantages for Procedure

Indications

1. Painful osteoporotic VCFs of the thoracic and lumbar spine resulting from primary or secondary osteoporosis.
2. Progressive low-energy osteopenic thoracolumbar VCFs that have occurred in the last 6 months with radiographic evidence of an ongoing fracture.
3. VCFs due to multiple myeloma and other lytic lesions [7, 11].

Y.-P. Lee (✉) and R.A. Keller
UCSD Department of Orthopaedic Surgery,
350 Dickinson Street, Ste 121, San Diego, CA 92103, USA
e-mail: yupo90025@yahoo.com

V.V. Patel et al. (eds.), *Spine Trauma*,
DOI: 10.1007/978-3-642-03694-1_20, © Springer-Verlag Berlin Heidelberg 2010

Fig. 20.1 (**a, b**) Anteroposterior (AP) and lateral radiographs of patient with L2 compression fracture

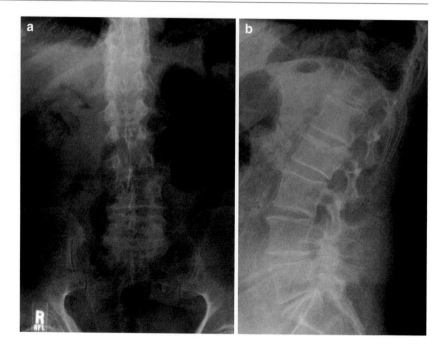

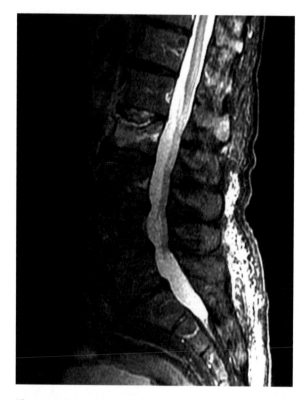

Fig. 20.2 Sagittal STIR MRI view of L2 compression fracture. It is recommended to obtain STIR (short tau inversion recovery) sequences on patients suspected of having acute compression fractures as the edema shows up better on these sequences

4. Traumatic compression fracture in conjunction with posterior pedicle screw fixation.

The advantage of kyphoplasty over vertebroplasty is a decreased incidence of cement leakage since the Polymethylmethacrylate (PMMA) is injected under low pressure, and increased potential for regaining vertebral body height.

20.4 Contraindications and Disadvantages for Procedure

Contraindications

1. Spine infections
2. Coagulopathies
3. Allergies against PMMA or contrast media
4. Burst fractures with significant retropulsion of bone into the spinal canal
5. Vertebral fractures with significant neurologic deficit
6. Solid metastases [11]
7. Relative: T1–T5 fractures if unable to visualize on X-ray

The disadvantage of kyphoplasty is additional equipment, anesthesia, and increased hospital costs [3].

20.5 Procedure

20.5.1 *Equipment Needed* (Fig. 20.3)

- C-arm fluoroscopy machine, ideally biplane fluoroscopy with two C-arms
- Scalpel
- 0.25% Marcaine with epinephrine
- 11-gauge Jamshidi needle
- Guide pin
- Cannula
- Mallet
- Inflatable bone tamp
- Hand held drill and bit
- PMMA, radiopaque contrast, liquid monomer
- 5 cc syringes
- Bone filling device (BFD)
- PMMA mixer
- Suture or Steri-Strip kit

20.5.2 Anesthetic and Neuromonitoring Considerations

General anesthesia or local anesthetic with intravenous sedation may be used for this procedure. Local anesthesia is safe and avoids the risks associated with general anesthesia. Also in case of proximity of the trocar or cement to the nerves, the patient may be able to report radicular pain. The disadvantage is that patients tend to move because of pain felt during certain surgical steps. This pain-induced movement increases the risk of neurologic injury and causes the surgical procedure to be more difficult, which increases the length of the surgery while causing discomfort to the patient. General anesthesia reduces the risk of movement during the procedure, creating surgical conditions, which are safe and comfortable to the patient. The negatives of general anesthesia are the inherent risks of general anesthesia and the recovery associated with it in older patients.

20.5.3 Patient Positioning and Room Setup

The patient is positioned prone, which allows natural extension of the thoracic and lumbar spine and also allows fluoroscopy to produce an image in multiple planes (Fig. 20.4). The use of a Jackson table would best facilitate patient positioning and fluoroscopic views. C-arm fluoroscopy (biplane fluoroscopy is ideal) should be positioned and tested to ensure all-important vertebral land marks can be identified prior to prepping. If the size of the room allows, placing the anteroposterior (AP) and lateral fluoroscopes on opposite sides of the patient facilitates the process.

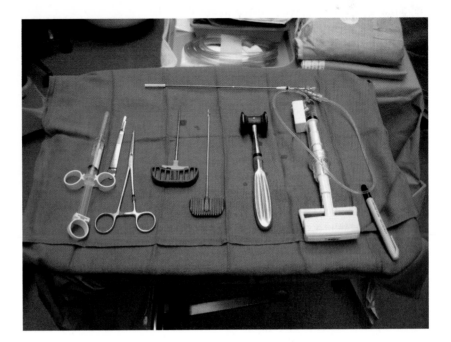

Fig. 20.3 View of instruments used

Fig. 20.4 Patient placed prone on Jackson table. Note how there is nothing underneath the table that may impede obtaining good radiographs

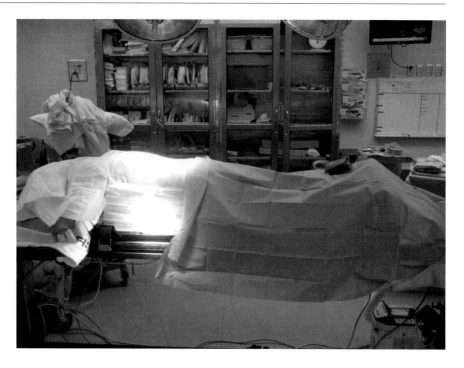

20.5.4 Surgical Approach

The vertebral body may be reached via a transpedicular or extrapedicular approach. One should be able to use a transpedicular approach from T10 to L5. It is more difficult to use a transpedicular approach above T9 due to the decrease in pedicle width in the superior vertebrae. In cases that involve vertebral bodies above T9, an extrapedicular approach may be preferable. The T5 vertebra is typically the most superior vertebra that can be treated with kyphoplasty.

Prior to beginning the procedure, it is important to obtain good AP and lateral images. It can be very difficult sometimes to get a good view of the pedicles in severely affected osteoporotic patients. Also, these patients may have some rotation of their vertebrae secondary to idiopathic or degenerative scoliosis. However, this step is crucial. On the AP view, the spinous process should be centered between the pedicles (Fig. 20.5). Also, the superior and inferior endplates should appear flat, not oval. On the lateral view, the superior and inferior endplates should appear flat and the pedicles should completely overlap (Fig. 20.6). If it is difficult to obtain a good AP image, take a lateral image and line up a guide pin so that it parallels the superior and inferior endplates. Then adjust the AP fluoroscope along this trajectory. Another technique to improve visualization of

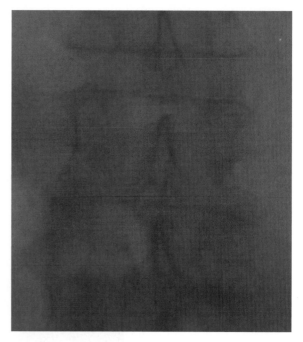

Fig. 20.5 AP view of the fractured L2 vertebra. Ideally, the spinous process should be centered between the pedicles. Also, the superior and inferior endplates should appear flat, not oval

the pedicles is to obtain an *en face* view of the pedicle. This is done by taking a 10° oblique view of the pedicle.

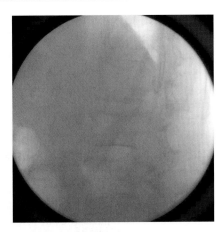

Fig. 20.6 Lateral view of the fractured L2 vertebra. The superior and inferior endplates should appear flat and the pedicles should completely overlap

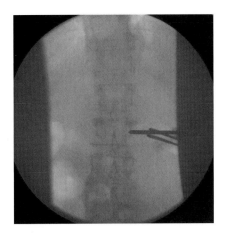

Fig. 20.7 Normally the starting point of the Jamshidi spinal needle should be directed to the superior–lateral corner of the pedicle on AP imaging. However, if the fracture is in the superior plate one should place the needle inferior to the midline to create an entry angle that directs the needle to the superior plane of the vertebral body as shown here

Begin the procedure with a small ~0.5-cm incision that is positioned approximately 1–2 cm lateral to the appropriate pedicle. An injection with 0.25% Marcaine with epinephrine helps to decrease bleeding. An 11-gauge Jamshidi spinal needle should be directed to the superior–lateral corner of the pedicle on AP imaging. If the fracture is in the superior plate one should place the needle inferior to the midline to create an entry angle that directs the needle to the superior plane of the vertebral body (Fig. 20.7). Conversely, if the fracture is in the inferior plate one should place the tool superior to the midline. One must also take the vertebral body height into account for needle placement. If the vertebral body height is 1.5 cm or less the needle should be aimed into the midpoint of the anterior cortex on a lateral view. If the height of the vertebral body is less than 9 mm, it is most likely untreatable with kyphoplasty. Prior to advancing the needle into the pedicle, a lateral view should be used to confirm that the needle is directed toward the vertebral body.

For thoracic VCFs from T9 and above, the pedicle may be too small for a transpedicular approach. In this instance the entry point is immediately superior and lateral to the pedicle, just medial to the rib head (or even through the rib head). With the extrapedicular approach, the pedicle is entered as it connects with the vertebral body slightly laterally. Be careful to not enter the pulmonary cavity laterally or violate the segmental artery inferiorly.

Advance the 11-gauge Jamshidi needle through the pedicle on the AP view. Once the tip of the needle is at the midpoint of the pedicle on the AP view (Fig. 20.8a), check a lateral view. At this point, the tip of the needle

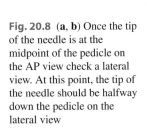

Fig. 20.8 (a, b) Once the tip of the needle is at the midpoint of the pedicle on the AP view check a lateral view. At this point, the tip of the needle should be halfway down the pedicle on the lateral view

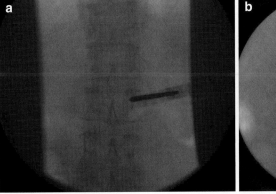

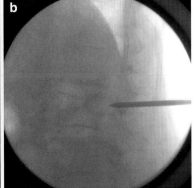

should be halfway down the pedicle on the lateral view (Fig. 20.8b). If it has not reached the midpoint of the pedicle yet, the trajectory is too lateral and needs to be redirected medially. If the tip of the needle is past the midpoint of the pedicle, it is too medial and needs to be redirected laterally. After you have made your adjustments, continue advancing your needle on the AP view until it is 1 mm lateral to the medial border of the pedicle. At this point, the tip of the Jamshidi needle should be 1–2 mm past the posterior cortex of the vertebral body. This ensures that you do not breach the medial wall of the pedicle and reduces the risk of cement extravasation into the canal. Once there, remove the stylet and insert a guide pin down the shaft of the needle until 1–2 mm of the guide pin can be seen on fluoroscopy (lateral view). While holding the guide pin in place, carefully remove the needle. Be sure to check AP and lateral views to assure the guide pin placement is correct. Advance the blunt dissector and cannula over the guide pin. This may require some force. If more force is required, tap it with a mallet gently to avoid fracturing the pedicle. Once again, confirm placement of the blunt dissector with AP and lateral views. Stop the advancement of the blunt dissector and cannula when the tip of the blunt dissector is a few millimeters into the vertebral body. Once the cannula is correctly placed, remove the blunt dissector and place the hand drill down the cannula. Use the drill bit to enter the vertebral body. When the drill is halfway across the vertebral body in the lateral view, one should check the AP view to make sure the drill is not too medial because the spinal cord could be threatened. The correct position is halfway between the pedicle and the spinous process. The final position of the bit should be just posterior to the anterior cortex of the vertebral body and halfway between the superior and inferior endplates. If necessary, angle the cannula to guide the drill to the correct position.

Once the drill has reached its appropriate position, remove it and insert the IBT through the same cannula. Repeat this procedure on the contralateral side. The IBT will be inflated with contrast medium in a dilution of 60% contrast mixed with saline. Once the IBT is in the correct position, inflate the IBT to 1 ml or 150 psi, whichever that comes first, with contrast medium using a manometer with a digital pressure gauge. With the inflation of the balloons, expansion of bone will create a cavity, thus reducing the pressure in the vertebral body. The balloon tamps should be alternately filled until the fracture is reduced or appropriate pressures are reached. As balloon volumes are increased above 2 cc, one should only introduce 0.5 cc or less until an optimal inflation or reduction of the fracture has been achieved (Fig. 20.9a, b). IBT inflation and performance is guided by (1) desired reduction; (2) proximity of IBT to cortical walls as seen by all fluoroscopic views; (3) pressure readings (readings should be below 220 psi as a rule of thumb, but may be higher, even up to 300 psi, if balloon placement is correct and vertebral stability is carefully monitored); (4) maximum rated volumes from the inflation syringe barrel are reached (4 cc for the 15-mm length or 6 cc for the 20-mm length). If any of these are reached, inflation should be stopped. With inflation, always use AP and lateral fluoroscopic views to ensure inflation of similar volumes and correct paths and proximities to cortices are accomplished.

After desired volume and reduction are obtained, deflate the IBT and remove by slowly pulling and rotating. If vertebral body height elevation has occurred, the surgeon may keep one balloon elevated while the other is removed and the cavity is filled with PMMA. Usually the balloon inflated to the higher pressure is left inflated.

Fig. 20.9 (**a**, **b**) As balloon volumes are increased above 2 cc, one should only introduce 0.5 cc or less until an optimal inflation or reduction of the fracture has been achieved. This typically occurs when the balloon abuts against the cortex of the superior endplate or the lateral cortex

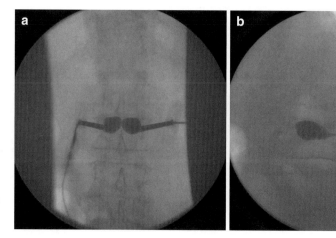

The PMMA should be mixed according to the instructions on the kyphoplasty kit and placed into the BFDs. Each BFD will hold up to 1.5 cc of PMMA. Once the bone cement is of a doughy consistency, it will be able to support the newly created vertebral body height and the other balloon may be removed.

When the vertebra is ready to be filled with bone cement, the BFD is inserted in the cannula to the anterior wall of the vertebral body. Confirm this placement with fluoroscopic views because improper placement can lead to leakage into the spinal canal. The cement cannula stylet is then used to gently push cement into the vertebral body. While pushing cement into the cavity, the cement cannula should be withdrawn to the level of the middle of the cavity. Continue injecting cement until the cavity is completely filled and there is some interdigitation of the cement with the bony trabeculae (Fig. 20.10). If a leak occurs anteriorly or through end plates, wait 90 s before continuing. The greatest risk is posterior leakage. If cement is getting close to the pedicle or 2–3 mm of the posterior edge of the vertebral body, injection should be stopped. Frequent checks with AP and lateral fluoroscopy are necessary to avoid cement leakage. Once the cement has been injected, replace the stylets to prevent cement from leaking back up the cannula.

After injection of an appropriate amount of void-filling cement, the cannulas should be twisted and removed once the cement has hardened. If the cement has set a little, you may need to slightly flex the cannula to break off cement of the distal tip. One should obtain final AP and lateral X-rays (Fig. 20.11a, b). The patient should be kept in the same position on the table until the cement has hardened. Normally this can be determined by waiting until the cement left in the mixing bowl has hardened. Once the bone cement has hardened, suture or Steri-Strip the wound [8].

In cases of traumatic compression fractures, kyphoplasty may sometimes be used to restore height in conjunction with a posterior fusion. However, it is important to obtain a CT scan to check for any retropulsion of

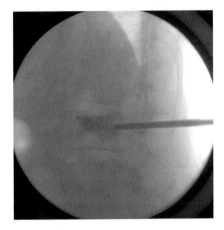

Fig. 20.10 Once the cement is mixed to a dough-like consistency, deflate the inflatable balloon tamp (IBT) and inject the cement until the cavity is completely filled and there is some interdigitation of the cement with the bony trabeculae

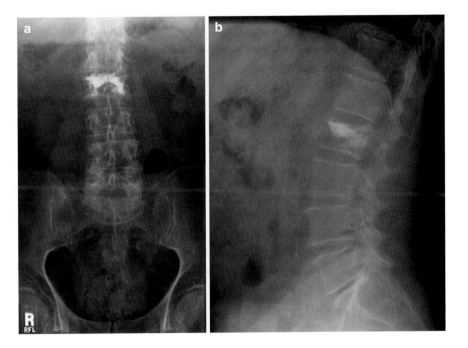

Fig. 20.11 (**a**, **b**) Final AP and lateral views of the L2 kyphoplasty

bony fragments or fissures in the posterior wall that may allow cement leakage in the canal. Kyphoplasty would be contraindicated in these cases. The steps for kyphoplasty in this scenario are essentially the same with the following changes. After the IBTs have been inflated and prior to injecting the PMMA, tap the cannula tract with the appropriate tap. Then, inject the PMMA when it has achieved a doughy consistency. After this, immediately place the pedicle screw down the pedicle before the PMMA hardens. Check AP and lateral views to ensure that no PMMA has migrated into the canal.

20.6 Technical Pearls and Pitfalls

20.6.1 Pearls

Take time to obtain good AP and lateral images. If you are having a difficult time obtaining a good AP, place a guide wire along the endplates of the vertebra on the lateral image to guide your AP view or use an *en face* view.

Angle the cannula as needed to help guide your drill to the desired position

If you can only get good views of one pedicle, consider a unipedicular approach. In this approach, you start more lateral than you do in extrapedicular approach. The tip of your drill and IBT should cross the midline and the spinous process on the AP view. It is important to do an extrapedicular approach for this technique because you will likely breach the medial pedicle wall if you try a transpedicular approach.

In a bipedicular approach is important to maintain the inflation of the highest pressure IBT while filling the contralateral side with bone cement to prevent shrinkage of elevated vertebral height.

If there is cement leakage prior to complete filling of the cavity, wait and allow the cement to harden. You may also reinsert the balloon and reinflate it to create a shell and then resume filling when the cement is harder.

In subacute fractures, it may be necessary to use the curette to soften the bone.

20.6.2 Intraoperative Complications and Bailout/Salvage Procedures

Cement leakage is the main cause of surgical complication with kyphoplasty. One intraoperative complication

that occurs is when a drill bit goes too far and breaches the anterior cortex of the vertebral body. This must be fixed prior to cementation to prevent leakage. The best way to plug an anterior cortical hole is by removing the drill, pass bone cement down the cannula with the bone filler device, and fill the defect. Normally, 2–3 cc are needed to fill a drill hole [8].

If epidural cement leakage should occur, a patient should be awakened from general anesthesia and the patient's neurological status should be assessed. If a new neurological deficit is found (due to spinal cord injury) decompression is mandated. Anterior or posterior approach to decompression will depend on many variables including location of cement, vertebrae level, and patient's ability to withstand a thoracotomy. If no neurological deficits exist, the patient should be observed closely.

If foraminal cement leakage should occur, it may cause radiculitis or weakness. If pain does not resolve posterior decompression is recommended.

If a puncture causes cerebrospinal fluid to leak, the hole should be packed with Gelfoam and PMMA should not be injected into the abandoned side.

If a patient appears to have neurological deficit in the recovery room, it could be because of bleeding that has resulted in an epidural hematoma. In this case, blood work should be done to immediately assess and correct coagulopathy. It should be followed by MRI or myelogram CT imaging to determine if the canal is compromised. If the canal is compromised, decompression is mandated [8].

20.7 Postoperative Considerations

20.7.1 Bracing, Activity, Follow-Up, Complications

Bracing is not usually required following kyphoplasty. Patients are mobilized approximately 6 h after the procedure [6]. Some patients may return from the hospital the same day while some elderly patients may require a 1–2 day hospital stay. Patients are encouraged to resume their normal daily activities as soon as tolerated, with the exception of weight-bearing activities. Weight-bearing activities should not be permitted for up to 6 weeks post-surgery in order to prevent fractures of untreated levels. Patients should have a 1-week follow-up to check the wound. A second week checkup should also be scheduled to determine need for physical therapy to increase trunk strength. Osteoporotic patients should start antiosteoporosis treatment/supplements. Osteoporotic patients should be reexamined at 3-month intervals to ensure no other fractures have developed [8].

There seems to be no significant long-term complications with kyphoplasty. There have been reports of VCFs adjacent to a kyphoplasty, however, it is not known if this is natural history or due to the kyphoplasty. Fribourg et al. reported that there is a 26% incidence of new fractures of other levels after kyphoplasty [4]. This incidence of new VCFs is most likely due to the severe osteoporoses most patients have who are treated with kyphoplasty [5].

References

1. Berruti A et al (2000) Incidence of skeletal complications in patients with bone metastatic prostate cancer and hormone refractory disease: predictive role of bone resorption and formation markers evaluated at baseline. J Urol 164(4):1248–1253

2. Charnley J (1970) The reaction of bone to self-curing acrylic cement. A long-term histological study in man. J Bone Joint Surg Br 52(2):340–353

3. Cloft HJ, Jensen ME (2007) Kyphoplasty: an assessment of a new technology. Am J Neuroradiol 28:200–203

4. Fribourg D, Tang C, Sra P et al (2004) Incidence of subsequent vertebral fracture after kyphoplasty. Spine 29(20): 2270–2276

5. Leslie-Mazwi T, Deen HG (2006) Repeated fracture of a vertebral body after treatment with balloon kyphoplasty case illustration. J Neurosurg Spine 4:270

6. Maestretti G, Cremer C, Otten P et al (2007) Prospective study of standalone balloon kyphoplasty with calcium phosphate cement augmentation in traumatic fractures. Eur Spine J 16(5):601–610

7. Mayer MH (2006) Minimally invasive spine surgery: a surgical manual. Springer-Verlag, Berlin, p 249

8. Resnick DK, Garfin SR (2005) Vertebroplasty and kyphoplasty. Thieme Medical Publishers, New York, pp 62–75

9. Riggs BL, Melton LJ 3rd (1995) The worldwide problem of osteoporosis: insights afforded by epidemiology. Bone 17(5 suppl):505S–511S

10. Saliou G, Lehmann P, Vallee JN (2008) Controlled segmental balloon kyphoplasty (a new technique for patients with heterogeneous vertebral bone density). Spine 33(7):E216–E220

11. Vaccaro AR, Albert TJ (2003) Spine surgery: tricks of the trade. Thieme, New York, p 94

Costotransversectomy

Kern Singh

21.1 Case Example

A 68-year-old woman with a history of breast carcinoma reports a gradual increase in low back pain most recently accompanied by a sudden inability to ambulate secondary to bilateral radicular pain and motor weakness. The patient also notes a 4-day history of inability to void with subsequent incontinence. Physical exam is significant for 3+/5 motor weakness in her lower extremities with decreased sensation to pinprick in the L3–L4 distribution.

Magnetic resonance imaging (MRI) of her lumbar spine demonstrates a lesion involving the entire L3 body with significant thecal sac compression (Fig. 21.1). On CT, the lesion extends out of the left L3 body (Fig. 21.2).

Because of her increasing pain, inability to ambulate and neurological deficits, the patient elected to undergo surgical intervention. In order to minimize her surgical morbidity, a posterolateral lumbar extracavitary approach was utilized to decompress her tumor and reconstruct her spine. This approach obviated the need for an anterior surgical exposure. A L1–L5 posterior instrumented fusion with an extracavitary L3 corpectomy and reconstruction was performed (Fig. 21.3).

21.2 Background

Various techniques have been described to treat compressive or pathologic lesions in the spine. Common surgical approaches include anterior, posterior, or combined anterior–posterior procedures. Anterior-only approaches allow for minimal removal of uninvolved bone, rapid removal of the lesion, effective reconstruction of the weight-bearing anterior column, and short-segment fixation. Anterior procedures come at the expense of iatrogenic morbidity. Faciezewski et al. in a review of 1,223 procedures (*Spine* 20:1592–1599, 1995) found an 11.5% complication rate directly attributed to anterior spinal surgery. Complications include vascular and neurological injury, infections, pulmonary complications, abdominal hernias, and genitourinary injuries. A posterior-only approach on the other hand may not theoretically remove the entire offending lesion; however, if multilevel lesions are present, a posterior approach is preferred. Finally, combined anterior–posterior approaches allow circumferential decompression and stabilization but at the cost of increased surgical time and two surgical incisions. With recent advances in techniques and instrumentation, a newer technique, the posterolateral lumbar extracavitary approach, provides excellent ventral decompression with safe visualization of the neural elements.

21.3 Indications and Advantages of the Procedure

21.3.1 Indications

- Infections
- Metastatic lesions
- Traumatic fractures with central canal stenosis
- Compressive lesions in the anterior spine

K. Singh
Department of Orthopaedic Surgery,
Rush University Medical Center,
1611 West Harrison Street,
Chicago, IL 60612, USA
e-mail: Kern.singh@rushortho.com

V.V. Patel et al. (eds.), *Spine Trauma*,
DOI: 10.1007/978-3-642-03694-1_21, © Springer-Verlag Berlin Heidelberg 2010

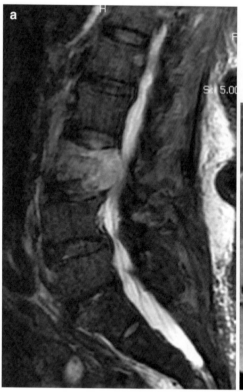
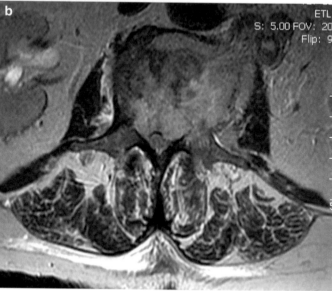

Fig. 21.1 (**a**) Preoperative sagittal STIR (Short T1 Inversion Recovery) MRI lumbar spine of a 68-year-old female with metastatic breast CA. Patient was noted to have complete destruction of the L3 vertebral body with significant collapse. (**b**) Preoperative axial images at the L3 level reveal significant soft-tissue compromise of the epidural space

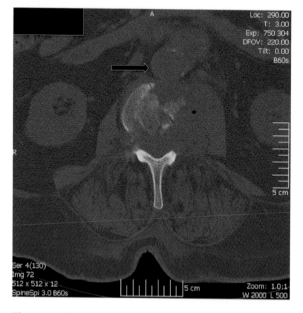

Fig. 21.2 CT lumbar spine of the same patient demonstrates destruction of the L3 vertebral body with soft-tissue extension to the left paravertebral region (*asterisk*). Of note, the aorta is calcified anterior to the spine (*arrow*)

21.3.2 Advantages of the Procedure

- All posterior incision obviating the need for anterior surgical approach
- Reconstruction of the anterior and middle column via posterior incision while simultaneously stabilizing the spine posteriorly
- No need for staged procedure
- Decrease surgical time compared to combined anterior–posterior procedure
- Minimizes vascular, neurological, reproductive, and visceral injuries associated with anterior procedures

21.4 Contraindications and Disadvantages of the Procedure

21.4.1 Contraindications

- None

Fig. 21.3 Anteroposterior (AP) (**a**) and lateral (**b**) lumbar spine radiographs reveal an extracavitary corpectomy at L3 with an expandable cage placement in the 68-year-old female with metastatic breast CA. The posterior spinal fusion was extended from L1 to L5. The patient was neurologically intact postoperatively and has had resolution of her symptoms with no recurrence at her most recent 2-year follow-up

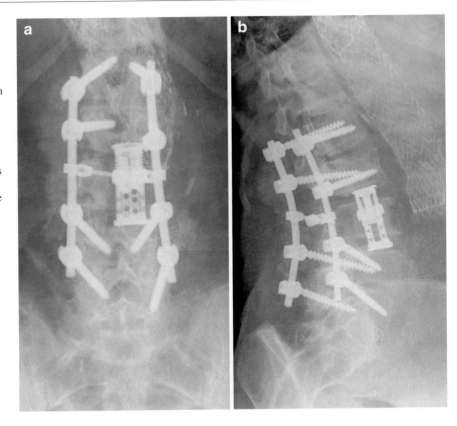

21.4.2 Disadvantages of the Procedure

- Technically difficult compared to a staged anterior–posterior procedure
- Potential for neurological injury, especially nerve root injury
- Inadequate decompression, resection of tumor, or removal of infected bone/disc
- Difficult spinal reconstruction

21.5 Procedure

21.5.1 Equipment Needed

- Jackson radiolucent surgical frame (Preferable to have a Jackson table that rotates)
- Pedicle screw and rod fixation system
- Typical spinal instrumentation set (Kerrison, Cobbs, Ronguers, etc.)
- Expandable vertebral cage
- Ring curettes
- C-arm

21.5.2 Anesthesia and Neuromonitoring

- General anesthesia
- Somatosensory evoked potentials (SSEP), motor evoked potentials (MEP), and possible electromyograph (EMG) for pedicle screw/nerve root stimulation

21.5.3 Surgical Procedure

Patient is positioned prone onto a Jackson radiolucent surgical frame. The face and boney prominences are well padded. The arms are abducted and flexed to minimize the risk of brachial plexopathy.

A standard midline posterior subperiosteal dissection is performed centered around the index level. The number of levels to be instrumented is variable depending on the bone quality, severity of deformity, and underlying pathology. For the typical procedure, we recommend two levels above and below the pathological level.

After the appropriate pedicle screws are placed (Fig. 21.4), a wide decompressive laminectomy at the

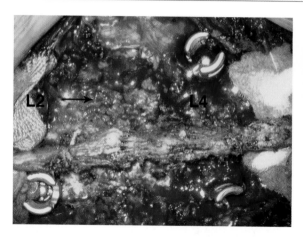

Fig. 21.4 Transpedicular screws are placed bilaterally into L2 and L4. The left L2–L3 facet capsule is identified (*arrow*) representing the L3 pedicle entrance. Typically, two levels of fixation, above and below, are performed

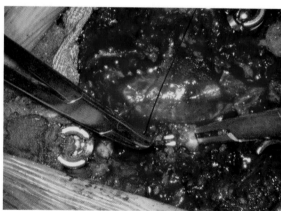

Fig. 21.6 In the thoracic spine, the exiting nerve can be sacrificed. In this picture, a hemostat is placed below the exiting nerve root. A 2.0 silk suture can be used to tie off the root

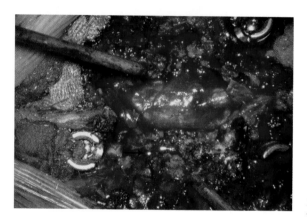

Fig. 21.5 A wide L2–L3 laminectomy and a complete facetectomy of the left L2–L3 (*arrow*) are completed. The contralateral facetectomy is labeled (*asterisk*)

index level as well as above and below the involved vertebrae is performed in the standard fashion. A unilateral complete facetectomy at the pathological level is also performed (Fig. 21.5). The extensive decompression is to allow for maximal cephalad–caudad working space between the roots, particularly critical during expandable cage placement.

The exiting nerve root on the side where the corpectomy will occur is identified. In the thoracic spine, the nerve can be sacrificed to improve visualization significantly at the pathological level (Fig. 21.6), but in the lumbar spine, all attempts should be made to preserve the integrity of the root. Next, a temporary unilateral rod is placed (contralateral to the side of the

pediculectomy/corpectomy). Gentle distraction is applied across the construct to allow a larger working window for the corpectomy. The segments are then locked in place to the rod for stabilization during decompression.

To begin the corpectomy, the transverse process of the affected vertebra is resected to the lateral edge of the vertebral body using a Kerrison rongeur. A Cobb elevator is then utilized for subperiosteal dissection (Fig. 21.7). A packing sponge is then placed around the vertebral body to minimize bleeding. A high-speed burr is then utilized to remove the lateral pedicle and vertebral body wall. The medial edge of the pedicle and dorsal wall of the body are left intact to protect the nerve root and spinal cord/cauda equina. Various sized ring curettes are then used to perform the discectomy above and below the level. The corpectomy is then completed with the use of high-speed burr and curved curette. Rotating/airplaning the Jackson table away from the surgeon allows improved access to the contralateral vertebral body wall. Care is taken to preserve the dorsal vertebral body cortex. Once the decompression is completed, the posterior vertebral body wall is depressed into the defect with the aid of a reverse-angled curette. Preservation of the posterior body wall allows for protection of the neural elements while the corpectomy ensues (Fig. 21.8).

Next, the expandable cage is inserted into the defect. The cage is first tightly packed with bone graft. The cage is initially placed parallel to the nerve root on the cephalad side of the affected level (Fig. 21.9).

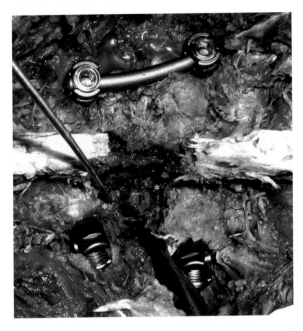

Fig. 21.7 After the laminectomy and facetectomy, the left L3 transverse process is resected. This allows for the skeletonization of the left L3 pedicle (*P*). A white asterisk (*asterisk*) denotes the L2 and L3 exiting nerve root. A Cobb elevator is seen on the lateral edge of the vertebral body

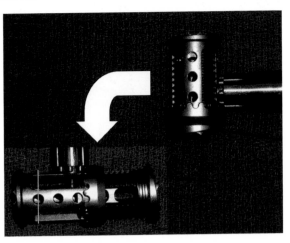

Fig. 21.9 The cage is then rotated 90° within the corpectomy site and expanded as demonstrated by the photograph

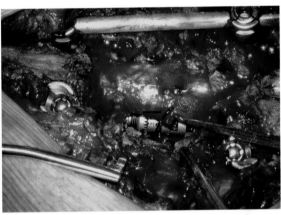

Fig. 21.10 After the cage is rotated 90°, the cage is fully engaged with it now being perpendicular with the adjacent endplates. The sacrificed thoracic exiting nerve root (*arrow*) is retracted for better visualization. Note, in the lumbar spine, the exiting nerve is preserved

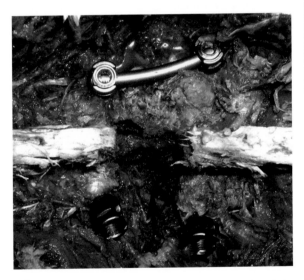

Fig. 21.8 The L3 vertebral body has been resected, and the large *black arrow* represents the defect. The *asterisk* denotes the L2 nerve root and the *plus sign* denotes the L3 nerve root

The nerve root is simultaneously retracted caudally. Once inside the defect, the cage is rotated 90° until it is perpendicular with the adjacent endplates (Fig. 21.10). Direct fluoroscopy is then taken to ensure the cage is appropriately engaging the endplates. Additional bone graft is then packed around the anterior and lateral portions of the cage (Fig. 21.11). The second rod is then inserted and slight compression is applied bilaterally across the segments. A final tightening of the setscrews is performed, and a cross-link is applied (Fig. 21.12). Radiographs are obtained to confirm adequate placement of the instrumentation and cage. Lastly, a posterolateral fusion is performed on the contralateral side where the laminectomies and facetectomies have not been done allowing for a scaffold for bone fusion.

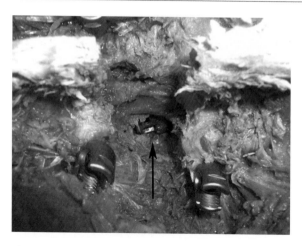

Fig. 21.11 The cage is then fully engaged within the corpectomy site with minimal retraction of the exiting nerve roots (*asterisk* L2 nerve root, + L3 nerve root)

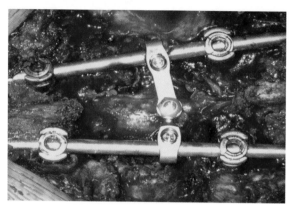

Fig. 21.12 The final instrumented construct after both rods and cross-link have been placed and tightened

21.6 Technical Pearls and Pitfalls

21.6.1 Pearls

- Careful subperiosteal dissection around the vertebral body is key to minimizing blood loss and potential inadvertent vascular injury in the anterior abdominal/thoracic cavity. Dissection is much more technically challenging in cases of infection as tissue planes become adherent.
- In cases of malignancy, discectomies are done prior to the corpectomy to ensure no local contamination.
- Logrolling the table away from the surgeon provides visualization across the midline to the contralateral vertebral body.

- An intact contralateral pedicle, transverse process, and vertebral body wall allow for increased osseous surface for bony fusion. Removal can be avoided except in cases of solitary metastasis or primary malignancy.

21.6.2 Potential Intraoperative Complications

- Exiting nerve root damage
- Excessive blood secondary to technical difficulty
- Inability to safely accomplish an anterior reconstruction secondary to excessive cage size

21.6.3 Salvage Procedure

- If bleeding is uncontrollable during the corpectomy, the surgeon should be prepared to convert to a combined anterior–posterior procedure to visualize the source of bleeding.
- If the cage is unable to be inserted, a staged anterior approach can be performed accomplishing the reconstruction.

21.7 Postoperative Considerations

21.7.1 Bracing

Bracing is usually not required; however, if fixation is a concern, a thoracolumbar orthosis with or without a thigh extension may be utilized until adequate bone consolidation is seen on radiographs.

21.7.2 Activity

Activity is usually not restricted postoperatively. Patients should be carefully observed in the immediate postoperative period to ensure patient is stable on his/her feet prior to ambulation as many of these patients preoperatively are weak.

21.7.3 Follow-Up

The typical postoperative course is 6 weeks, 3, 6 months, 1, 2 years. Radiographs are taken at each visit to ensure adequate bony healing and instrumentation position.

21.7.4 Potential Postoperative Complications

- Dislodgement of the cage
  - The surgeon should contemplate a revision anterior surgery to correct the position of the cage if it compromises stability.
- Recurrence of infection or malignancy

  - Symptoms suggesting recurrence of a primary tumor, metastasis, or osteomyelitis should prompt further imaging and consideration of an anterior vs. revision posterior approach for debridement.
- Nerve injury
  - If there are no signs of nerve function return at 6 week, an electromyograph (EMG) should be ordered to determine the potential for neural recovery.

Reference

1. Faciszewski T, Winter RB, Lonstein JE, Denis F, Johnson L (1995 Jul 15) The surgical and medical perioperative complications of anterior spinal fusion surgery in the thoracic and lumbar spine in adults. A review of 1223 procedures. Spine (Phila Pa 1976) 20(14):1592–1599

George M. Whaba and Nitin N. Bhatia

22.1 Introduction

Thoracolumbar and lumbar injuries represent the majority of spinal fractures, with injuries between T11 and L1 being the most frequent [11]. Despite the frequency of these injuries, there remains considerable controversy regarding the most appropriate treatment. An understanding of the underlying anatomy and biomechanics, as well as familiarity with the clinical and radiographic assessment of the initial trauma, will help guide the surgeon toward the optimal management of the patient.

22.2 Anatomic and Biomechanical Considerations

The thoracolumbar junction is a transitional zone between the mobile lumbar spine and the relatively rigid thoracic spine. It also represents a transitional zone between the kyphosis of the thoracic spine and the lordosis of the lumbar spine [27]. This results in the increased susceptibility to injury of the thoracolumbar junction. Moreover, the short ribs at T11 and T12 do not articulate with the sternum and do not provide the same protection as the remainder of the thoracic cage. Vertebral bodies at this level are smaller than their lumbar counterparts and are less able to withstand traumatic loads.

N.N. Bhatia (✉) and G.M. Whaba
Department of Orthopaedic Surgery,
UC Irvine Medical Center,
101 The City Drive South, Orange, CA 92868, USA
e-mail: bhatian@uci.edu

Facet joints in the lumbar spine are oriented in the sagittal place, which allows greater flexion and extension, but limits motion in rotation. Thus any rotatory displacement at the thoracolumbar region should raise suspicion for a facet dislocation of fracture-dislocation [25]. This is in contrast to the facets joints in the thoracic spine, which are oriented in the coronal plane and provide increased stability by limiting flexion and extension, as well as anterior translation [21].

The ligamentous structures of the thoracolumbar spine are also crucial in providing stability and must be considered when evaluating an injured spine. The anterior longitudinal ligament (ALL) and the posterior longitudinal ligament (PLL) are the primary ligaments. The ALL originates from the occiput and becomes thicker and broader as it descends to the anterior sacrum. In contrast, the PLL attaches broadly to the foramen magnum and the cervical spine and descends posteriorly to the sacrum [2]. The primary biomechanical effect of the ALL is to resist extension, while the PLL resists flexion. The ligamentum flavum connects adjacent laminae, while the interspinous ligament and supraspinous ligament connect adjacent spinous processes. Together, these posterior ligaments act together as a restraint against hyperflexion [15]. Additionally, the lumbar facet capsules, which are more robust than those found in the thoracic spine, contribute significantly to stability in rotation and bending. Finally, the annulus fibrosus of the intervertebral disc, as well as the paraspinal musculature, also contributes to stability.

The lordosis of the lumbar spine shifts the center of gravity posteriorly. Flexion forces may place the spine in a sagittal neutral position. As a result, axial loads can result in a burst-type fracture pattern without significant anterior wedging [15]. This finding is in contrast to the kyphotic thoracic spine, which places the

V.V. Patel et al. (eds.), *Spine Trauma*,
DOI: 10.1007/978-3-642-03694-1_22, © Springer-Verlag Berlin Heidelberg 2010

center of gravity anteriorly and predisposes to anterior compression and wedging.

Consideration of the neural elements is also critical. The spinal cord terminates at the conus medullaris at L1 in adults. Below this level, the nerve roots of the cauda equina have a relatively large canal within which to travel. Moreover, the nerve roots are far more resistant to blunt trauma than the spinal cord. Thus even a displaced burst fracture with significant canal compromise can demonstrate surprisingly minimal neurological deficits in the lumbar spine. In contrast, the spinal cord has less space available as it travels through the thoracic spinal canal, and it is much less forgiving to even mild trauma.

22.3 Evaluation and Initial Management of the Trauma Patient

The evaluation and initial management of a patient with a suspected spine injury will consist of a standard trauma protocol with clinical examination, medical stabilization, and radiographic evaluation. This assessment provides the surgeon with the necessary data regarding the patient and injury, which will allow selection of the optimal operative and nonoperative interventions. Since many of these topics are covered in greater detail elsewhere in this text, a brief overview follows.

The initial clinical evaluation must consist of the standard trauma primary survey, as prescribed by the Advanced Trauma Life Support protocol. This primary survey focuses on immediately identifying any life-threatening injuries, and beginning resuscitation if appropriate. Airway, breathing, circulation, disability, and environment are the five components of the primary surgery. Relevant to spine trauma, immobilization and protection of the cervical spine are included in the assessment of the airway. Thoracolumbar trauma is often associated with thoracic and abdominal injuries. These include hemo or pneumothorax, liver or splenic lacerations, aortic injuries, and bowel injuries. Hemorrhage in the thorax, abdomen, or pelvis can produce life-threatening hypovolemic shock if not addressed quickly, with crystalloid solution and blood products if necessary. If a spinal cord injury is present, neurogenic shock may also occur due to the loss of sympathetic tone. It is distinguished from hemorrhagic

shock by the presence of relative brachycardia in the setting of hypotension. This situation requires vasopressors to elevate the patient's blood pressure. Neurogenic shock is less commonly seen with injuries below the thoracolumbar junction versus cervical and upper thoracic injuries [23]. Regardless of the specific cause, hypotension must be treated aggressively to prevent secondary injury to the spinal cord due to hypoperfusion.

Once the patient has been stabilized, the secondary survey can be performed. The spine must be examined by both inspection and palpation. The patient is log-rolled sideways while maintaining spine precautions, as the neck is carefully held in a neutral position. All spinous processes are palpated to assess for tenderness, step-offs, or widening, any of which may suggest injury to the posterior elements [23]. Sometimes the step-off or interspinous gap is the only clue to serious segmental instability. During the secondary survey, a more detailed neurologic evaluation can be performed to identify any deficits, and if necessary, determine the level of spinal cord injury. The American Spinal Injury Association Impairment Scale is a validated method to reliably classify and monitor the patient's level and severity of spinal cord injury. A complete spinal cord injury is one that has total loss of motor and sensory function caudal to the level of injury. Any residual voluntary motor or sensory function below the injury level would classify the lesion as an incomplete spinal cord injury. In order to confirm the presence of a complete spinal cord lesion, the clinician must ensure that the patient has recovered from spinal shock. Spinal shock is a phenomenon of flaccid paralysis due to disruption of all spinal cord function below the level of an acute injury. The return of reflexes below the injury level, such as the bulbocavernosus reflex, signifies the resolution of spinal shock and usually occurs within 48 h [23].

The importance of the clinical evaluation needs to be emphasized. The mechanism of the injury and the history can be much valuable to clue the surgeon into looking for occult injury, i.e., falling from a height may lead to aortic injuries and multiple level injuries. Likewise, visualizing the patient for bruises can be very helpful in the obtunded patient to specifically rule out visceral injuries such as splenic injuries, which are easily missed in the wake of neurogenic shock. Therefore, it is vital to inspect the whole torso and then palpate every level of the spine, feeling for crepitus, step-off, and bruising. Do not forget to palpate the anterior aspect of the cervical spine as retropharyngeal swelling and tenderness might point to an occult hyperextension injury with relatively normal X-rays.

It is also important to palpate the sternum and consider the cheat wall and extension of the thoracic spine. Sternal fractures are often missed and, if not diagnosed, the severity of a "benign compression fracture" in the thoracic area is underestimated. In these cases the injury is part of the thoracic dislocation and is usually accompanied with severe internal organ damage including esophageal tears.

The pelvis is just as important, and in blast injuries, spinopelvic dislocations are often missed if not perceived as such during the clinical exam. It is difficult to image these areas, and therefore, the key to interpreting the images lies in the clinical assessment of the patient.

Radiographic studies add critical information in identifying and defining bony and ligamentous injuries. Moreover, they allow for classification of these injuries, provide guidance in selecting the appropriate treatment, and are crucial for preoperative planning if surgical intervention is indicated. If a spinal injury is identified, imaging of the entire spine should be obtained, since multiple noncontiguous spinal injuries can be as common as 4.5–15.2% [7, 13, 26]. AP radiographs allow for evaluation of coronal and rotation alignment. Coronal translations and disruption of the normal interpedicular distance are findings that would indicate severe trauma. On lateral radiographs, the clinician can evaluate sagittal alignment and potential loss of vertebral body height.

Computed tomography (CT) is very effective in defining bony anatomy and injury. Thin slices (2 mm) should be performed to provide the necessary amount of detail, especially in areas of injury. Axial cuts are helpful in examining the integrity of the middle column, which helps distinguish compression fractures from burst fractures, as well as assess for canal compromise due to bony fragments. These cuts also show excellent detail of the posterior elements, which may reveal injuries such as laminar fractures, facet fractures, or dislocations. Sagittal and coronal reconstructions may allow for evaluation of alignment in greater detail than that provided by plain radiographs. Reconstructions are also helpful in identifying fractures or translational deformities that are oriented in the same plane as the axial cuts. Three-dimensional reconstruction can provide valuable information in patients with complex posttraumatic deformity.

Magnetic resonance imaging (MRI) provides visualization of important soft tissue structures that are not seen using other imaging modalities. Trauma to the spinal cord or conus medullaris can be identified by edema, represented by areas of increased signal intensity on T2-weighted images. MRI can also show injuries to spinal ligaments, such as the posterior ligamentous complex. The integrity of these ligaments may determine the success of various treatment options. Finally, MRI can reveal acute intervertebral disc injuries, although herniations producing canal compromise are much less common in the thoracolumbar spine relative to the cervical spine [23].

22.4 Classification of Thoracolumbar and Lumbar Spine Injuries

Numerous classification systems for thoracolumbar and lumbar fractures have been devised over the past few years, all with their own strengths and limitations. The ideal system would be simple and consistent between different observers, yet comprehensive and inclusive of the great variability that is seen in these injuries. The perfect classification scheme would also reflect clinical and radiologic characteristics, as well as reflect the ligamentous and neurologic injuries that are associated with the spine trauma. Finally, this system should have prognostic value and assist in treatment decision making [19]. Unfortunately, most available classifications focus predominately on fracture pattern, and no ideal system exists. A few of these classification schemes are in wide use and merit special consideration.

In 1983, Denis popularized a classification system involving a three-column model, based on his radiographic review of 412 thoracolumbar injuries. The anterior column consists of the ALL, anterior annulus fibrosus, and anterior vertebral body. The middle column contains the posterior vertebral body, posterior annulus fibrosus, and the PLL. The posterior column consists of posterior bony arch, interspinous and supraspinous ligaments, facet capsule, and ligamentum flavum. Moreover, Denis went on to classify injuries as "minor" injuries, which do not lead to acute instability, and "major" injuries, which do produce instability. Minor injuries include isolated fractures of the transverse processes and spinous processes. Major injuries were divided into compression fractures, burst fractures, seat belt-type injuries, and fracture-dislocations. These categories were further separated into additional subtypes. Denis also classified instability as (1) mechanical, with risk of progressive kyphosis, (2) neurologic, indicating risk of deterioration in a previously intact patient, and (3) combined [8, 9]. This classification system introduced the importance of the middle column and stressed its role as the distinguishing feature between compression fractures and burst fractures. However, a primary disadvantage is the disconnection between injury patterns and treatment options, with no additional benefit being contributed by its added complexity of having so many fracture subtypes.

McAfee modified the Denis classification, based on CT studies of 100 patients with thoracolumbar injuries, based on the mode of failure of the middle column: compression, distraction, and translation [17]. This approach was particularly useful at the time it was published, when the available modes of fixation were limited to distraction rods, compression rods, and sublaminar fixation [19]. Thus each failure mode could be paired with an appropriate method of fixation. With modern fixation techniques, this distinction may be less relevant. However, McAfee also simplified the Denis system into six categories of injuries: (1) wedge-compression fractures, (2) stable burst fractures, (3) unstable burst fractures, (4) Chance fractures (bony), (5) flexion-distraction injuries, and (6) translation injuries (fracture-dislocations). As noted above in the Denis scheme, burst fractures were characterized by injury to both the anterior and middle columns. Unstable burst fractures were defined as having disruption of the posterior column as well. McAfee described a Chance fracture as a horizontal fracture pattern parallel to the axial plane. Other flexion-distraction injuries were grouped separately. Translation injuries were defined as "those in which the alignment of the neural canal has been disrupted" and typically represent a failure in shear of all three columns [17]. This category would include injuries described by other authors as fracture-dislocations and pure-dislocations. Another important aspect of McAfee's study

was the finding that stable injuries (compression fractures and stable burst fractures) were far less likely to be associated with neurologic deficits.

McCormack developed a classification system that attempted to aid in treatment decision making. Based on a study of 28 surgically managed patients with unstable thoracolumbar injuries, a load-sharing classification was developed to grade the comminution of thoracolumbar fractures and provide guidance about the need to provide anterior support. By quantifying the vertebral body comminution, fragment displacement, and kyphosis of a particular fracture, the authors were able to assess the load transfer ability of the anterior and middle columns in the immediate postoperative period. Each factor was graded as mild (1 point), moderate (2 points), or severe (3 points) [18]. A subsequent retrospective review of 51 thoracolumbar fracture patients by Parker found that patients with less severely comminuted fractures (load-sharing classification score <7 points) were treated successfully with short-segment posterior instrumentation. They suggest that more severe injuries would benefit by adding anterior reconstruction [20]. Notable limitations of this system include its omission of ligamentous injuries and neurologic deficits [19].

The most structured and comprehensive classification system to date was introduced by Magerl, in conjunction with the AO group, based on a collaborative multicenter study reviewing 1,445 patients with thoracolumbar injuries [16]. This system utilizes the principles of the well-known 3-3-3 AO extremity fracture classification scheme. Based primarily on pathomorphology, they defined three primary injury types: (A) compression, (B) distraction, and (C) torsion. Each type is further subdivided into three additional groups. These groups are each separated yet again into three more subgroups, and even further as necessary. The system implies an increasing severity of injuries, from A1 to C3. The strength of the AO/Magerl classification, its comprehensiveness, also turned out to be its greatest weakness. The initial report includes 53 specific injury types, demonstrating the complexity of the system [16, 19]. A subsequent study found the mean interobserver agreement to be 67%, when limited to just classification of the primary injury types (A, B, C). This reliability declined even further when additional subgroups were added [3].

22.5 Spinal Stability and General Principles of Management

The goals of management for any spinal trauma include maximizing neurologic recovery, reducing and stabilizing the spinal column, and enabling early mobilization and rehabilitation. Assessing the stability of a spinal injury is the key to determining the most appropriate management. Stability was defined by Whitesides as the ability to tolerate stress without any progressive deformity or neurologic compromise [29]. Similarly, White and Panjabi defined instability as the inability "under physiologic loads to maintain relationships between vertebrae in such a way that neither damage nor subsequent irritation to the spinal cord or nerve roots, and, in addition, there is no development of incapacitating deformity or pain" [28]. Even with these widely accepted definitions, much controversy exists regarding the optimal management for many thoracolumbar and lumbar injuries. However, certain general principles can be helpful in guiding clinical practice.

Neurologic compromise is seen by most authors as evidence of instability and is typically considered an indication for surgery, especially when accompanied by ongoing neural compression. Given the relatively large amount of canal space available in the lumbar spine, a significant amount of instability and displacement is necessary to cause injury to the cauda equina [1]. As noted above, the concept and importance of "neurologic instability" date back to Denis' initial report of his classification scheme [9]. Related to the consideration of neurologic deficit is the evaluation of canal compromise. Spinal decompression may be indicated in patients with incomplete neurologic deficits and significant canal compromise [6]. Canal compromise greater than 50% is frequently cited as an indication for surgical decompression, but little data support this figure as a universal rule. Moreover, even patients with complete neurologic injuries can benefit from stabilization procedures, which would allow faster mobilization and rehabilitation [24].

The second important component of clinical stability is mechanical stability, which Denis also discussed [9]. Denis focused on the importance of the middle column and suggested that injuries to two or more columns result in instability. Currently, a common approach to determining stability involves evaluation of the posterior ligamentous complex. A spine injury involving multiple columns and associated with disruption of the posterior elements would be considered mechanically unstable, and surgical fixation would generally be indicated (Fig. 22.1).

Regardless of which classification system is used, the key to decision making is identifying the injured structures involved and determining the severity of each injury. This contributes to the evaluation of both mechanical and neurologic instability and clarifies which treatment options would most benefit the patient. McAfee's modification of the Denis system is appealing because it can provide a helpful framework for approaching these traumas. He essentially described two broad categories of injuries: stable and unstable. Stable injuries that consist of compression fractures and stable burst fractures can be treated nonoperatively. Unstable injuries, such as unstable burst fractures, flexion-distraction injuries (including Chance fractures), and fracture-dislocations, typically require surgical stabilization [17, 19].

Compression fractures involve a flexion-compression mechanism of injury, associated with a flexion moment around an axis in the middle column. In contrast, axial loading is the primary mechanism in burst fractures, with flexion usually playing a smaller role. Burst fractures represent more significant trauma, with extension of the injury into the middle column vs. the isolated anterior column involvement seen with compression fractures. Consideration of the posterior osteoligamentous complex is critical in the evaluation of these injuries. Certain criteria have been cited in the literature as suggestive of significant posterior element disruption. Although controversial, these criteria are considered by some authors as indications for surgical intervention: greater than 50% loss of anterior body height, greater than 25° of kyphosis, or interspinous distance widening [4, 5, 22, 24]. When necessary, MRI can provide additional data regarding the integrity of the posterior elements. Classically, compression fractures are considered stable injuries. The majority are treated nonoperatively, with or without bracing, depending on the severity of the fracture. With conservative management, close radiographic follow-up, including weight-bearing radiographs, is crucial to confirm the lack of kyphotic progression.

The same principles and criteria apply regarding evaluation of posterior osteoligamentous disruption in burst fractures. A burst fracture can be associated with either mechanical instability due to posterior column injury or neurologic instability with the presence of neurologic deficits. Although there is a lack of prospective data definitively supporting most treatment algorithms for

Fig. 22.1 L1 burst fracture:
(**a**) Lateral x-ray showing
loss of anterior vertebral
body height and retropulsion
of the superior-posterior
fragment of the L1 body;
(**b**) axial CT scan showing
three-column involvement
resulting in instability

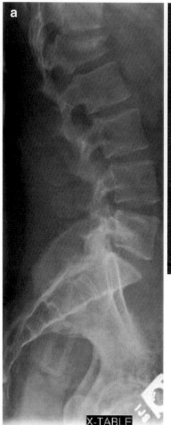
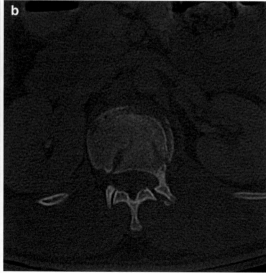

burst fractures, authors agree that an incomplete spinal cord injury and significant ongoing neural compression are strong indications for surgical intervention. Stable burst fractures are treated in the same manner as stable compression fractures, with appropriate bracing and close radiographic follow-up. Nonoperative treatment of neurologically intact patients with stable thoracolumbar burst fractures has lower complication rates than surgical intervention on this subset of patients with at least equivalent clinical results [30]. While the rate of nonunion in nonoperatively treated burst fracture patients is not documented in the literature, it is unlikely to be high. Symptomatic nonunion of the anterior and middle columns in a burst fracture can also be an indication for surgical intervention [5]. Kyphotic collapse and pain are the more common unfavorable outcomes, based on the natural history of the injury.

Flexion-distraction injuries, including Chance fractures, are associated with high-energy traumas that produce flexion with an apex within or anterior to the vertebral body, resulting in distraction across the entire spinal segment. An in vitro study by Hoshikawa on porcine thoracolumbar spines showed that larger flexion angles at the time of injury produce a more anterior motion axis of fracture (MAF) [14]. Thus even an axial compression load can produce a flexion-distraction injury if the MAF is anterior enough. These injuries frequently demonstrate disruption of the posterior osteoligamentous complex, horizontal fractures through the lamina and vertebral body, and facet joint fractures and/or dislocations. Neurologic deficits are very common in this setting. Moreover, bowel perforations and other abdominal injuries are also frequently seen in these patients. In treating a purely osseous flexion-distraction injury (bony Chance fracture) in a patient with no neurologic deficits, there may be consideration of nonoperative management with bracing until fracture healing [5, 19]. Most other injuries in this category require surgical stabilization. Typically, the ALL is intact and provides same stability by serving as a tension band in conjunction with posterior fixation [22]. For that reason, an anterior surgical approach may destabilize the injury further by disrupting the ALL, and posterior stabilization may be preferred.

Fracture-dislocations are typically associated with similar high-energy mechanisms as those seen in flexion-distraction injuries, but are distinguished by the presence of translation. This translational shear component results in a devastating and destabilizing injury to all three columns and a very high rate of neurologic deficit [19]. Abdominal injuries are also highly prevalent with this pattern [15]. Surgical intervention is recommended for most patients in this category, even those with complete neurologic deficits, in order to restore mechanical stability. Posterior instrumentation and fusion following reduction, with or without decompression, is the typical treatment of choice. In cases with minimal anterior and middle column involvement, short-segment transpedicular fixation has shown good results [12]. Conversely, injuries that demonstrate significant vertebral body comminution, or canal compromise from fragment retropulsion, may be appropriate for combined anterior and posterior approaches or longer posterior-only constructs [5].

Extension injuries were not included in the classification system by McAfee, primarily because they are relatively rare in the thoracolumbar spine [17]. However, Denis did describe it as a subtype of his fracture-dislocation category ("shear type of fracture-dislocation") [9]. This pattern is more likely to be seen in patients who have underlying spinal pathologies, such as ankylosing spondylitis [22]. In this setting, there is ossification of the ligamentous structures leading to a profound loss of flexibility in the involved spinal levels. As a result, even a seemingly minor trauma can result in significant disruption of the injured segment [15]. A typical pattern will demonstrate injury of the anterior column through distraction, such as ALL disruption and anterior end plate avulsion fracture, along with compression of the posterior elements. More severe cases may involve complete three-column disruption with translation. These injuries are highly unstable, often associated with neurologic impairment, and typically require surgical management [10].

22.6 Summary

Thoracolumbar and lumbar injuries are highly variable and complex, and their management remains controversial. There continues to be disagreement regarding the classification of injuries, indications for surgical intervention, timing of surgery, and the specific surgical strategies optimal for a given injury. However, there is clarity with respect to the goals of management for these patients. These goals focus on maximizing neurologic recovery, restoring spinal stability, and promoting early mobilization and rehabilitation. An appreciation of the anatomy and biomechanics of the injury and a basic framework from which to approach these injuries will guide the surgeon toward the optimal management for achieving these goals with the patient (Table 22.1).

Table 22.1 AO classification system for spinal injuries.

A. Compression injury

A1: Impaction fracture
     A1.1 End plate impaction
     A1.2 Wedge impaction
     A1.3 Vertebral body collapse

A2: Split fracture
     A2.1 Sagittal split fracture
     A2.2 Coronal split fracture
     A2.3 Pincer fracture

A3: Burst fracture
     A3.1 Incomplete burst fracture
     A3.2 Burst-split fracture
     A3.3 Complete burst fracture

B. Distraction injury

B1: Posterior ligamentary lesion
     B1.1 With disk rupture
     B1.2 With type A fracture

B2: Posterior osseous lesion
     B2.1 Transverse bicolumn
     B2.2 With disk rupture
     B2.3 With type A fracture

B3: Anterior disk rupture
     B3.1 With subluxation
     B3.2 With spondylolysis
     B3.3 With posterior dislocation

C. Rotation injury

C1: Type A with rotation
     C1.1 Rotational wedge fracture
     C1.2 Rotational split fracture
     C1.3 Rotational burst fracture

C2: Type B with rotation
     C2.1 B1 Lesion with rotation
     C2.2 B2 Lesion with rotation
     C2.3 B3 Lesion with rotation

References

1. Bernhardt M, White AA, Panjabi MM (2006) Biomechanical considerations of spinal stability. In: Herkowitz HN, Garfin SR, Eismont FJ et al (eds) Rothman-Simeone the spine, 5th edn. Saunders-Elsevier, Philadelphia

2. Bertram C, Prescher A, Furderer S et al (2003) Attachment points of the posterior longitudinal ligament and their importance for thoracic and lumbar spine fractures. Orthopade 32:848–851

3. Blauth M, Bastian L, Knop C et al (1999) Inter-observer reliability in the classification of thoraco-lumbar spinal injuries. Orthopade 28:662–681

4. Bohlman HH (1985) Treatment of fractures and dislocations of the thoracic and lumbar spine. J Bone Joint Surg Am 67: 165–169

5. Bono CM, Rinaldi MD (2006) Thoracolumbar trauma. In: Spivak JM, Connolly PJ (eds) Orthopaedic knowledge update: spine, 3rd edn. American Academy of Orthopaedic Surgeons, Rosemont

6. Bradford DS, McBride GG (1987) Surgical management of thoracolumbar spine fractures with incomplete neurologic deficits. Clin Orthop Relat Res 218:201–216

7. Calenoff L, Chessare JW, Rogers LF et al (1978) Multiple level spinal injuries: importance of early recognition. AJR Am J Roentgenol 130:665–669

8. Denis F (1983) The three column spine and its significance in the classification of acute thoracolumbar spinal injuries. Spine 8:817–831

9. Denis F (1984) Spinal instability as defined by the three-column spine concept in acute spinal trauma. Clin Orthop Relat Res 189:65–76

10. Denis F, Burkus JK (1992) Shear fracture-dislocations of the thoracic and lumbar spine associated with forceful hyperextension (lumberjack paraplegia). Spine 17:156–161

11. Gertzbein SD (1992) Scoliosis Research Society. Multicenter spine fracture study. Spine 17:528–540

12. Glaser JA, Estes WJ (1998) Distal short segment fixation of thoracolumbar and lumbar injuries. Iowa Orthop J 18:87–90

13. Henderson RL, Reid DC, Saboe LA (1991) Multiple non-contiguous spine fractures. Spine 16:128–131

14. Hoshikawa T, Tanaka Y, Kokubun S et al (2002) Flexion-distraction injuries in the thoracolumbar spine: an in vitro study of the relation between flexion angle and the motion axis of fracture. J Spinal Disord Tech 15:139–143

15. Koulouris G, Ting AYI (2007) BMW imaging of thoraco-columbar spinal injury. In: Schwartz ED, Flanders AE (eds) Spinal trauma, 1st edn. Lippincott Williams & Wilkins, Philadelphia

16. Magerl F, Aebi M, Gertzbein SD et al (1994) A comprehensive classification of thoracic and lumbar injuries. Eur Spine J 3:184–201

17. McAfee PC, Yuan HA, Fredrickson BE et al (1983) The value of computed tomography in thoracolumbar fractures. An analysis of one hundred consecutive cases and a new classification. J Bone Joint Surg Am 65:461–473

18. McCormack T, Karaikovic E, Gaines RW (1994) The load sharing classification of spine fractures. Spine 19: 1741–1744

19. Mirza SK, Mirza AJ, Chapman JR et al (2002) Classifications of thoracic and lumbar fractures: rationale and supporting data. J Am Acad Orthop Surg 10:364–377

20. Parker JW, Lane JR, Karaikovic EE et al (2000) Successful short-segment instrumentation and fusion for thoracolumbar spine fractures: a consecutive 41/2-year series. Spine 25: 1157–1170

21. Singer KP, Willen J, Breidahl PD et al (1989) Radiologic study of the influence of zygapophyseal joint orientation on spinal injuries at the thoracolumbar junction. Surg Radiol Anat 11: 233–239

22. Singh K, Kim D, Vaccaro AR (2006) Thoracic and lumbar spinal injuries. In: Herkowitz H, Garfin S, Eismont FJ, Bell G (eds) Rothman-Simeone the spine, 5th edn. Saunders-Elsevier, Philadelphia

23. Spivak JM, Vaccaro AR, Cotler JM (1995) Thoracolumbar spine trauma: I. Evaluation and classification. J Am Acad Orthop Surg 3:345–352

24. Spivak JM, Vaccaro AR, Cotler JM (1995) Thoracolumbar spine trauma: II. Principles of management. J Am Acad Orthop Surg 3:353–360

25. Sullivan JD, Farfan HF (1975) The crumpled neural arch. Orthop Clin North Am 6:199–214

26. Vaccaro AR, An HS, Lin S et al (1992) Noncontiguous injuries of the spine. J Spinal Disord 5:320–329

27. Vaccaro AR, Kim DH, Brodke DS et al (2004) Diagnosis and management of thoracolumbar spine fractures. Instr Course Lect 53:359–373

28. White AA, Panjabi MM (1978) Clinical Biomechanics of the Spine, 1st edn. JM Lippincott, Philadelphia

29. Whitesides TE Jr (1977) Traumatic kyphosis of the thoracolumbar spine. Clin Orthop Relat Res 128:78–92

30. Wood K, Buttermann G, Mehbod A et al (2003) Operative compared with nonoperative treatment of a thoracolumbar burst fracture without neurological deficit: a prospective, randomized study. J Bone Joint Surg Am 85:773–781

Posterior Instrumentation for Thoracolumbar and Lumbar Fracture Dislocation

23

Christian P. DiPaola and Brian K. Kwon

23.1 Case 1

A 38-year-old, otherwise healthy, male, fell about 30 ft. from a tree. He presented with a GCS of 15, and complete motor/sensory loss below T6 (deemed to be a T6 ASIA A spinal cord injury). His initial CT scan is shown and revealed a T6 fracture dislocation with an apparent flexion distraction mechanism. He also had facet fractures at T8 and T9 and spinous process fractures at T9 and T10 (Fig. 23.1a–c).

A posterior approach to the thoracic spine was performed in anticipation of placing pedicle screw instrumentation across the injury. Operative findings of extensive closed degloving and complete ligamentous injury at T5–9 were present. Instrumentation was thus performed from T3 to T11. A side-loading pedicle screw system (SiLo®, Medtronic Spine and Biologics, Memphis TN) was used to correct the deformity and stabilize the injured motion segments. After screws were inserted at all levels (Fig. 23.2), two rods were contoured to approximate the native thoracic kyphosis and were secured to the distal screws. The proximal screws were then reduced to the rod using the rod-screw "persuaders", thus thereby realigning the fracture dislocation and partially correcting the segmental kyphosis. Postoperative X-rays demonstrate realignment and

fixation of the spine from an all-posterior approach (Fig. 23.3a, b).

23.2 Background

The management of thoracolumbar injuries has evolved substantially over the past 3 decades, aided by an increased understanding of spinal biomechanics, improved methods of imaging and classification, and the explosive growth of spinal instrumentation technology. However, the basic principles of restoring stability and decompressing neural elements remain the same. While tremendous advances have been made in methods for accessing the anterior column of the thoracolumbar spine and both reconstructing and stabilizing it, posterior pedicle screw instrumentation remains the mainstay of thoracolumbar fixation.

This chapter discusses the use of posterior instrumentation systems for thoracolumbar fracture dislocations and burst fractures with severe bony retropulsion into the canal requiring decompression. Fracture dislocations are characterized by sagittal and/or coronal translation or rotational deformity and are typically associated with obvious disruption of the posterior ligamentous complex (PLC) (with resultant instability). Burst fractures are axial loading injuries that, in the purest sense, compromise the anterior and middle column only, and incite bony retropulsion into the spinal canal. The PLC may, in such cases, be intact. More commonly, however, a combination of axial loading and flexion serves to disrupt the PLC as well as the anterior column, leaving these highly unstable (and to some extent, on the verge of becoming a fracture dislocation). In both these scenarios, neurologic compromise is common.

B.K. Kwon (✉)
6th Floor Blusson Spinal Cord Center,
Department of Orthopaedics,
University of British Columbia, 818 W. 10th St,
Vancouver, BC, V5Z1M9, Canada
e-mail: brian.kwon@vch.ca

C.P. DiPaola
University of Massachusetts Medical Center,
119 Belmont St, Worcester, MA 01605, USA

V.V. Patel et al. (eds.), *Spine Trauma*,
DOI: 10.1007/978-3-642-03694-1_23, © Springer-Verlag Berlin Heidelberg 2010

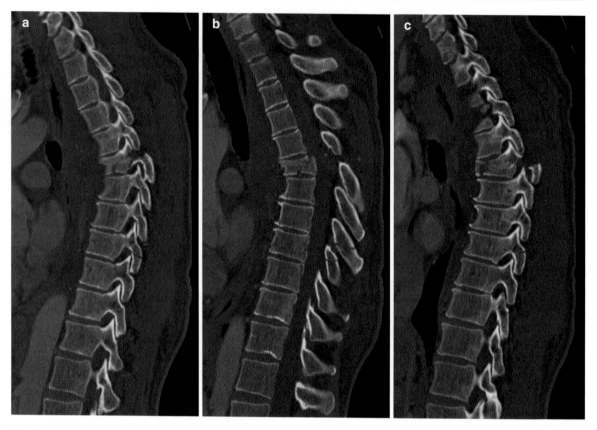

Fig. 23.1 (**a–c**) Saggital reconstruction of thoracic spine CT demonstrating facet fractures (**a, c**), spinous process fractures (**b**), and T6 fracture dislocation with segmental kyphosis (**a–c**)

23.3 Classification and Indications

A number of thoracolumbar fracture classification systems have been described through the years, all of which attempt to characterize the morphology and assess the stability of the injury using injury mechanism, physical exam, radiographic findings, and most recently, neurologic status [7, 11, 15, 22]. Recently a thoracolumbar fracture injury classification has been devised that incorporates three aspects of the patient presentation to guide treatment. The key elements include (1) The morphology of the injury based on imaging studies, (2) The integrity of the PLC, and (3) The neurologic status of the patient [36–40, 42]. This classification system (described in depth in the cited articles) allows critical elements of the patient assessment to be communicated quickly and concisely to help the surgeon understand the injury and aid in treatment decision making.

By virtue of their translational or rotational malalignment, thoracolumbar fracture dislocations are, generally speaking, best treated with posterior pedicle screw instrumentation [42]. The ability to correct severe translation or rotational malalignment is difficult (if not impossible in some cases) from the anterior approach alone. Basic deformity correction principles mandate a posterior approach with pedicle screw fixation in such cases. Biomechanically, the posterior pedicle screw instrumentation is better able to resist shear and rotational forces at play in these injuries [42]. For distractive injuries characterized primarily by PLC disruption, posterior instrumentation is ideally suited for restoring the posterior tension band.

More controversial, however, is the role of posterior instrumentation in patients with thoracolumbar burst fractures in the setting of (1) Severe bony retropulsion and a neurologic deficit, or (2) PLC disruption or severe anterior and middle column comminution causing mechanical instability. The questions here are more complex: *Can posterior instrumentation achieve adequate ventral decompression of the thecal sac? And can posterior instrumentation alone provide sufficient*

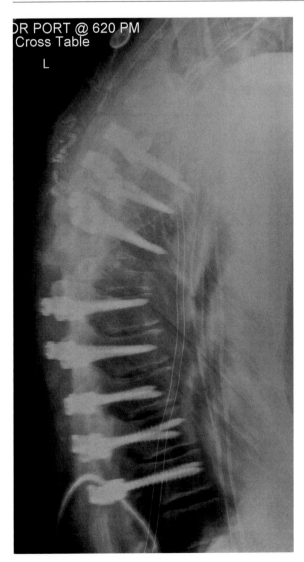

R PORT @ 620 PM
Cross Table

L

Fig. 23.2 Intraoperative radiograph prior to reduction and fixation with rods. Note the loss of vertebral body height at T6 and segmental kyphosis

Patients with complete thoracic spinal cord injury with little chance of recovery may also benefit from posterior instrumentation and fusion for immediate stabilization, maintenance of alignment, and easier nursing care [42]. An all-posterior approach in the polytrauma patient also is beneficial in that it avoids violation of the intrathoracic or intraabdominal space which may be injured as well [42].

23.4 Contraindications

There are few specific contraindications to posterior instrumentation in thoracolumbar fracture dislocations. In thoracolumbar burst fractures, one could argue that in cases where the PLC is intact, there is little reason to approach the spine posteriorly and potentially disrupt it. However, there may be reasons in such cases to avoid an anterior approach. In general, stabilization achieved with fixation allows for immediate patient mobilization, the benefits of which are obvious in the multi-trauma situation. Physiologic instability and the inability to ventilate while in the prone position may, however, make it impossible to technically perform the surgery. Indirect reduction and posterior stabilization of burst fractures may be more difficult after 72 h postinjury [10, 44]. This appears to happen because the mobility of the structures (i.e., bony fragments, disks, and ligamentous structures) decreases over time in the early phases of fracture healing. Indirect reduction techniques also tend to be less successful in patients with greater than 67% canal compromise [16]. Also, patients with a "reverse cortical sign" showing a fracture fragment that is 180° rotated are not appropriate for this technique.

stability in the setting of severe anterior and middle column comminution? To address the first question, indirect reduction of the retropulsed burst fragments has been shown to be achievable by distraction and ligamentotaxis [1, 7, 42]. This technique can reduce the extent to which bony retropulsion has compromised the canal by as much as 50%, but typically achieves somewhat less than this [10, 19, 35]. Some of the potential limitations of this technique are related to the kyphosis that can be induced with distraction, and the potential for failing to decompress the neural elements with an incomplete reduction of the burst fragment.

23.5 Advantages

The obvious advantage of the posterior approach is its familiarity to all spine surgeons, the relative ease at placing pedicle screw instrumentation, and the biomechanical strength of posterior pedicle screw constructs. The approach avoids potential injury to intraabdominal or retroperitoneal structures that are at risk during anterior exposures and the morbidity of performing a thoracotomy and/or taking down the diaphragm to access injuries at the thoracolumbar junction.

Fig. 23.3 (**a, b**) Postoperative radiographs after posterior reduction and fixation of the fracture. Partial restoration of alignment and kyphotic correction were able to be achieved

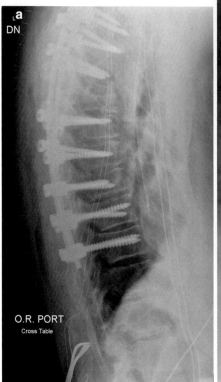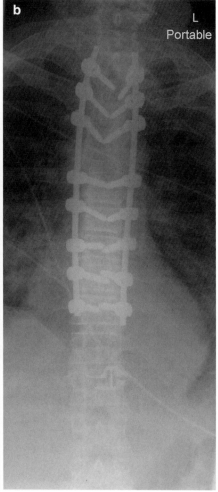

23.5.1 Disadvantages

The main disadvantage of the posterior approach in thoracolumbar burst fracture management is the possibility of failing to adequately decompress the neural elements when depending on ligamentotaxis and indirect reduction of the burst fragment, particularly after 72 h postinjury. Direct visualization of the burst fragment and its removal is not possible with this technique, unless a posterolateral or transpedicular approach is employed. Also, to achieve stability, short segment fixation constructs have historically not been sufficient, and additional levels may need to be instrumented in order to provide adequate biomechanical rigidity. Whether the addition of levels in a posterior construct is worse than the morbidity of a thoracoabdominal approach and take-down of the

diaphragm to perform a shorter segment anterior construct is unknown.

23.6 Surgical Technique

23.6.1 Positioning

When thoracolumbar instability is known or suspected, strict spine immobilization is the rule. The safety of log-rolling patients with thoracic and/or lumbar spinal instability has come into question due to the amount of motion generated [31, 32]. Surgical positioning is a maneuver that can potentially cause neurologic deterioration in the patient with an unstable spine. There are multiple reports that describe the onset of electrophysiologic perturbations (some associated with neurologic deterioration) in the operating room immediately after supine to prone positioning [2, 3, 14, 24]. It has recently been shown that the Jackson table turning method from supine to prone on the operating table generates significantly less thoracolumbar spine motion than a standard log-roll [13]. The Jackson technique involves sliding the supine patient to the Jackson table with a slider board. The patient is secured to the table with a strap across the body, just below the elbows. The ventral aspect of the carbon fiber frame with the respective headrest, chest rolls, and leg pads (Fig. 23.3a) is suspended over the patient by securing it to the top rung of the metal H-frame at each end of the bed. The pads are adjusted along the length of the patient and straps are prepared to secure the patient. The frame is then lowered to tightly squeeze the patient into the frame. At this point, it may become difficult, if not impossible, to ventilate the patient and so the team must be prepared to quickly finish securing the patient with straps, so that the turning may proceed. It is also wise to ensure that the anesthetic team is ready for this turn, as it is not infrequent that – at this moment when they become unable to ventilate the patient – they also suddenly realize that their intravenous and monitoring lines will be intractably twisted and tangled up when the patient is turned. The team should be ready to secure the straps, and all lines, cables, chest tubes, and the catheters should be positioned (or disconnected) so that they do not delay the turn once the patient has been squeezed into the frame (Fig. 23.3b). When ready, the team unlocks the bed at the head and feet of the table and turns the table assembly 180° (Fig. 23.3c) [13]. Final padding of all bony prominences is performed. The arms are padded appropriately at the cubital tunnel and care is taken to not abduct the shoulders greater than 90° to protect the brachial plexus (Fig. 23.3d). There are many devices to choose for holding the head, but it is important to limit pressure to the face and eyes to decrease the risk of pressure ulcers or blindness. The senior author prefers using the Mayfield head clamp for prone cases planned greater than 3 h as this keeps the eyes and face fully free of direct pressure and allows one to position the neck in a neutral position. It is generally easiest to apply the Mayfield head clamp prior to transfer to the operating table. The Mayfield clamp holder assembly is then attached to the clamp prior to rotation.

23.7 Equipment

Depending on the preference of the surgeon, extent of injury, and physiologic state and habitus of the patient, the surgeon should consider the use of fluoroscopy or plain film X-ray throughout the case. This can be helpful for confirmation of levels at the beginning of the case and for use in locating and confirming pedicle screw insertion sites and trajectory. Also, red blood cell sparing devices such as Cell Saver® should be considered to possibly limit allogeneic transfusion. Blood should be available for transfusion as needed, as well because the polytrauma patient is at risk for hematologic compromise. Particularly when operating early on patients with thoracolumbar fracture dislocations, the intraoperative blood loss can be substantial, and the surgeon is well served to be ready for this.

- Fluoroscopy
- Neuromonitoring
- Fracture/Jackson table
- Pedicle screw system
- Bone graft if needed
- Laminectomy set
- Dural repair equipment/supplies
- Rod cutter
- Rod benders
- Hooks and wires as needed for bailout

A pedicle screw system that allows correction of angular deformity independently from distraction is ideal as it allows optimization of lordosis and vertebral height separately.

23.8 Neuromonitoring

Multiple types of neurologic monitoring are available including SSEP, MEP, and EMG. It is beyond the scope of this chapter to discuss the technique and role of each type of monitoring. If available, these techniques may be valuable in detecting neurologic changes as spinal manipulation or pedicle screw insertion occurs. No technique, however, is 100% sensitive and a perfect electrophysiologic system for checking the accuracy of pedicle screw placement in the thoracolumbar spine is lacking.

23.9 Approach

A standard midline posterior approach to the region of the injury is typically employed. A subperiosteal exposure is performed, exposing out as far lateral as the transverse processes. Care should be taken not to disrupt the interspinous ligaments and facet capsules of the spinal levels adjacent above and below the extent of the fusion. This may protect the adjacent segment from decompensating in the future. Wiltse-type parasagittal muscle-splitting approaches, and more recently, percutaneous "minimally invasive" techniques have been described. These alternative approaches are not appropriate for fractures in which there is a need to directly decompress the spinal cord posteriorly or when a dural tear requiring repair is suspected. They also rely much more heavily on intra-operative fluoroscopy for proper screw placement. Their role in fracture surgery has yet to be fully defined, but the potential for this technology to limit the extent of soft tissue disruption around the spine has been demonstrated by some surgeons, and the popularity of this technology will undoubtedly increase in the future [28, 43].

For severe fracture dislocations, or fractures that have significant posterior element disruption, the surgeon may wish to expose the spine above and below the zone of injury and instrument these levels first. This approach may help limit blood loss as it is likely that the greatest amount of bleeding will occur in the zone of injury around the dislocation. Once the injured area is exposed, the surgeon should be wary of plunging with the cautery around the region of posterior element disruption or lamina fracture. This will help protect against inadvertent entrance into the spinal canal. At this point, the spine surgeon should also be prepared to encounter traumatic dural tears and CSF leakage. Proper supplies such as microsurgical instruments and small gage monofilament (6-0) suture should be available along with fibrin glue and dural patch material.

23.9.1 Pedicle Screw Insertion

Insertion of thoracic and lumbar pedicle screws requires extensive knowledge of the complex anatomy of the spine. Anatomic landmarks need full exposure and recognition. Intraoperative imaging (i.e., fluoroscopy, radiography, or image guidance) may help with the accurate placement of pedicle screws, but ultimately, the safe insertion of screws relies heavily on the surgeon's appreciation for the anatomy. Thoracic pedicle dimensions from T4–T8 tend to be the smallest and thus are most challenging regions to successfully place pedicle screw instrumentation [8, 47]. A number of methods have been described for the proper placement of thoracic pedicle screws. Common methods of insertion involve identification of the transverse process, pars, and superior and inferior articular facet. A starting point is located at a point where the superior border of the transverse process converges with the lamina along the lateral border of the articular facet. This is typically in line with or just slightly medial to the pars (Fig. 23.4) [8, 47]. Osteotomy of the inferior articular process exposes the superior articular process that lies directly anteriorly as the facet joint is coronally aligned. This maneuver may help to identify the medial-lateral borders of the superior articular process, but is not typically necessary. The transverse process often needs to be burred or rongeured to access the entry point. It may also be helpful to remove dorsal bone from the thoracic transverse process as the prominence of this structure can push the surgeon's hand too far medially causing a lateral

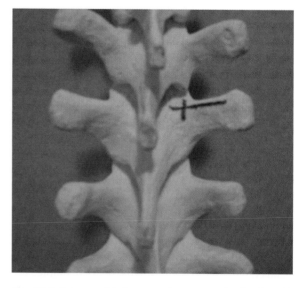

Fig. 23.4 Spine model demonstrating entry point for thoracic pedicle screw

misdirection of screw trajectory. The pedicle is bluntly probed with a 3 mm thoracic pedicle probe. The probe can be straight or curved. If the probe is curved, then for the initial 20 mm of insertion the probe tip should be angled laterally to avoid medial pedicle perforation. After about 20 mm, the vertebral body should be entered with the tip pointed medially. Aberrant screw placement lateral to the pedicle (and body) can put the more ventral vascular structures at risk in the thoracic spine (Fig. 23.5). Medial misdirection can damage the spinal cord and inferior misplacement can injure nerve roots.

In order to insert lumbar pedicle screws, similar anatomical structures must be identified. The lumbar transverse process, pars, and superior articular process are exposed and visualized. The intersection point of a line that splits the midline of the transverse process and intersects the pars and superior articular process is defined as the entry site. A portion of the superior articular process can be burred or rongeured, so that the pedicle can be entered with a pedicle probe. Figure 23.6 demonstrates a foam bone model with screws inserted in representative lumbar pedicles. Note the anatomy and convergence of landmarks.

There are multiple manufacturers that offer pedicle screw instrumentation systems that can fit the needs of the spine trauma surgeon. In general, these systems can be described as either top loading monoaxial and polyaxial screw systems, or side loading systems with

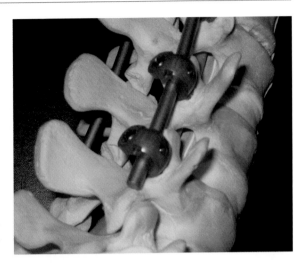

Fig. 23.6 Pedicle screw instrumentation is noted in the lumbar spine model

or without sagittal variability (these screws can be considered a type of monoaxial screw system). Monoaxial screw systems offer somewhat more powerful reduction capabilities compared to polyaxial screws, although the fixed head of the monoaxial screws requires a more technically precise placement [42].

With polyaxial screw systems, lordosis reduction is achieved by reduction of the screw heads to a precontoured rod meant to match normal thoracolumbar kyphosis and lordosis as necessary. Various systems have reduction instruments that allow rods to be coaxed into the screw heads before final tightening of set screws. Cross connectors can also be added to provide greater torsional stability to the construct. This is especially important in the case of fracture dislocations [42].

Side-loading screw systems such as the Synthes USS® and Medtronic Silo® are useful for correcting kyphosis at the injury level. The Synthes USS® system has "sticks" that attach to the end of the pedicle screw, making them function effectively like a Schantz pin. As these side-loading screws are monoaxial in nature, they can be placed in relative kyphosis, with the anticipation that reducing the screws into a lordotic or straight rod will bring the fracture into a more lordotic position. An example of how this can be achieved with the Synthes USS® system is illustrated in (Fig. 23.7). Note how the screws are placed in relative kyphosis initially, and when reduced to the rod, the normal alignment is restored across the thoracolumbar junction. Distraction across the screws can also help to

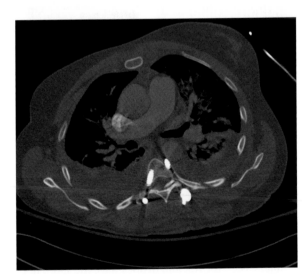

Fig. 23.5 Postoperative chest CT demonstrates aberrant lateral screw breach, which may put the aorta at risk

Fig. 23.7 Posterior management of L1 burst fracture. (**a**) Intraoperative X-ray of a patient with an L1 burst fracture that had canal compromise. Note the relative kyphosis of initial spinal alignment. Screws with "stick" handles applied are demonstrated here. The positioning is in kyphosis for the purpose of demonstrating a burst fracture with kyphotic alignment. (**b**) The screws are reduced to a rod that is neutral across the thoracolumbar junction. This reduces the kyphotic deformity across L1

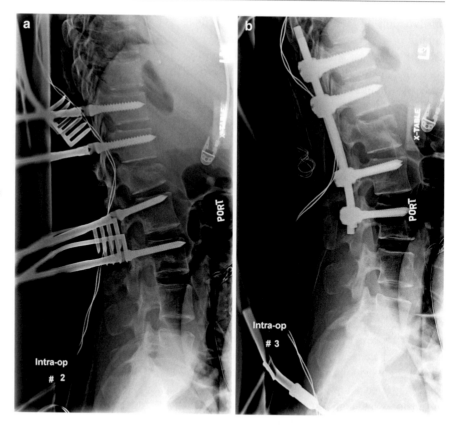

reduce a retropulsed burst fragment, as long as the posterior longitudinal ligament is intact and still attached to the burst fragment. One should be aware, however, of the potential to induce kyphosis with such a distraction maneuver. One of the difficulties of the USS side-loading system is that the rod-screw angle is fixed at about 90°. The Silo side-loading screw system employs a sagittal "rocking saddle mechanism" (Fig. 23.8) that facilitates rod reduction into the screws and enables the sagittal alignment of the screws to be altered once the rod has been captured (Fig. 23.9a, b). Care should be taken, especially with monoaxial screw systems, to avoid overaggressive manipulation of the rod into the screw if the patient has poor bone quality. Generally, patients with low energy injuries should be assumed to have poor bone quality until proven otherwise.

The extent of instrumentation (number of levels instrumented) is often determined by a judgment of relative fracture stability and bone quality. Typically, it is advised to instrument at least two levels above and below the fracture, so that the forces invoked in supporting the deformity correction and providing

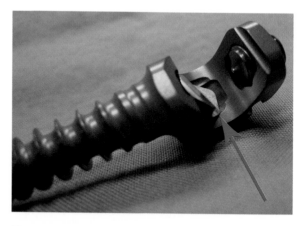

Fig. 23.8 Medtronic "uniaxial" type screw is shown. Note the side-loading head with a sagittal "rocker" type mechanism that allows for angular correction in the sagittal plane (*arrow*)

immediate stability are distributed among the screws [42]. The poorer the bone quality or greater the extent of injury (i.e., for fracture dislocation), the more necessary it will be to obtain additional points of fixation [9, 46]. Short segment fixation (i.e., one level above

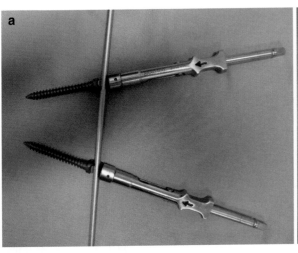
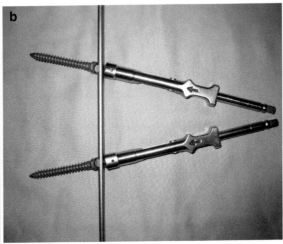

Fig. 23.9 Pedicle screws attached to "stick" type handles that are used for vertebral distraction and manipulating the vertebral bodies into lordosis. The sagittal rocking saddle within the Silo screw head allows for manipulation of the vertebral bodies into a more lordotic alignment once the rod has been captured. This can be very helpful in a kyphotic deformity. An example is shown here where the screws are in a kyphotic alignment and the rod is reduced into the screws (**a**). Then, with the sticks attached, the screws can be distracted (to achieve ligamentotaxis) and brought into a more lordotic position (**b**)

and below the level of injury) has been used successfully with selected fractures in which restoration of the posterior tension band is the only requirement. It is still not possible to completely predict which fractures will be treated successfully with short segment fixation, but it appears that the greater the anterior load sharing capability of the anterior and middle column, the more likely the chances of successful treatment with short segment fixation [27]. It has been shown that lower lumbar burst fractures may be more likely to be amenable to short segment pedicle screw fixation [23]. The benefit of this technique is also that lumbar motion segments are spared, which theoretically decreases the likelihood of adjacent segment disease.

23.9.2 Fusion

The ultimate goal of instrumenting the spine is to establish immediate stability to facilitate fracture healing and bony fusion. There are multiple options to enhance bony fusion. Once instrumentation has been performed, the facets and transverse processes are decorticated with the aid of a burr, rongeur, or osteotome. Local bone from the laminectomy or facet osteotomy can also be used in the fusion bed. Iliac crest autograft, harvested from the posterior ileum, remains the gold standard for posterior spinal fusion in the setting of trauma. However, the morbidity of harvesting iliac crest autograft has been well established [4, 17] and thus alternative biologic products are currently on the market such as recombinant human BMPs that may also be useful alternatives or adjuncts to autograft. It should be noted that the efficacy and safety of these products have yet to be fully determined in thoracolumbar trauma, and their application in this regard is off-label.

The decision to fuse or not to fuse and the extent to which fusion is performed in the setting of fracture has not been fully elucidated. Some authors prefer to place bone graft and generate fusion at every instrumented level [42]. While other studies have shown no true clinically significant difference in groups of patients that have been treated with instrumentation alone vs. instrumentation and bony fusion, for thoracolumbar fractures [41].

23.10 Technical Pearls

- For optimal reduction and canal decompression with indirect measures, surgery is best performed within 72 h [10, 42].
- When a pedicle hole is difficult to find, a small laminotomy can be made to palpate the pedicle

medially just below the superior facet. Also, the pedicle can be palpated laterally with a Penfield 4 just lateral to the superior facet (in the thoracic spine) [42, 47].

- When thoracic pedicles are too small to accommodate screws they may be cannulated from a lateral extrapedicular approach [42, 47].
- Laminar hooks or sublaminar wires may be used to supplement pedicle screw constructs in osteoporotic bone [42].
- T4–T8 pedicle dimensions tend to be the smallest and thus it may be most difficult to safely insert pedicle screws in this region.
- Cut the rod slightly longer than templated because distraction maneuvers to regain vertebral body height will necessitate more length [42].
- Typically, when lamina fractures occur in conjunction with burst fractures, the possibility of dural tears or entrapped nerve roots must be addressed [5, 12, 45].
- If after a reduction and realignment of the spine decompression is inadequate, open decompression may be needed (Chap 4).

23.10.1 Pitfalls

- Avoid short segment fixation (i.e., one level above and below the fracture) in fractures with severe anterior column disruption. It typically does not provide adequate stabilization of the fracture unless one additionally performs some form of augmentation/reconstruction of the anterior column [42].
- Control blood loss fastidiously [42].
- Avoid violation of the anterior vertebral body due to risk of vascular or visceral injury. Avoid violation of the medial pedicle due to risk of spinal cord injury.

23.11 Intraoperative Complications

The incidence of iatrogenic neurologic deficit with the use of pedicle screw instrumentation is reported to be about 1%. This may occur as a result of misplaced screws or because of manipulation of the spinal cord or nerve roots [21]. Visceral or vascular structures are at risk during pedicle screw insertion if screws are inserted too laterally or anteriorly [42]. Specific awareness of vascular structures is particularly important due to their proximity to pedicle screw insertion trajectories. Aberrant left-sided thoracic and upper lumbar pedicle screw insertion can put the aorta at risk acutely or due to chronic attritional injury [20, 33, 34] (Fig. 23.8).

Dural tears have been associated with the presence of lamina fractures in thoracolumbar trauma [5, 12, 45]. An all-posterior approach is ideal for exploration and repair of these tears as needed.

Unrecognized fractures preoperatively can become apparent intraoperatively. Always be prepared to instrument additional levels as needed.

Screw pullout of pedicle fracture may occur intraoperatively, especially when the patient has osteopenia or osteoporosis. It has been shown in multiple studies that resistance to loosening and pullout of pedicle screws is directly related to bone mineral density [18, 25, 26].

23.12 Bailout and Salvage Procedures

When pedicle screws lose fixation intraoperatively or when anatomy precludes the use of pedicle screw fixation in particular segments of the spine, other supplemental means of fixation can be employed. Sublaminar wires and interspinous process cables can be used to gain additional stability. Pedicle hooks and sublaminar claws can also be used as points of fixation.

23.13 Postoperative Course

23.13.1 Bracing

There is no good data or literature to support the use of braces postoperatively after the treatment of thoracolumbar trauma. It is at the discretion of the surgeon as to whether the patient will tolerate a brace (i.e., it may be difficult to brace a polytrauma with multiple abdominal, thoracic, and/or extremity injuries). Braces may be used to supplement, but do not substitute for proper internal fixation. If there is a concern for ongoing instability, an anterior procedure or bedrest can be considered.

23.13.2 Activity

Patients are typically allowed to participate in activities as tolerated as long as the surgeon feels that fixation is adequate. Patients are encouraged to mobilize, and when comfortable, an upright X-ray is performed to demonstrate maintenance of appropriate spinal alignment with weight bearing.

23.13.3 Follow-Up

The senior author prefers having the dressing changed on post-op day 3 or sooner, if it becomes soiled or saturated. After that point a dressing should be maintained for 10–14 days or until staples or sutures are ready to be removed. Patients are typically seen back at 3 month intervals in the first postoperative year and then at longer intervals as needed. Each patient's postoperative clinical follow-up should be tailored by their individual needs and clinical scenario. If wound health or fixation concerns are more worrisome, more regular follow-ups may be warranted.

23.14 Complication Management

The management of complications requires judicious follow-up and anticipation of signs and symptoms. Infection has been reported to occur in about 10% operatively treated thoracolumbar fractures [29, 30]. Persistent wound drainage is often the first sign of spinal wound infection. The senior author prefers an aggressive approach to wound management with early irrigation and debridement and administration of culture specific antibiotics as necessary in such cases. Following CRP and ESR can help gage a patient's response to treatment.

References

1. Aebi M, Thalgott JS, Webb JK (1998) AO ASIF Principles in spine surgery. Springer, Berlin
2. Anderson RC, Dowling KC, Feldstein NA, Emerson RG (2003) Chiari I malformation: potential role for intraoperative electrophysiologic monitoring. J Clin Neurophysiol 20(1):65–72
3. Anderson RC, Emerson RG, Dowling KC, Feldstein NA (2001) Attenuation of somatosensory evoked potentials during positioning in a patient undergoing suboccipital craniectomy for Chiari I malformation with syringomyelia. J Child Neurol 16(12):936–939
4. Arrington ED, Smith WJ, Chambers HG, Bucknell AL, Davino NA (1996) Complications of iliac crest bone graft harvesting. Clin Orthop Relat Res (329):300–309
5. Aydinli U, Karaeminogullari O, Tiskaya K, Ozturk C (2001) Dural tears in lumbar burst fractures with greenstick lamina fractures. Spine 26(18):E410–E415
6. Bucholz RW, Gill K (1986) Classification of injuries to the thoracolumbar spine. Orthop Clin North Am 17(1):67–73
7. Chang KW (1992) A reduction-fixation system for unstable thoracolumbar burst fractures. Spine 17(8):879–886
8. Cinotti G, Gumina S, Ripani M, Postacchini F (1999) Pedicle instrumentation in the thoracic spine. A morphometric and cadaveric study for placement of screws. Spine 24(2):114–119
9. Coe JD, Warden KE, Herzig MA, McAfee PC (1990) Influence of bone mineral density on the fixation of thoracolumbar implants. A comparative study of transpedicular screws, laminar hooks, and spinous process wires. Spine 15(9):902–907
10. Crutcher JP Jr, Anderson PA, King HA, Montesano PX (1991) Indirect spinal canal decompression in patients with thoracolumbar burst fractures treated by posterior distraction rods. J Spinal Disord 4(1):39–48
11. Denis F (1983) The three column spine and its significance in the classification of acute thoracolumbar spinal injuries. Spine 8(8):817–831
12. Denis F, Burkus JK (1991) Diagnosis and treatment of cauda equina entrapment in the vertical lamina fracture of lumbar burst fractures. Spine 16(8 suppl):S433–S439
13. DiPaola CP, DiPaola MJ, Conrad BP, Horodyski M, Del Rossi G, Sawers A, Rechtine GR 2nd (2008) Comparison of thoracolumbar motion produced by manual and jackson-table-turning methods. Study of a cadaveric instability model. J Bone Joint Surg Am 90(8):1698–1704
14. Epstein NE, Danto J, Nardi D (1993) Evaluation of intraoperative somatosensory-evoked potential monitoring during 100 cervical operations. Spine 18(6):737–747
15. Ferguson RL, Allen BL Jr (1986) An algorithm for the treatment of unstable thoracolumbar fractures. Orthop Clin North Am 17(1):105–112
16. Gertzbein SD, Crowe PJ, Fazl M, Schwartz M, Rowed D (1992) Canal clearance in burst fractures using the AO internal fixator. Spine 17(5):558–560
17. Goulet JA, Senunas LE, DeSilva GL, Greenfield ML (1997) Autogenous iliac crest bone graft. Complications and functional assessment. Clin Orthop Relat Res (339):76–81
18. Halvorson TL, Kelley LA, Thomas KA, Whitecloud TS 3rd, Cook SD (1994) Effects of bone mineral density on pedicle screw fixation. Spine 19(21):2415–2420
19. Harrington RM, Budorick T, Hoyt J, Anderson PA, Tencer AF (1993) Biomechanics of indirect reduction of bone retropulsed into the spinal canal in vertebral fracture. Spine 18(6):692–699

20. Hernigou P, Germany W (1998) Evaluation of the risk of mediastinal or retroperitoneal injuries caused by dorsolumbar pedicle screws. Rev Chir Orthop Reparatrice Appar Mot 84(5):411–420

21. Katonis P, Christoforakis J, Kontakis G, Aligizakis AC, Papadopoulos C, Sapkas G, Hadjipavlou A (2003) Complications and problems related to pedicle screw fixation of the spine. Clin Orthop Relat Res (411):86–94

22. McAfee PC, Yuan HA, Fredrickson BE, Lubicky JP (1983) The value of computed tomography in thoracolumbar fractures. An analysis of one hundred consecutive cases and a new classification. J Bone Joint Surg Am 65(4):461–473

23. McLain RF (2006) The biomechanics of long versus short fixation for thoracolumbar spine fractures. Spine 31(11 suppl): S70–S79, discussion S104

24. Ofiram E, Lonstein JE, Skinner S, Perra JH (2006) "The disappearing evoked potentials": a special problem of positioning patients with skeletal dysplasia: case report. Spine 31(14):E464–E470

25. Okuyama K, Abe E, Suzuki T, Tamura Y, Chiba M, Sato K (2000) Can insertional torque predict screw loosening and related failures? An in vivo study of pedicle screw fixation augmenting posterior lumbar interbody fusion. Spine 25(7): 858–864

26. Okuyama K, Abe E, Suzuki T, Tamura Y, Chiba M, Sato K (2001) Influence of bone mineral density on pedicle screw fixation: a study of pedicle screw fixation augmenting posterior lumbar interbody fusion in elderly patients. Spine J 1(6):402–407

27. Parker JW, Lane JR, Karaikovic EE, Gaines RW (2000) Successful short-segment instrumentation and fusion for thoracolumbar spine fractures: a consecutive 41/2-year series. Spine 25(9):1157–1170

28. Rampersaud YR, Annand N, Dekutoski MB (2006) Use of minimally invasive surgical techniques in the management of thoracolumbar trauma: current concepts. Spine 31(11 suppl):S96–S102, discussion S104

29. Rechtine GR 2nd, Cahill D, Chrin AM (1999) Treatment of thoracolumbar trauma: comparison of complications of operative versus nonoperative treatment. J Spinal Disord 12(5):406–409

30. Rechtine GR, Bono PL, Cahill D, Bolesta MJ, Chrin AM (2001) Postoperative wound infection after instrumentation of thoracic and lumbar fractures. J Orthop Trauma 15(8):566–569

31. Rechtine GR, Conrad BP, Bearden BG, Horodyski M (2007) Biomechanical analysis of cervical and thoracolumbar spine motion in intact and partially and completely unstable cadaver spine models with kinetic bed therapy or traditional log roll. J Trauma 62(2):383–388, discussion 388

32. Rechtine GR, Del Rossi G, Conrad BP, Horodyski M (2004) Motion generated in the unstable spine during hospital bed transfers. J Trauma 57(3):609–611, discussion 611–2

33. Sarlak AY, Buluc L, Sarisoy HT, Memisoglu K, Tosun B (2008) Placement of pedicle screws in thoracic idiopathic sco-

liosis: a magnetic resonance imaging analysis of screw placement relative to structures at risk. Eur Spine J 17(5):657–662

34. Sjostrom L, Jacobsson O, Karlstrom G, Pech P, Rauschning W (1993) CT analysis of pedicles and screw tracts after implant removal in thoracolumbar fractures. J Spinal Disord 6(3):225–231

35. Sjostrom L, Karlstrom G, Pech P, Rauschning W (1996) Indirect spinal canal decompression in burst fractures treated with pedicle screw instrumentation. Spine 21(1): 113–123

36. Vaccaro AR et al (2006) Reliability of a novel classification system for thoracolumbar injuries: the Thoracolumbar Injury Severity Score. Spine 31(11 suppl):S62–S69, discussion S104

37. Vaccaro AR, Kim DH, Brodke DS, Harris M, Chapman JR, Schildhauer T, Routt ML, Sasso RC (2004) Diagnosis and management of thoracolumbar spine fractures. Instr Course Lect 53:359–373

38. Vaccaro AR et al (2006) Assessment of injury to the posterior ligamentous complex in thoracolumbar spine trauma. Spine J 6(5):524–528

39. Vaccaro AR et al (2005) A new classification of thoracolumbar injuries: the importance of injury morphology, the integrity of the posterior ligamentous complex, and neurologic status. Spine 30(20):2325–2333

40. Vaccaro AR et al (2005) The thoracolumbar injury severity score: a proposed treatment algorithm. J Spinal Disord Tech 18(3):209–215

41. Wang ST, Ma HL, Liu CL, Yu WK, Chang MC, Chen TH (2006) Is fusion necessary for surgically treated burst fractures of the thoracolumbar and lumbar spine? A prospective, randomized study. Spine 31(23):2646–2652, discussion 2653

42. Whang PG, Vaccaro AR (2007) Thoracolumbar fracture: posterior instrumentation using distraction and ligamentotaxis reduction. J Am Acad Orthop Surg 15(11):695–701

43. Wild MH, Glees M, Plieschnegger C, Wenda K (2007) Five-year follow-up examination after purely minimally invasive posterior stabilization of thoracolumbar fractures: a comparison of minimally invasive percutaneously and conventionally open treated patients. Arch Orthop Trauma Surg 127(5):335–343

44. Willen J, Lindahl S, Irstam L, Nordwall A (1984) Unstable thoracolumbar fractures. A study by CT and conventional roentgenology of the reduction effect of Harrington instrumentation. Spine 9(2):214–219

45. Wing P, Aebi M, Denis F, Harris M, Meyer PR Jr (1999) Management of an unstable lumbar fracture with a laminar split. Spinal Cord 37(6):392–401

46. Wittenberg RH, Shea M, Swartz DE, Lee KS, White AA 3rd, Hayes WC (1991) Importance of bone mineral density in instrumented spine fusions. Spine 16(6):647–652

47. Zeiller SC, Lee J, Lim M, Vaccaro AR (2005) Posterior thoracic segmental pedicle screw instrumentation: evolving methods of safe and effective placement. Neurol India 53(4):458–465

F. Cumhur Oner

24.1 Background

There is growing evidence that surgical reduction and fixation may enhance the chances of neurologic recovery in traumatic thoracolumbar (TL) fractures [1]. Although there seems to be no strong relation between the canal encroachment and the neurologic injury or recovery patterns [2], many surgeons feel that patients may benefit from clearance of the canal. The most common traumatic fracture type causing neurologic impairment in thoracolumbar (TL) junction is the burst fracture. In this fracture type, usually the upper endplate fails under the compressive forces in the intervertebral disc and burst out circumferentially. This typically causes a splaying of the pedicles and thrust of a bone fragment from the posterior wall section of the upper endplate into the vertebral canal. The amount of canal encroachment visible on CT or MR images may vary and is probably not directly related to the initial impact and compression on the dural sac or the neurologic damage. The most reliable way to remove all the encroaching fragments is a (partial) corpectomy via an anterior approach. However, this requires a highly invasive approach, which may not be feasible to perform on an emergency basis in frequently poly-traumatized patients. Evidence from cervical trauma studies (STASCIS) suggests that timing of surgery may be a crucial factor in the neurologic prognosis [3]. Surgical techniques, which allow the surgeon a quick reduction, decompression, and stable fixation may prove more beneficial than delayed surgery with more complete decompression.

Fixation and reduction using pedicle screw constructs is a common and reliable surgical technique especially with dedicated trauma instrumentation allowing independent dekyphosing and distraction. If the surgery is performed within the first day after trauma, substantial reduction is usually possible. There has been a considerable amount of debate on the issue of whether indirect reduction of the encroaching fragment is possible by distraction [4]. The data are conflicting and most surgeons do not rely on indirect reduction alone in patients with neurologic injury. Many techniques have been described to perform direct decompression from a posterior or posterolateral route. Growing acquaintance of the spine surgeons with osteotomies including pedicle subtraction osteotomy may facilitate the adoption of these techniques. The technique described here is the preferred method of the author and allows a stepwise procedure until the surgeon is satisfied with the achieved reduction and decompression.

24.2 Technique

This technique is especially useful if the patient can be operated on within the first 24 h after trauma. It is best applied in the thoracolumbar junction (Th10-L2) with burst fractures with or without posterior ligamentous complex injury (Fig. 24.1). Put the patient prone between chest and pelvic support. Make sure that the abdomen is free (Fig. 24.2). Take anteroposterior (AP) and lateral views and mark the fractured vertebra. Use a standard midline posterior approach allowing free access to the fractured vertebra, one level cranial, and one level caudal. Use a dedicated fracture reduction system, which allows one to perform dekyphosing and distraction maneuvers independently (Fig 24.3). Put

F.C. Oner
University Medical Center Utrecht, HP G 05.228, 85500,
3508 GA Utrecht, The Netherlands
e-mail: f.c.oner@umcutrecht.nl

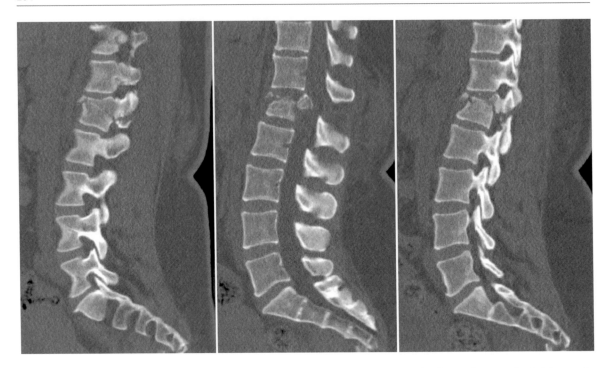

Fig. 24.1 A typical burst fracture with Posterior Ligamentary Complex (PLC) injury causing incomplete neurologic injury at the thoracolumbar (TL) junction

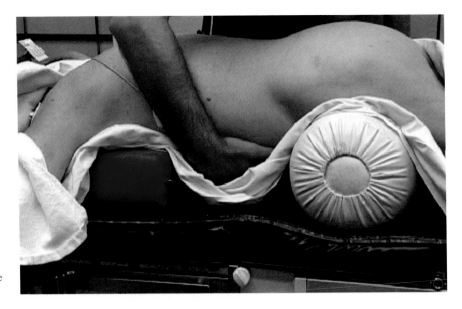

Fig. 24.2 Put the patient prone between chest and pelvic support and make sure that the abdomen is free

the longest and thickest diameter pedicle screws in the pedicles of the cranial and caudal vertebras, preferably getting purchase of the anterior cortex. Perform laminectomy starting between the laminas of the cranial and the fractured vertebra, that is, from cranial to caudal as the most significant compression is typically at the level of the upper endplate. Splitting of the spinous

process and entrapment of the dura is common in burst fractures. Starting the laminectomy from the cranial end will allow freeing of the uninvolved dura and first then freeing of the entrapped dura without further damage. Probe the foramina between the cranial and the fractured vertebras to make sure that there is no dural entrapment. Insert the rods to the screws and reduce the

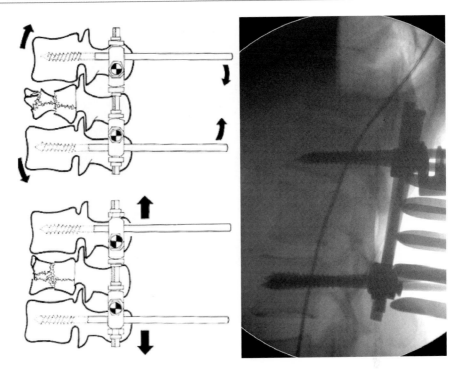

Fig. 24.3 A dedicated TL spinal trauma reduction system should allow dekyphosing and distraction maneuvers to be performed independent of each other

fracture by dekyphosis and distraction (Fig 24.4). Use preferably a system with an offset between the screws and the rods such that the rod lies medial to the facet joints. If the fracture is a real burst-type injury, the anterior longitudinal ligament should be intact and should prevent over-distraction. Reduction of the fracture is the most important part of the decompression, so maximal restoration of the anatomy of the motion segment should be aimed. Confirm the reduction with lateral fluoroscopy. Remove the facet joint between the cranial and fractured vertebra of the right or left side depending on which side the fracture fragment is causing the most compression on the CT or MR images. Expose the nerve root and the posterolateral corner of the disk. Do not excise or damage the disk. A curved dura probe can now be gently inserted between the disk and the ventral dura (Fig. 24.5). In this way, it is possible to feel the compressing fragment and visualize it on lateral fluoroscopic images. A curved bone tamp can in the same way, be inserted in this space. Tap gently with the tamp (Fig. 24.6). Usually there is a void ventral to the fragment after the reduction of the fracture. In this case, the fragment can be tamped back easily. Remove the tamp and check the reduction with the dura probe (Fig. 24.7). If the reduction is not sufficient, remove the pedicle taking care not to move the fracture fragment as this may cause more damage to the dural sac. Drilling

the pedicle with a high-speed burr is usually the safest way to achieve this. When the pedicle is removed, the fracture fragment is exposed from the posterolateral angle. In the same way as in a pedicle subtraction osteotomy a cavity can then be created with curettes ventral to the displaced fragment (the so-called eggshell procedure) and the fragment can be tapped into that cavity using the curved bone tamp (Fig. 24.7). The same procedure can be used from the contralateral pedicle if necessary. The operation is completed by a posterolateral fusion using iliac crest bone.

In cases with high degree of comminution, it is usually possible to achieve good reduction of the fragment without pedicle subtraction technique. However, in that case there is usually a substantial defect in the vertebral body after reduction. In this case, balloon-assisted endplate reduction technique can be used to restore the load-sharing capacity of the anterior column [5] (Fig. 24.8).

24.3 Equipment Needed

- Pedicle screw systems that allow independent distraction and reduction of kyphosis
- Jackson table

Fig. 24.4 Start laminectomy between the cranial uninvolved vertebra and the fractured vertebra. After freeing of the dura install the rods and perform the reduction by dekyphosing followed by distraction. After reduction, remove the facet joint on the side with the most severe compression

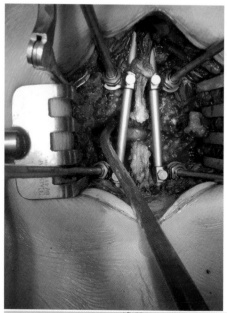

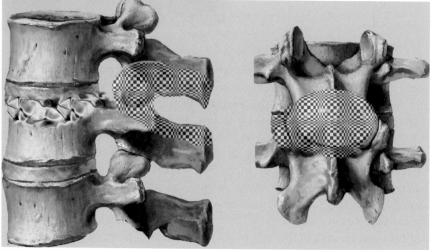

- Neuromonitoring
- Curved probe, for example, Woodson or panfield 4
- Curved tamp for reducing bone fragments
- Fluoroscopy
- Bone graft harvest tools or bone graft substitute
- Dural repair tools and suture

24.4 Anesthesia/Neuromonitoring

- Neuromonitoring compatible anesthesia

24.5 Pearls

- Watch for traumatic dural entrapment or tears
- Nerve roots can also be trapped in fractures
- Dekyphosing should be performed before distraction

24.6 Pitfalls

- Severe instability should be carefully positioned on the table

Fig. 24.5 Insert a curved dura probe to palpate the fracture fragment. Check the position of your probe on lateral fluoroscopy images

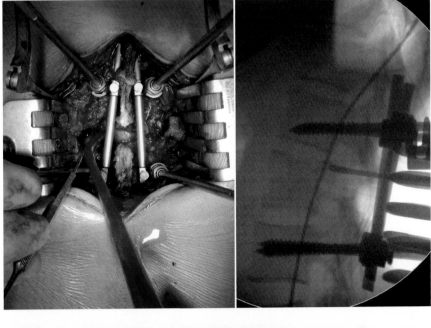

Fig. 24.6 Insert a curved bone tamp into the same space and tap gently the fragment ventrally

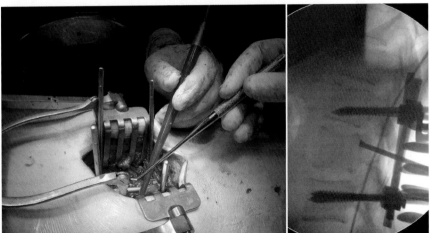

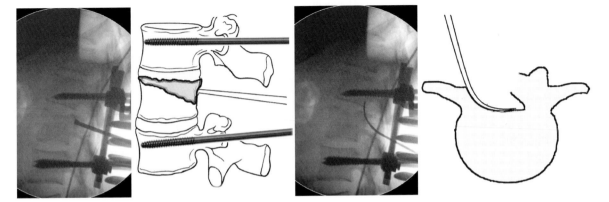

Fig. 24.7 After reduction, check with the curved dura probe. If the reduction is not sufficient, perform the same procedure from the contralateral side. If the reduction is still not satisfactory, remove the pedicle to get access to the vertebral body and remove the cancellous bone underlying the fragment (*shaded area*) in order to push the fragment into the created cavity just like in a pedicle subtraction osteotomy

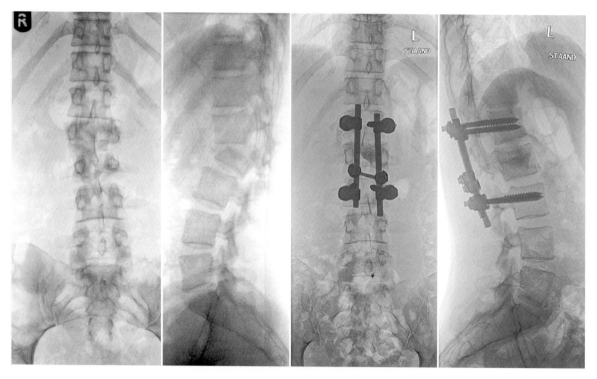

Fig. 24.8 If there is much comminution, balloon-assisted end-plate reduction technique can be added after the reduction to create anterior support as in this case of a young lady with ASIA-A cauda equina injury. She was operated on within 6 h after trauma and recovered almost completely

- Be prepared for an anterior approach if adequate reduction cannot be performed

24.7 Intraoperative Complications

- Dural tear – be prepared for repair or drain placement
- Poor screw purchase – be prepared for anterior instrumentation or cementation of screws

24.8 Bailout

- Anterior corpectomy and/or instrumentation. Can be staged
- Bracing
- Additional level instrumentation

24.9 Bracing

- Thoraco-Lumbo-Sacral Orthosis (TLSO) as needed

24.10 Potential Complications

- Nonunion and/or rekyphosis. Be prepared for anterior procedure

References

1. Dai LY, Jiang SD, Wang XY, Jiang LS (2007) A review of the management of thoracolumbar burst fractures. Surg Neurol 67:221–231
2. Fehlings MG, Vaccaro A, Aarabi B, Shaffrey C, Harrop J, Dvorak M, Fisher C.G., Rampersaud YR, Massicotte EM,

Lewis S (2008) A prospective, multicenter trial to evaluate the role and timing of decompression in patients with cervical spinal cord injury: initial one year results of the STASCIS study. AANS annual meeting 28 April 2008. Abstract 48885

3. Oner FC, Verlaan JJ, Verbout AJ, Dhert WJ (2006) Cement augmentation techniques in traumatic thoracolumbar spine fractures. Spine 31(11 suppl):S89–S95. (http://aans.org)

4. Stadhouder A, Buskens E, de Klerk LW, Verhaar JA, Dhert WA, Verbout AJ, Vaccaro AR, Oner FC (2008) Traumatic thoracic and lumbar spinal fractures: operative or nonoperative treatment: comparison of two treatment strategies by means of surgeon equipoise. Spine 33(9):1006–1017

5. Verlaan JJ, Diekerhof CH, Buskens E, van der Tweel I, Verbout AJ, Dhert WJ, Oner FC (2004) Surgical treatment of traumatic fractures of the thoracic and lumbar spine: a systematic review of the literature on techniques, complications, and outcome. Spine 29(7):803–814

Anterior Treatment of Thoracolumbar Burst Fractures

25

Gene Choi, Eric Klineberg, and Munish Gupta

25.1 Case Example

A 46-year-old male was riding an all-terrain vehicle at about 30 mph when he lost control and fell backward off the vehicle, landing on his buttocks and back. He immediately experienced severe back pain and was brought to the nearest hospital for evaluation, and then transferred to a tertiary referral center for treatment of an L1 burst fracture. On evaluation, he complained of severe low back pain, along with numbness and tingling in his lower extremities, but no weakness, or loss of bowel or bladder control. He was tender to palpation over the thoracolumbar junction with no palpable step-off or interspinous widening. His motor exam was normal, and he had decreased sensation in the L4, L5, and S1 dermatomes. He had no other associated injuries.

Anteroposterior (AP) and lateral radiographs and computed tomography (CT) scan of the thoracolumbar spine revealed a burst fracture of the L1 vertebral body with 40% loss of height, 15° of kyphosis, and 60% canal compromise (Figs. 25.1–25.4). The patient was brought to the operating room to undergo an L1 anterior corpectomy and fusion from T12 to L2 with instrumentation.

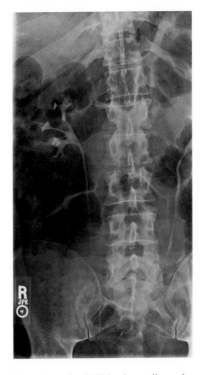

Fig. 25.1 Anteroposterior (AP) lumbar radiograph

25.2 Background

Thoracolumbar fractures constitute the majority of traumatic spine injuries. Most of these injuries occur at the thoracolumbar junction. The transition from lumbar lordosis to thoracic kyphosis, along with the relative mobility of the lumbar spine compared to the thoracic spine makes this region vulnerable to axial load forces. Burst fractures in this region result from excessive axial loading, causing compressive failure of the anterior and middle columns. Neurologic deficits can result from retropulsed fragments of bone or disc into the spinal

M. Gupta (✉) and E. Klineberg
Department of Orthopaedic Surgery, University of California Davis, 4860 Y Street, Suite 3800, Sacramento, CA 95817, USA
e-mail: munish.gupta@ucdmc.ucdavis.edu

G. Choi
Orthopedic and Spine Surgery, Riverside Medical Clinic, 7117 Brockton Ave, Riverside, CA 92506

V.V. Patel et al. (eds.), *Spine Trauma*,
DOI: 10.1007/978-3-642-03694-1_25, © Springer-Verlag Berlin Heidelberg 2010

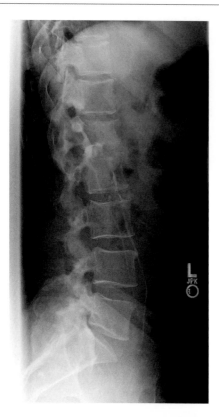

Fig. 25.2 Lateral radiograph

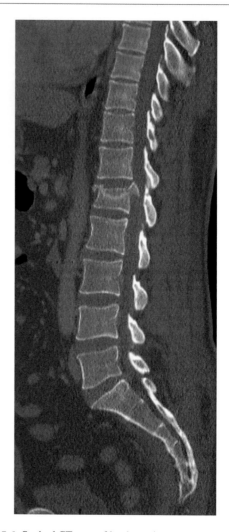

Fig. 25.4 Sagittal CT scan of lumbar spine

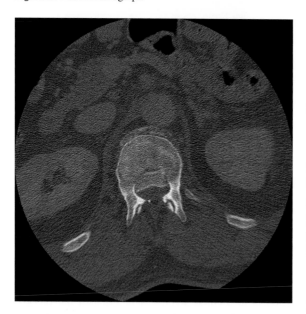

Fig. 25.3 Axial CT image of L1 vertebra

include canal compromise greater than 50%, vertebral body comminution with greater than 30° of kyphosis, greater than 50% loss of vertebral body height, and the presence of neurologic deficits with cord or root compression. Surgical management of these injuries can involve anterior, posterior, and combined approaches.

25.3 Indications and Advantages for Procedure

canal. The treatment of these injuries is dependent on the presence of instability or neural compromise. The generally accepted criteria for operative treatment

The main advantages of the anterior approach are that it allows direct visualization and decompression of the neural elements, and that it allows for direct reconstruction of anterior column support with a load-sharing construct. In patients with incomplete neurologic injury, anterior treatment may result in improved neurologic recovery when compared to posterior treatment alone. The anterior approach also allows for better correction of kyphotic deformity, especially in the presence of significant comminution or subacute injuries that may not be correctable with posterior surgery alone. It can also be used in cases where posterior surgery has not obtained adequate canal reduction with incomplete neurologic recovery.

25.4 Contraindications and Disadvantages for the Procedure

In general, a stand-alone anterior procedure should not be used in the presence of posterior column distraction or a distraction injury to the posterior ligamentous complex. Physical examination findings of tenderness and swelling over the posterior spine along with the presence of interspinous widening or stepoff can indicate injury to the posterior elements. Imaging studies should be evaluated for more subtle signs of posterior disruption, such as facet joint widening seen with a CT scan or increased signal with magnetic resonance imaging (MRI). Fracture–dislocations usually require posterior reduction and stabilization, followed by an anterior procedure if further decompression or stability is required. Combined anterior and posterior procedures should also be considered in the presence of poor bone quality, as in the case of osteoporosis, infection, or tumors.

Concomitant injuries can also influence the choice of anterior treatment. Patients with injury to the chest or abdomen may not tolerate an anterior thoracolumbar exposure. Patients with pulmonary compromise or morbid obesity may also limit the ability to use an anterior approach.

25.5 Procedure

25.5.1 Preoperative Planning

- CT scans should be evaluated carefully for evidence of any posterior injury that might require additional posterior fixation. The width of the vertebral bodies

can be measured to help estimate screw lengths needed for bicortical purchase.
- The position of the aorta should also be noted. In most cases, a left-sided approach is utilized, as this avoids the vena cava and the need to retract the liver. In situations where the aorta has a far left-sided position or because of concomitant injuries, a right-sided approach can be considered.
- The type of fixation to be used should be decided beforehand. A cage or femoral allograft can be used to restore the anterior column, and various plate–screw or rod–screw constructs are available. In the presence of a fracture, we prefer to use a titanium cage and rod–screw construct.

25.5.2 Patient Positioning

- The patient is placed in the lateral decubitus position. We use a beanbag with suction and multiple pillows to help maintain position. Radiolucent bolsters can also be used. Care must be taken to ensure a true lateral position is obtained. Taping the pelvis can help prevent the patient from rolling, along with ensuring the beanbag is well conformed along the pelvis prior to being placed on suction (Fig. 25.5).
- The patient's thoracolumbar junction should be positioned over the table break and the table flexed to "open up" the operative side to aid in the approach. This should be done prior to placing the beanbag on suction.
- An axillary roll should be placed, and the hip and knee flexed on the operative side to relax the psoas muscle.

25.5.3 Surgical Approach

- The planned incision should be marked out prior to draping to allow palpation of the ribs and spine. The approach is usually through the bed of the rib two levels above the injured level. For an L1 burst fracture, the T11 rib bed is utilized.
- A standard anterolateral approach to the thoracolumbar spine is utilized. The incision is made over the rib, which is exposed along its entire length. Subperiosteal dissection around the rib can first be

Fig. 25.5 Patient positioning

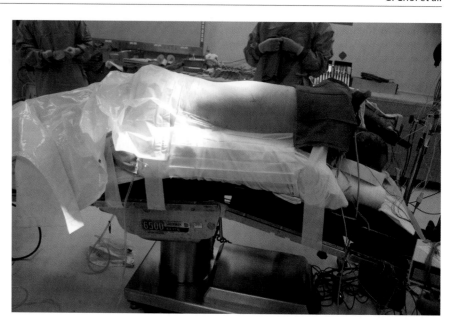

started using an elevator circumferentially around the rib, then passing a laparotomy pad around the rib and running it along its length using a sawing motion. This will effectively and quickly perform the dissection around the rib. The rib is then cut anteriorly at its cartilaginous junction and posteriorly as close to the rib head as possible. The rib bed is incised using electrocautery by making a small starter incision first, then inserting a finger and cutting over it to protect the underlying structures (Fig. 25.6). A self-retaining rib retractor is then placed.

- The diaphragm is cut along its periphery leaving a small cuff remaining for closure. The edge of the

diaphragm can be marked with suture to aid in closure (Fig. 25.7). A malleable retractor is then placed to protect the anterior structures.
- The psoas muscle is then stripped from the lateral aspect of the vertebral bodies using a Cobb elevator and electrocautery (Fig. 25.8).
- Once the lateral aspects of the vertebral bodies are exposed, the involved vertebra is usually obvious due to deformity or hematoma. An intraoperative X-ray with a needle or similar instrument placed within the disc space above or below the involved vertebra can be used to verify the level.
- The overlying pleura is divided at the level of the fracture and at the adjacent levels. The segmental

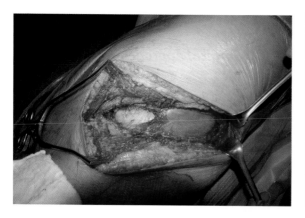

Fig. 25.6 Incising the rib bed

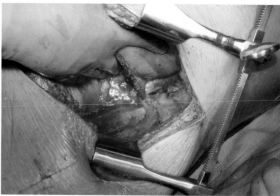

Fig. 25.7 Cutting the diaphragm

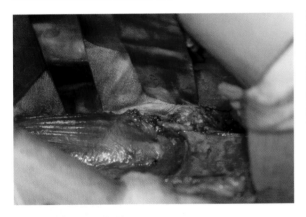

Fig. 25.8 The psoas muscle overlying the spine

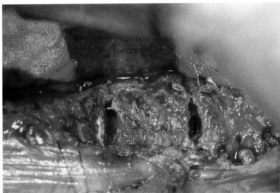

Fig. 25.10 After performing the discectomies

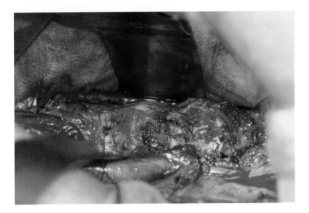

Fig. 25.9 Completed exposure of the spine

vessels are isolated and ligated at the fractured vertebra and above and below.

- Using a Cobb elevator and Bovie electrocautery, the adjacent vertebral bodies are exposed posteriorly to identify the pedicle and the neural foramen. In the lumbar spine, this involves carefully elevating the psoas muscle off of the body from anterior to posterior. In the thoracic spine, this requires resection of the rib head (Fig. 25.9).
- Exposure is then performed anteriorly to the anterior longitudinal ligament.
- The fractured body is then exposed in similar fashion. Discectomy is then performed both above and below the involved vertebra. The annulus is incised using a scalpel or Bovie electrocautery. The disc material is the removed using Leksell and pituitary rongeurs. The cartilaginous endplates are then elevated off of the bony endplate using a wide sharp Cobb elevator. Care should be taken to avoid

damaging the bony endplate. The anterior longitudinal ligament should be left intact (Fig. 25.10).

- Once most of the cartilage has been removed, there is usually some left along the posterior margin of the endplate. This can be removed by using a straight curette, scraping toward the posterior longitudinal ligament, and then along it using a twisting action. This should be performed from the near side proceeding to the contralateral side.
- Once the discectomies are completed, the corpectomy is performed. Using the exposed pedicle and foramen as a guide to the posterior margin of the body, an osteotome is placed approximately 10 mm anterior to the base of the pedicle and parallel to the posterior margin. The osteotome is then used to cut the vertebral body, separating most of the anterior and central body, leaving the posterior margin intact. The osteotome should not pass distal to the contralateral wall of the body.
- The osteotomized fragments are removed using a Leksell rongeur and kept for use as autograft. The remaining cancellous bone is then removed using large curettes and rongeurs until a thin shell of bone is left anteriorly and along the contralateral wall. Bleeding is controlled using bone wax and Gelfoam (Fig. 25.11).
- Decompression of the spinal canal is then performed by carefully peeling the fragments anteriorly using a sharp 45° up-angled long handle curette (Fig. 25.12). This is usually performed with the surgeon on the patient's posterior side. Epidural bleeding is usually encountered at this time, which can be controlled using thrombin-soaked Gelfoam. The dura can be seen bulging into the corpectomy site as

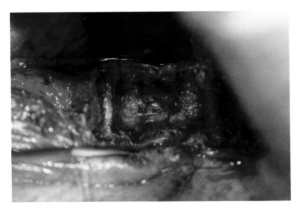

Fig. 25.11 After the initial corpectomy

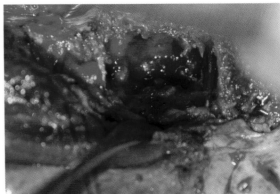

Fig. 25.13 The decompressed cord

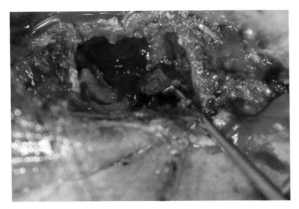

Fig. 25.12 Removing the retropulsed fragments

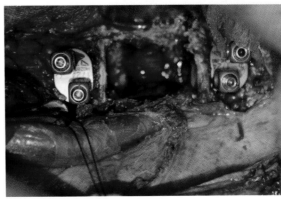

Fig. 25.14 Placement of the screws used in the Kaneda system

decompression proceeds. Any remaining posterior wall that is not fractured can be removed using a Kerrison rongeur. The decompression is adequate when the dura is exposed from pedicle to pedicle and disc space to disc space. This can be confirmed by gently palpating the contralateral pedicle using a Freer elevator or similar instrument. At this time, a large piece of thrombin-soaked Gelfoam can be placed over the dura to help control epidural bleeding (Fig. 25.13).

- In our practice, we use a titanium expandable cage to restore the anterior column along with a screw–rod construct for additional support.
- The screws are placed directly laterally, using the endplates as a guide to ensure they are placed parallel. The lateral aspect of the vertebral bodies should be smoothed using a rongeur or high-speed burr. The holes for the screws are started with an awl and then deepened using a straight probe until

the second cortex is breached. A ball-tipped probe is used to measure length (Fig. 25.14).

- Once the screws are placed, the deformity is reduced by having an assistant pushing anteriorly along the posterior spine at the apex of the deformity. A lamina spreader can also be used to aid reduction.
- The size of cage needed is then measured and the cage is placed in the center of the endplates and expanded until good contact with the endplates is obtained with the deformity reduced (Fig. 25.15). Bone graft is then packed into the cage. Rib bone harvested during the approach can be cut to size and placed around the cage as well (Figs. 25.16 and 25.17).
- Radiographs are taken to confirm reduction and proper placement of the cage and screws. Rods are then sized, placed, and the setscrews tightened with gentle compression across the screws applied (Fig. 25.18).
- The pleura is repaired over the hardware as well as possible. A chest tube is placed, the diaphragm is

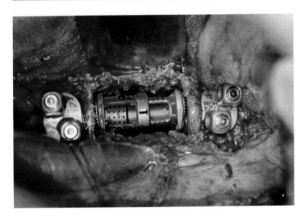

Fig. 25.15 Placement of the titanium cage

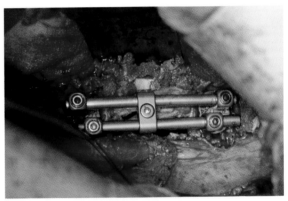

Fig. 25.18 Placement of the rods

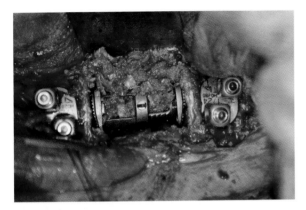

Fig. 25.16 Bone graft packed in and in front of the cage

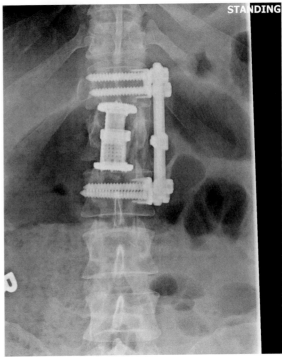

Fig. 25.19 Postoperative AP radiograph

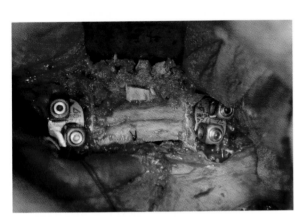

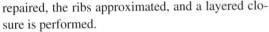

Fig. 25.17 Harvested rib placed around the cage

repaired, the ribs approximated, and a layered closure is performed.

- Once the patient is able, standing AP and lateral radiographs are obtained (Figs. 25.19 and 25.20).

25.6 Technical Pearls and Pitfalls

- Removing the rib head from the thoracic vertebra accomplishes two goals: allows identification of the neural foramen and pedicle, and creates a flat surface for later placement of a plate or rod and screw construct.

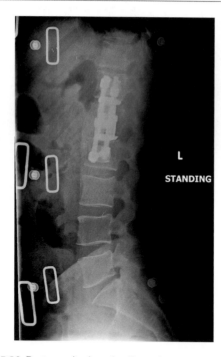

Fig. 25.20 Postoperative lateral radiograph

- Identifying the pedicle is the key to identifying the posterior margin of the vertebral body and the neuroforamen.
- An osteotome can be used to quickly separate the retropulsed posterior fragments from the remaining body.
- A 45° up angle curette is a good tool for carefully separating the retropulsed fragment from the posterior longitudinal ligament and the dura. A complete decompression should be performed, as this is the main goal for an anterior procedure.
- If using a screw–rod construct, the screws should be placed first so that an unobstructed view of the endplates can guide placement. Bicortical screw purchase is required to maximize rigidity of the construct.
- Pushing anteriorly along the posterior spine helps aid in reduction of the deformity and placement of a cage. If using an expandable cage, this can be used to maximize cage height and therefore reduction of the kyphosis.
- Leave both the anterior rim and contralateral wall of the fractured vertebra intact.
- Sharp curettes and Cobb elevators are critical to making the procedure easier.
- It is extremely important to maintain the patient orientation/position on the table to avoid inadvertent entry into spinal canal.

25.7 Postoperative Considerations

- A thoracolumbosacral brace is fitted once the chest tube is removed.
- Ambulation is progressively increased.
- The brace is worn for 12 weeks.

Recommended Reading

Bradford DS, McBride GG (1987) Surgical management of thoracolumbar spine fractures with incomplete neurologic deficits. Clin Orthop 218:201–216

Dunn HK (1984) Anterior stabilization of thoracolumbar injuries. Clin Orthop 189:116–124

Ghanayem A, Zdeblick T (1997) Anterior instrumentation in the management of thoracolumbar burst fractures. Clin Orthop 335:89–99

Kaneda K, Abumi K, Fujiya M (1984) Burst fractures with neurologic deficits of the thoracolumbar-lumbar spine: results of anterior decompression and stabilization with anterior instrumentation. Spine 9:788–795

Kaneda K, Taneichi H, Abumi K et al (1997) Anterior decompression and stabilization with the Kaneda device for thoracolumbar burst fractures associated with neurologic deficits. J Bone Joint Surg Am 79:69–83

Wood KB, Bohn DK, Mehbod A (2005) Anterior versus posterior treatment of thoracolumbar burst fractures without neurological deficit: a prospective randomized study. J Spin Dis Tech 18:S15–S23

Wood KB, Butterman G, Mehbod A et al (2003) Operative compared with nonoperative treatment of a thoracolumbar burst fracture without neurological deficit: a prospective randomized study. J Bone Joint Surg Am 85:773–781

Anterior and Posterior Surgery and Fixation for Burst Fractures

Yasutsugu Yukawa

26.1 Case Example

A 15-year-old woman fell from a height of 20 ft., sustaining an L1 burst fracture (Dennis [3] type B) with ASIA-C neurological deficit. Plain anterior–posterior (AP) and lateral radiographs demonstrate L1 burst fracture with widening of the pedicles, lamina separation, and widening between T12 and L1 spinous processes. Sagittal and axial computed tomography (CT) images show retropulsed fragment into the spinal canal with encroachment >50% (Fig. 26.1a–d). Magnetic resonance (MR) imaging demonstrates spinal canal encroachment and conus medullaris compression. Combined posterior–anterior surgery was performed (Fig. 26.1e). During surgery the posterior ligamentous complex was found to be completely torn (Fig. 26.1f). The patient started her rehabilitation with Thoraco-lumbo-sacral orthosis (TLSO) on the second day following the surgery. Six months later, her X-rays and CT scan showed bony union with good alignment and complete canal clearance (Fig. 26.1g–k). Her neurological state improved to ASIA-D. The patient returned to school with minimal restrictions in her activities of daily living (ADL).

26.2 Background

The thoracolumbar region is a common site for spinal injuries. The rigid thoracic segment and the mobile lumbar spine create a junction with concentration of stresses that accounts for the higher likelihood of injuries between T10 and L2 compared with the other areas of the spine. Thoracolumbar burst fractures result in two aspects: loss of trunk support and neural injury of the spinal cord, conus medullaris and/or cauda equina. There is still significant controversy regarding not only the need for surgical vs. nonsurgical management of thoracolumbar burst fractures, but also the approach and type of surgery if operative intervention is chosen. No definitive treatment algorithm has yet been universally accepted for this spinal trauma. However, operative treatment has been found to be effective. The two main goals of surgeries for thoracolumbar burst fractures are the adequate decompression of the spinal canal to maximize neurologic recovery and the creation of spinal stability to prevent painful deformity and potential future neurologic deterioration.

We have used combined surgery with short segment posterior instrumentation followed by anterior decompression and strut grafting in the treatment of thoracolumbar burst fractures [12]. The posterior construct is composed of pedicle screws, infralaminar hooks and rods system. The posterior/anterior combined procedure has several merits; 360° fracture observation, direct canal decompression, rigid fixation with posterior instrumentation, and anterior strut reconstruction [4, 5, 11]. On the other hand, this surgery has a few demerits: the need for two separate skin incisions and the relatively high invasiveness. This procedure ablates the need for circular incision of the diaphragm, thus the invasiveness is comparable to that of sole anterior surgery. The direct decompression potentiates good neural recovery and the rigid fixation promotes a high union rate and lower instrumentation failure rate. Combined surgery with posterior instrumentation followed by anterior decompression and strut grafting

Y. Yukawa
Department of Orthopaedics, Chbu Rosai Hospital,
1-10-6 Komei, Minato-ku, Nagoya, 455-0019, Japan

V.V. Patel et al. (eds.), *Spine Trauma*,
DOI: 10.1007/978-3-642-03694-1_26, © Springer-Verlag Berlin Heidelberg 2010

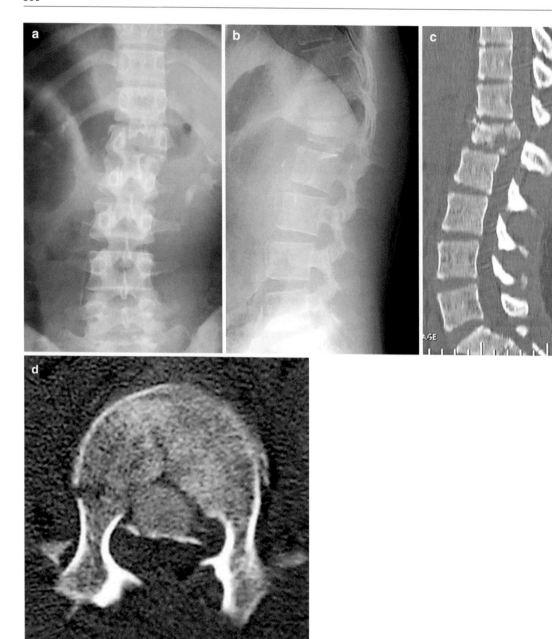

Fig. 26.1 A representative case. (**a**, **b**) Preoperative posterior–anterior (PA) and lateral X-rays. (**c**, **d**) Preoperative sagittal and axial CT scans. (**e**) Preoperative sagittal MR T2 image. (**f**) Intraoperative findings, posterior ligamentous complex was completely torn. (**g**, **h**) postoperative PA and lateral X-ray. (**i**, **j**) Postoperative sagittal and axial CT scan. (**k**) Postoperative sagittal MR T2 image

yields good fracture reduction, a high fusion rate, and a high neurological recovery rate, in the treatment of thoracolumbar burst fractures.

This chapter introduces posterior/anterior combined surgery in the treatment of thoracolumbar burst fractures at the levels between T11 and L3, and describes its

Fig. 26.1 (continued)

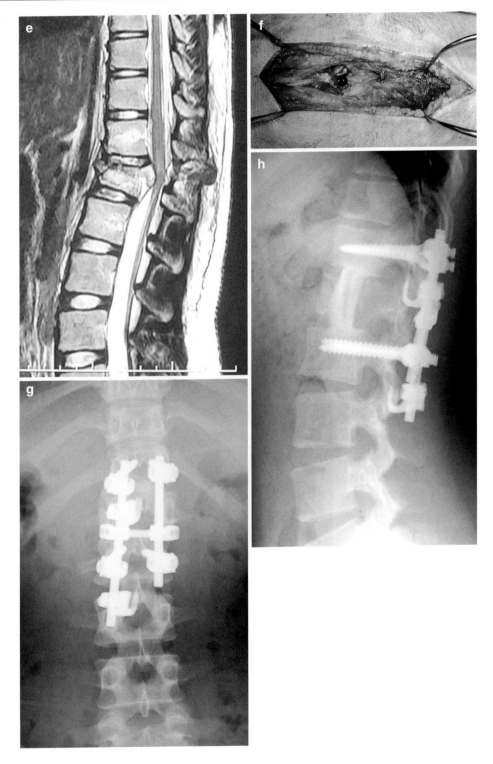

Fig. 26.1 (continued)

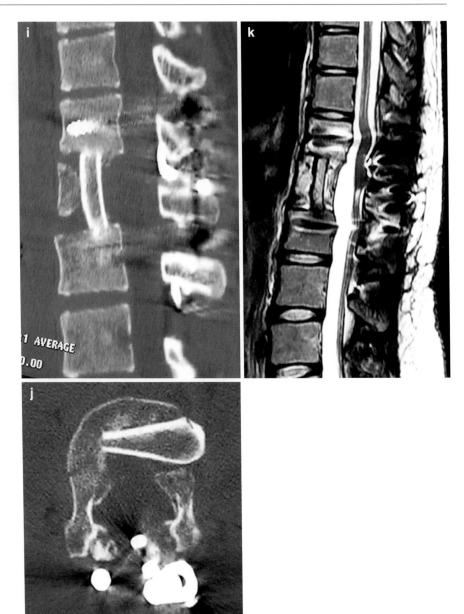

indications, procedural steps, technical pitfalls, and postoperative course in detail.

26.3 Indications and Advantages for Procedure

Stability of the vertebral column in the thoracolumbar region is dependent on the integrity of the osseous and ligamentous components. Once these structures are disrupted, the stability of the vertebral column becomes compromised, resulting in an unstable spine.

The indication for this surgery is a fracture between T11 and L3 with at least one of the following three criteria: neurological deficits, significant encroachment into the spinal canal by the retropulsed osseous fragments [6], or severe vertebral damage with kyphotic deformity.

1. Incomplete neurologic deficit.
2. Canal compromise; stenotic ratios T11, 12: 35%, L1: 45%, L2: 55%.
3. Segmental kyphotic deformity; >20°, anterior body height <50%.

The ideal indication for this surgery is unstable burst fracture combined with posterior column injury (three-column injury by Denis [3]).

The anterior or lateral approach allows direct spinal canal decompression and visualization. As the posterior reduction and fixation is achieved first in this surgery, the anterior decompression can be performed under stable condition; thus, the decompression procedure itself is unlikely to induce iatrogenic neural deterioration. Direct decompression provides better neural recovery than indirect decompression [1, 9].

This procedure requires the dissection of only the injured vertebral body and its two adjacent discs except in cases of T12 and L1 contiguous burst fractures, differentiating it from stand-alone anterior decompression and fixation that needs the dissection of three vertebral levels. The diaphragm can be kept intact in the treatment of single level burst fractures with the combined approach. Postoperative respiratory complications are rarely seen as an extrapleural approach without the application of diaphragmatic dissection.

Posterior/anterior combined fixation provides the strongest possible fixation, thus allowing the shortest fixation with maintenance of alignment. Furthermore, the adjacent segments are only mildly affected. As the candidates for this treatment are relatively young, preservation of motion segments are very important for their future.

26.4 Contraindications and Disadvantages of the Procedure

If a patient has a history of previous thoracic surgery or retroperitoneal surgery, the contralateral approach should be selected. Elderly patients with significant pulmonary dysfunction or patients with abdominal aortic aneurysms are not candidates for this procedure.

Disadvantages of this surgery are the need for two skin incisions for two separate surgical procedures and its relative invasiveness. The surgery may seem highly invasive; however, it is comparable to stand-alone anterior surgery [7, 12].

26.4.1 Preoperative Imaging

Complete sets of radiographs are needed in all patients for decision-making and surgical planning. These include preoperative plain radiographs (AP and lateral views), CT scans, and magnetic resonance imaging (MRI). Occasionally flexion and extension X-rays are necessary to assess the integrity of the posterior ligament complex. The posterior ligamentous complex should be examined in the obtained images in order to assess whether the fracture is a three-column injury.

26.4.2 Timing of Surgery

The indication for emergent surgical intervention in thoracic and lumbar trauma is progressive neurologic deficit in an unstable fracture pattern with significant spinal cord compression. Studies have shown, however, that even delayed decompression of persistent thoracolumbar spinal cord compression can be beneficial in terms of improved neurologic status [8].

26.5 Procedure

26.5.1 Equipment Needed

A pedicle screw system in which hooks can be easily used at the same level should be selected.

A self-retaining thoracotomy or abdominal retractor used in general surgery is necessary for the anterior procedure. A flexible surgical table is also crucial.

Unless the spine surgeon is familiar with anterior surgery, the assistance of a thoracic or general surgeon to access the anterior thoracolumbar spine is preferred.

26.5.2 Anesthetic and Neuromonitoring Considerations

Intubation with a double-lumen tube is preferred, so that the left and the right main stem bronchi can be ventilated separately in cases of T11 and 12 burst fractures. This initiation allows unilateral lung collapse for adequate exposure of the spine later during anterior surgery.

Patients with spinal injuries need to maintain adequate spinal cord blood flow throughout the surgery. This requires careful monitoring by the anesthesiologist, as well as clear communication from the surgeon informing his expectations, anticipated blood loss, and the time of surgery.

Neurological deterioration is the most feared complication of the surgery. Neurological injury is not simply a by-product of the surgery itself. It can occur preoperatively during transfer of the patient to the operating table, and with neck extension for intubation or patient positioning. Prevention of further neurological injury is the most important surgical perspective. Therefore, intraoperative neurophysiological monitoring of spinal cord and spinal nerve root function is gaining popularity to reduce the incidence of new or additional neurological impairment during surgery. Technological advances in neurophysiological instrumentation permit the neurophysiologist to monitor somatosensory (SSEPs), transcranial electrically stimulated motor-evoked potentials (MEPs), and both spontaneous and stimulated electromyography in a single test protocol all displayed simultaneously. Intraoperative neurophysiological monitoring should be considered an integral adjunct to the surgical management of the spine-injured patient [10].

26.5.3 Posterior Surgery

- *Patient positioning and room setup for posterior surgery*

  First, the patient is set prone on the Hall frame for posterior surgery (Fig. 26.2a). After prone positioning, the patient is secured to the table with wide tapes. Typically, the arms are abducted at the shoulder and flexed at the elbow to prevent

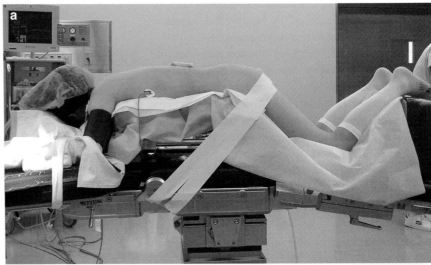

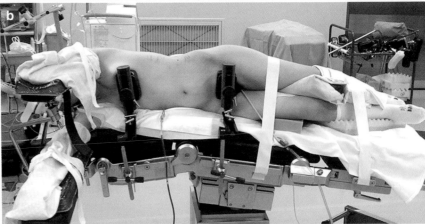

Fig. 26.2 (**a**) Body position during posterior surgery. (**b**) Body setting during anterior surgery

compression or entrapment of the neurovascular structures. Finally, and most importantly, care must be taken to appropriately protect the face in the prone position to avoid skin breakdown or undue pressure to the eyes resulting in loss of vision. This prone position produces a gentle reduction force to correct the kyphotic deformity.

- *Surgical approach – posterior approach*
The posterior midline skin incision is used. The spinous processes are identified and a subperiosteal dissection is performed to expose three levels of the dorsal surface of the spine centered on the fracture level. Care must be taken to avoid damage to dura or nerves that may be pinched in lamina fractures. Retractors are placed on the paraspinal muscles to maintain exposure of the dorsal spine. Subperiosteal dissection beyond the facets to the transverse processes provides the necessary exposure for pedicle screw insertion.
- *Reduction technique*
First the patient is set prone on the Hall frame, and the kyphotic deformity is reduced by body position. The reduction by instrumentation is described in the next section.
- *Posterior fixation technique*
Posterior instrumentation is performed using both pedicle screws and infralaminar hooks.

After adequate dissection to expose the posterior aspect of three levels, instrumentation is performed. Usually three laminae and two facets are exposed on each side and the facet capsules are removed and the articular cartilage is denuded by a fine curette for facet fusion. The insertion points for the pedicle screws are shown in the bone model (Fig. 26.3a). Two pedicle screws are inserted bilaterally in the upper and lower vertebrae adjacent to the lesion after careful probing. The combination of two pedicle screws and one infralaminar hook is used in each level cranial and caudal to the fracture. An infralaminar hook is inevitably used in the same level as pedicle screws. Usually an infralaminar hook is used in the side with less canal encroachment. Ideal reduction is achieved by positioning and manual reduction rather than instrumentation. Some compression force is used between the upper and lower levels to reduce the kyphotic deformity

(Fig. 26.3b, c). Occasionally, retropulsed fragments can be reduced indirectly by the application of distractive forces (ligamentotaxis) and the realignment of the kyphotic curvature. After radiographic confirmation of the alignment and implant position, the transverse connecter is added. The wound is then closed in layers with the suction tube inserted in the standard fashion.

26.5.4 Anterior Surgery

- *Patient positioning and room setup for anterior surgery*
After the posterior surgery, the patient is repositioned in the lateral decubitus position with the right side appropriately padded against the table with an axillary roll, the anterior surgery being performed via a left-sided approach (Fig. 26.2b). The left hip is flexed at approximately 30° to relax the psoas major muscle. The right side of the waist is also supported with adequate padding. Care should be taken to pad the common peroneal nerve at the level of the fibular neck. The ribs on the left side in the extrapleural approach, the space between the left 12th rib and the iliac crest in the retroperitoneal approach are spread open by flexure of the table for maximum exposure.
- *Anterior approach*
An extrapleural approach for T11, T12, or retroperitoneal approach for L1–3 is utilized to expose the injured vertebra. The left-side approach is favored for several anatomical reasons. On the left side, the aorta can be mobilized and manipulated more easily than the thin-walled vena cava. In addition, retroperitoneal dissection around the liver on the right side can be avoided.

(a) *Extrapleural approach for T11, T12*
An extrapleural approach with removal of the rib one or two levels superior to the injured level is performed to expose the lower thoracic spine (T11 and 12). The incision is centered over the left rib one or two levels superior to the injured level. Then the latissimus dorsi and the serratus anterior are divided with the cautery. The periosteum of the selected rib is identified and incised. Subperiosteal dissection

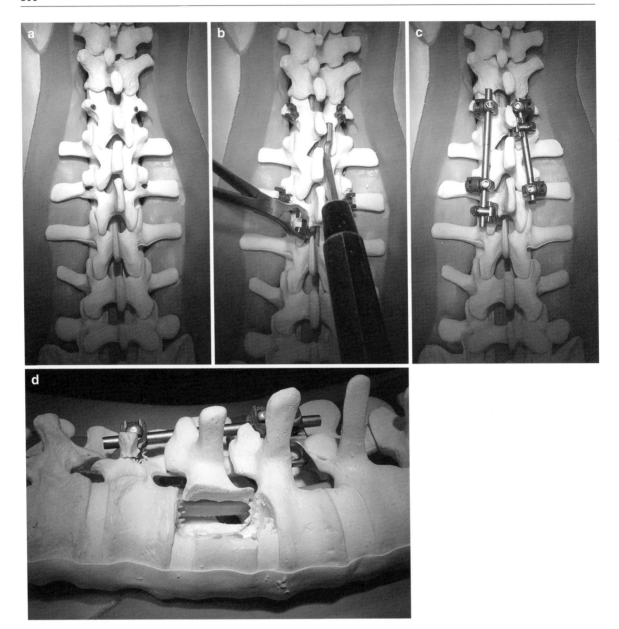

Fig. 26.3 Surgery on bone model. (**a**) Pedicle screw insertion points at T12 and L2 level. (**b**) Hook trial inserted at T12 lamina. (**c**) Combination of two pedicle screws and infralaminar hook at each of T12 and L2 level. (**d**) Complete decompression after resection of the vertebral body and the adjacent discs

proceeds to the proximal and the distal borders of the rib, detaching the intercostal muscles, then advanced around its inner and under surface. The rib is excised with a rib cutter at its maximal length in order to facilitate tissue handling in the retropleural space. Careful and blunt dissection of the parietal pleura away from the intercostal muscle is required. After creating enough retropleural space, a rib-spreading retractor is inserted. Deflation of the left lung with a double-lumen endotracheal tube is helpful for the following steps. The desired level should be confirmed by inserting a marker needle into the disc space followed by radiographic or fluoroscopic imaging. The segmental intercostal artery and veins are cut after clipping or ligation of both ends on the left wall of the injured vertebra.

If the pleura is inadvertently damaged in this procedure, it can be repaired with absorbable sutures.

However, if the damage is irreparable, the procedure should be converted from extrapleural to transthoracic approach with special considerations in the type of drainage and the postoperative course.

(b) *Retroperitoneal approach for L1–3*

In the lateral position, the incision is placed just below the 12th rib. The Latissimus dorsi, the external and internal obliques, and the transversus abdominis muscles are divided. On dissecting the fascia transversalis, the peritoneal layer is exposed. The peritoneum is bluntly dissected away from the diaphragm and abdominal wall, developing the retroperitoneal space. The peritoneum is packed away with protecting sponges and self-retaining retractors. The diaphragm is now visible attached to the proximal end of the psoas major and the T12–L1 disc. The left vertebral wall is covered with the psoas muscle. The muscle is divided longitudinally in the middle into anterior and posterior portions. The desired level should be confirmed by inserting a marker needle into the disc space followed by radiographic or fluoroscopic imaging. Segmental lumbar vessels are identified and ligated at the mid portion of the vertebral body. The psoas muscle and the periosteum are detached from the vertebrae and the adjacent discs, and retracted to expose the vertebral body laterally. The left-lateral wall of the injured vertebrae is now visible.

When the 11th (or 12th) rib head gets in the way of dissection of L1 and L2, the interfering rib could be broken at its base bluntly or by sharp dissection to secure enough working space.

- *Anterior fixation technique*

Surgical space is developed with the extrapleural approach for T11, 12, or the retroperitoneal approach for L1–3. After ligation or clipping of the segmental vessels, subperiosteal dissection exposes the left side of the vertebral body, the adjacent discs, and the pedicle. Intervertebral disc excision can be undertaken using a scalpel or cautery with Cobb elevators and ring curettes. This exposure also allows corpectomy. The intervertebral discs and the cartilaginous end plate cephalad and caudad to the injured level are almost fully excised, taking care not to damage the adjacent intact bony endplates. Vertebral body resection is performed after the rough resection of the vertebral discs, as it invites considerable bleeding from the bone marrow. First

we resect 2 cm width from the left-cortical wall, and the cancellous bone is removed from the center of the vertebral body by curettes, rongeurs, or osteotomes to the depth of the opposite pedicle. The posterior vertebral body is sliced vertically by an osteotome and the posterior wall is thinned gradually. When the floating bony fragments are left alone, they are removed in a piece-meal fashion using a curette. The vertebral body and the displaced fragments into the spinal canal are removed completely until the base of the contralateral pedicle is well visualized (Fig. 26.3d, 26.4). The posterior longitudinal ligament is often found to be disrupted or attenuated as a result of the original trauma, but it is not resected to avoid bleeding from the epidural venous plexus. After complete decompression, the length of the resulting gap is measured from the vertebral end plate above to the end plate below. A tricortical iliac crest bone graft is obtained. The strut bone graft is placed into the gap between the upper and lower vertebral bodies, parallel to the axis of the thoracolumbar spine. A small incision in the attachment of the diaphragm to the T12–L1 disc is used in cases of T12 or L1 burst fractures, but the diaphragm is usually kept intact. The psoas muscle is sewn back together in the retroperitoneal approach. The wound is then closed in layers and drained in the standard fashion.

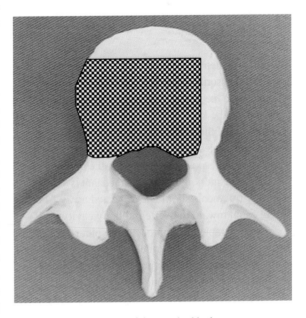

Fig. 26.4 Resection area of the vertebral body

The defect of the iliac crest is usually reconstructed with the resected rib or a bone spacer. Allografts can be used as substitutes to the tricortical iliac crest. In such case, autogenous bone graft chips from local site should be used in combination.

26.6 Technical Pearls and Pitfalls

26.6.1 Pearls

Concomitant usage of pedicle screws and infralaminar hooks in same level makes the fixation very strong and reduces the occurrence of instrumentation failure [2].

The rib head inserting into the superior aspect of the same named vertebral body is also a very important landmark to identify the correct surgical level.

Excision of the adjacent discs and the cartilaginous endplates should be done before the final decompression of the posterior vertebral wall, to avoid excessive epidural bleeding and neurological deterioration.

Epidural bleeding is not easy to control directly, but thrombostatic agents such as Gelfoam and Avitene can be used. To reduce the total bleeding from the surgery, it is important to finish the corpectomy expeditiously. Finally, the tight closure of the psoas major muscle is effective to reduce postoperative bleeding.

26.6.2 Pitfalls

Shift in the patient's position during surgery might cause anatomical disorientation and increases the possibility of iatrogenic neurologic damage. Spatial orientation must always be kept in mind. Appropriate positioning and fixation of this position should not be taken lightly. The entire surgical team is responsible and must reassess the patient's position throughout the operation.

A pushing motion into the spinal canal is very risky; the bony fragments should be dissected away from the spinal canal toward the vertebral body cavity.

In the extrapleural approach, the pleura should be meticulously inspected to rule out tears. If not repaired, the tube drainage would not function properly and pleural effusion might occur.

Undersized strut graft gives less stability and induces graft migration and postoperative kyphotic deformity. To measure accurately the distance between the two endplates and appropriate graft size is critical. It is also important to preserve the adjacent subchondral end plates.

26.7 Potential Intraoperative Complications

Intraoperative complications include problems related to the particular approaches to the spine, patient positioning on the surgical table, and neurological deterioration.

- Posterior surgery: instrument migration, iatrogenic neurological deficit
- Anterior surgery: iatrogenic neurological deficit, pseudomeningocele, major vessel injury, chylothorax, atelectasis, and pleural effusion

26.8 Bailout/Salvage for Procedure Failure

Traumatic or iatrogenic dural tears should be repaired through laminectomy when encountered in the posterior surgery. This can be technically difficult in the anterolateral decompressive procedure and may require the use of a fascial patch and/or lumbar cerebrospinal fluid drain.

If neurological deterioration is detected postoperatively, there is essentially nothing that could be done other than to give high-dose steroids (NASCIS II) and verify that there is no cord compression.

Prophylaxis is the concept that must be applied continuously throughout the operation.

26.9 Postoperative Considerations

26.9.1 Bracing

Hard corset (TLSO) is applied for about 3 months.

26.9.2 Activity

Ambulation and rehabilitation protocols are initiated on the day of drain removal, usually from 2 to 5 days following surgery.

26.9.3 Follow-Up

Patients with paralysis are transferred to a rehabilitation unit after several days following surgery. For these patients, prevention of secondary diseases, optimization of function, and reintegration into the community are paramount.

Usually patients are instructed to visit the clinic and take follow-up X-rays at 1, 3, 6, 12, 24 months after surgery, when the procedure is properly done.

26.9.4 Potential Complications

Postoperative complications fall into four broad categories, including general medical complications, problems associated with the specific surgical approaches and positioning, postoperative infection, and instrumentation failure following pseudoarthrosis. As the fixation is very rigid, instrumentation failure or pseudoarthrosis is very rare.

26.9.5 Treatments/Rescue for Complications

Early ambulation of patients with paralysis or multisystem trauma is important to prevent pulmonary complications, skin breakdown, deep vein thrombosis, and pulmonary embolism.

Diagnosis of postoperative infections requires a high index of suspicion. Infections following posterior surgical approaches are generally more common than after anterior approaches. Wound drainage and unexplained fever are usually the earliest signs of infection. CT scan imaging may demonstrate an abscess at the operative site. Early irrigation, debridement, and appropriate antibiotic usage are the hallmarks of successful treatment of this complication.

Once loss of fixation is noted on follow-up radiographs, the surgeon should take immediate steps to prevent further implant displacement or malalignment. This may include reoperation at the same site with revision of the instrumentation and/or stabilizing the spine from alternative surgical approaches.

References

1. Bradford DS, McBride GG (1987) Surgical management of thoracolumbar spine fractures with incomplete neurologic deficits. Clin Orthop Relat Res 218:201–216
2. Chiba M, McLain RF, Yerby SA, Moseley TA, Smith TS, Benson DR (1996) Short-segment pedicle instrumentation. Biomechanical analysis of supplemental hook fixation. Spine 21(3):288–294
3. Denis F (1983) The three column spine and its significance in the classification of acute thoracolumbar spinal injuries. Spine 8(8):817–831
4. Ebelke DK, Asher MA, Neff JR, Kraker DP (1991) Survivorship analysis of VSP spine instrumentation in the treatment of thoracolumbar and lumbar burst fractures. Spine 16(8 Suppl):S428–S432
5. Gertzbein SD, Court-Brown CM, Jacobs RR, Marks P, Martin C, Stoll J, Fazl M, Schwartz M, Rowed D (1988) Decompression and circumferential stabilization of unstable spinal fractures. Spine 13(8):892–895
6. Hashimoto T, Kaneda K, Abumi K (1988) Relationship between traumatic spinal canal stenosis and neurologic deficits in thoracolumbar burst fractures. Spine 13(11):1268–1272
7. Kaneda K, Taneichi H, Abumi K, Hashimoto T, Satoh S, Fujiya M (1997) Anterior decompression and stabilization with the Kaneda device for thoracolumbar burst fractures associated with neurological deficits. J Bone Joint Surg Am 79(1):69–83
8. Kostuik JP (1988) Anterior fixation for burst fractures of the thoracic and lumbar spine with or without neurological involvement. Spine 13(3):286–293
9. McAfee PC, Bohlman HH, Yuan HA (1985) Anterior decompression of traumatic thoracolumbar fractures with incomplete neurological deficit using a retroperitoneal approach. J Bone Joint Surg Am 67(1):89–104
10. Schwartz DM (2003) Intraoperative neurophysiological monitoring during post-traumatic spine surgery. In: Vaccaro AR (ed) Fractures of the cervical, thoracic and lumbar spine. Marcel Dekker, New York, pp 373–383
11. Shiba K, Katsuki M, Ueta T, Shirasawa K, Ohta H, Mori E, Rikimaru S (1994) Transpedicular fixation with Zielke instrumentation in the treatment of thoracolumbar and lumbar injuries. Spine 19(17):1940–1949
12. Yukawa Y, Kato F, Ito K et al (2006) Anteroposterior combined surgery for thoracolumbar burst fractures – anterior decompression, strut grafting and posterior instrumentation with pedicle screws and laminar hook. Paper presented at ASIA-ISCoS Combined Meeting, Boston, USA, 25–28 June 2006

Percutaneous/Minimally Invasive Treatment for Thoracolumbar Fractures

27

Neel Anand, Eli M. Baron, and Mark Dekutoski

27.1 Case Report

A 36-year-old female sustained a motor vehicle collision. At the time she was a restrained driver of a truck which collided head on with a car. She was brought to the trauma center on a spine board. She did not experience loss of consciousness.

She complained of severe back pain. Neurologic examination revealed normal sensation and strength throughout her lower extremities with the exception of her fractured right leg, which could not be assessed. CT scan of her chest/abdomen/pelvis and subsequent lumbar spine CT scan revealed the patient to have an L3 burst fracture with significant comminution and posteriorly displaced fragment into the spinal canal. Additionally, the patient was noted to have disruption of the L3–4 facet joint on the right (Fig. 27.1).

Given the comminution of the vertebral body with large fragments in the spinal canal and the disruption of the posterior ligamentous complex, surgery was recommended. The patient underwent two-stage surgery. She underwent lateral retroperitoneal approach to the spine and L3 corpectomy with the placement of a poly-ether-ether ketone expandable cage and staple, screw, and rod construct (Fig. 27.2). Posteriorly, she underwent minimally invasive spinal fixation using percutaneous technique (Fig. 27.3).

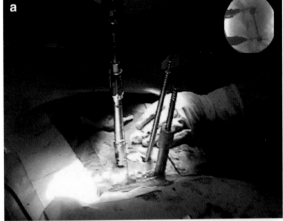

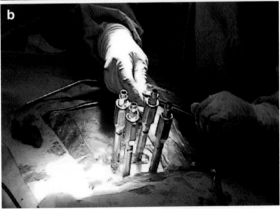

Fig. 27.1 (**a, b**) Axial and sagittal reconstruction CT scan demonstrating L3 unstable burst fracture. Note the facet disruption on the right and the significant canal compromise

N. Anand (✉) and M. Dekutoski
Department of Surgery, Cedars Sinai Medical Center, Cedars Sinai Institute for Spinal Disorders, Los Angeles, CA, USA
Neel.Anand@cshs.org

E.M. Baron
Department of Orthopedic Surgery, Mayo Clinic Graduate School of Medicine, Gonda 14, 200 First Street Southwest, Rochester, MN, USA

27.2 Background

Segmental fixation, specifically with pedicle screws and rods, has become the primary technique for fixation of thoracolumbar fractures [2]. Traditionally, this

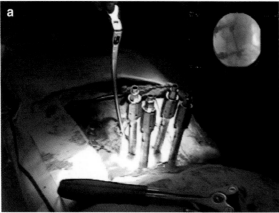

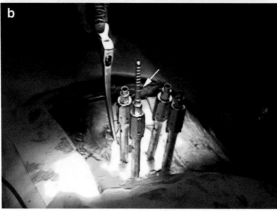

Fig. 27.2 (**a, b**) Lateral and AP fluoroscopic image demonstrating polyether-ether ketone cage and staple/screw/rod construction status post L3 corpectomy

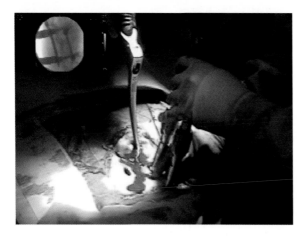

Fig. 27.3 Lateral and AP fluoroscopic post-op images demonstrating circumferential reconstruction, showing percutaneous pedicle screws placed after corpectomy/cage placement and staple/screw/rod construction

has been performed with or without fusion via open surgical technique. Nevertheless, open surgical technique is associated with high morbidity, high infection rates, and mean blood loss of greater than 1,000 cc [13]. Rechtine reported an infection rate as high as 10% [9]. Given the muscle damage associated with paraspinal muscle stripping procedures [3–5, 12, 14], minimally invasive techniques have been developed. They are associated with theoretically lower blood loss, less muscle damage, and overall reduced morbidity [16].

27.3 Indications

Indications for minimally invasive posterior fusion and minimally invasive posterior stabilization without fusion have been proposed, including

1. Creation of a posterior tension band following anterior reconstruction over fused segments (posterior technique without fusion).
2. Restoration of the posterior tension band over unfused segments (e.g., osteoporotic burst fracture following cement augmentation or burst fracture with questionably intact posterior ligaments).
3. Stabilization without fusion (e.g., osseous flexion distraction or boney Chance).
4. Stabilization with focal posterior fusion (e.g., ligamentous flexion distraction injury).
5. Percutaneous stabilization for multiple spine injuries in polytrauma.
6. Ankylosing spondylitis.
7. Alternative to bracing.
8. Where bracing is not practical: for example, when a patient has numerous associated pelvic or chest wall injuries or is excessively obese [1].

27.4 Advantages

Advantages of the minimally invasive surgical technique include reduced blood loss, reduced morbidity, and possibly reduced infection rates, given the reduction in tissue trauma [8]. Nevertheless, an open approach may be technically more feasible, especially if a direct decompression or open reduction technique is considered (e.g., transpedicular vertebrectomy and cage placement).

Additionally, minimally invasive pedicle screw placement is highly fluoroscopy dependent, theoretically increasing operating room staff, surgeon, and patient radiation exposure. Nevertheless, as image guidance becomes more available, this disadvantage may disappear.

27.5 Equipment

Equipment needed for minimally invasive posterior spinal fixation includes a posterior percutaneous fixation system, a fluoroscopy unit, Jamshidi (PAK) needles, and a radiolucent operating table. For the purposes of this discussion, we will refer to the Medtronic CD Horizon Longitude system (Medtronic Sofamor Danek, Memphis, TN). We recommend a Jackson table (Mizuho OSI, Union City, CA), as it is radiolucent and allows the legs to be positioned in extension to maintain lordosis [7]. For anesthetic purposes, total intravenous anesthesia is recommended if neurophysiologic monitoring is going to be used. We use this practice routinely in the thoracic spine, but not necessarily in the lumbar spine. A single C-arm is necessary if image guidance is not available.

27.5.1 Procedure

The patient is positioned in prone on the Jackson table (Fig. 27.4). Attention is paid to the table to ensure that all bony prominences are padded and that the abdomen remains suspended. With females, we prefer to

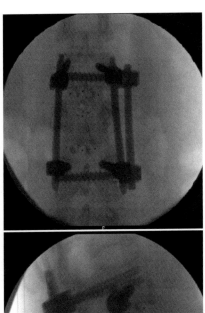
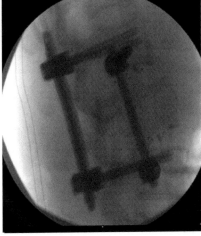

Fig. 27.5 A 15 blade is placed on the skin by the lateral border of the pedicle as confirmed on AP fluoroscopy. An incision is then made

rest the breasts on the actual chest bolster, as this provides for additional lordosis. The legs are maintained in extension.

An AP fluoroscopic image is obtained and we mark the lateral borders of the pedicles with a no. 15 blade (Fig. 27.5). Although some have advocated a more lateral incision for minimally invasive pedicle screw placement [11], in our experience, an incision by the lateral border of the pedicle on AP imaging is actually more conducive to instrumentation placement. While obtaining an AP image, it is important to have the end plate squared without any parallax.

After injecting subcutaneously with lidocaine with epinephrine, an incision should be made large enough to accommodate the housing of any screw extender used with the minimally invasive system. Two adjacent

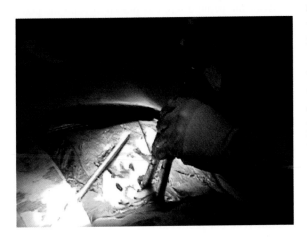

Fig. 27.4 A patient is positioned prone on a Jackson table. The legs are extended to maximize lumbar lordosis

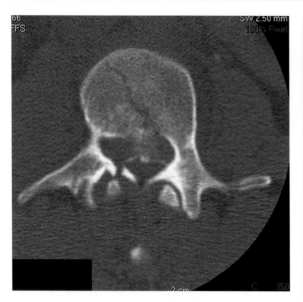

Fig. 27.6 AP fluoroscopy is then used to guide Jamshidi (PAK) needle placement

pedicles can be accessed via a single 35–40 mm incision. This is followed by the placement of a Jamshidi needle into the upper outer quadrant of the pedicle (Fig. 27.6). Using directed pressure, a mallet, and AP fluoroscopic guidance, the Jamshidi needle is advanced into the pedicle, with care taken not to advance across the medial border. The Jamshidi needle is placed approximately 30 mm into the bone, without crossing the medial border of the pedicle. All Jamshidi needles to be used in the procedure are placed.

Subsequently, the C-arm is swung to the lateral position. A lateral fluoroscopic image is obtained.

The Jamshidi needles at this point should be beyond the base of the pedicles and contained within the vertebral body. Subsequently, guide wires are placed in the holes and the Jamshidi needles are removed (Fig. 27.7). Great care should be taken not to dislodge the guide wire while removing the Jamshidi needles.

Serial dilators are then used (Fig. 27.8). Dilation proceeds upwards, from a small to a medium and a final dilator is typically used. The small and medium dilators are removed. The pedicles and proximal vertebral body are tapped with a cannulated tap (Fig. 27.9). Subsequently, the dilators are removed and the cannulated pedicle screw is placed (Fig. 27.10). All these are done under lateral fluoroscopy. Great care should be taken to avoid advancement of the guide wire or its backward

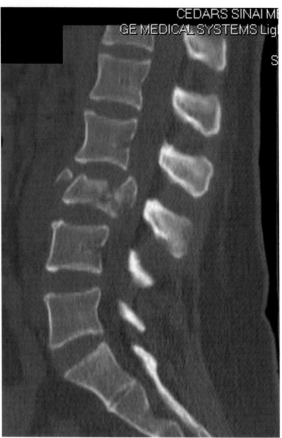

Fig. 27.7 Lateral fluoroscopic imaging is used to confirm Jamshidi needle placement and stylets are removed followed by the placement of guide wires

movement while removing the tap. It is important to have full control of the guide wire at all times.

After the pedicle screw is placed beyond the pedicle, the guide wire is removed. It may be necessary to use a Kocher or a needle driver in a levering action to remove the guide wire while doing so.

After the screws are placed, the screw extenders are all lined up. Subsequently, a rod measuring device is used to measure an appropriately sized rod (Fig. 27.11).

An additional small incision is made rostral to the proximal pedicle screw. A rod is then passed using free-hand technique through the screw head extenders of the proximal and caudal screws (Fig. 27.12). The placement of the rod is confirmed with the rod tester (Fig. 27.13). Additionally, fluoroscopic guidance is useful. With our preferred rod screw system, palpable engagement is confirmed with the rod tester.

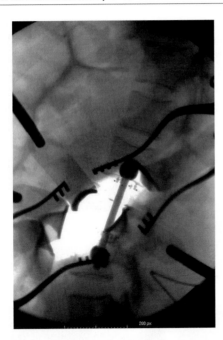

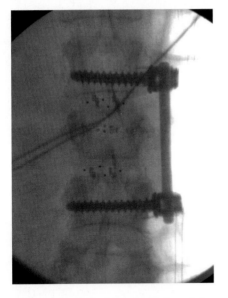

Fig. 27.8 The Jamshidi needles are then removed and serial dilators are used to dilate muscle around the guide wires

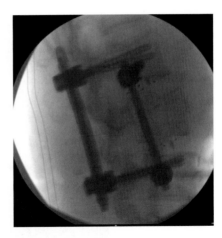

Fig. 27.10 Dilators and tap are removed and a cannulated pedicle screw is placed over a guide wire using lateral fluoroscopic guidance

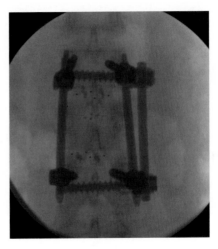

Fig. 27.11 Screw extenders are aligned and a measuring device is used to select an appropriately sized rod

Fig. 27.9 A cannulated tap is used with lateral fluoroscopic guidance over the guide wire to drill/tap through the pedicle into the proximal vertebral body

Subsequently, the rod is reduced (Fig. 27.14). This is done serially, with the screw extenders being reduced to equal depth. In this example the extender is reduced to 8 mm first, followed by reduction all the way as indicated

by the RD label in the reduction window. Subsequently, a suction trephine is used to remove any tissue in the screw head. Final locking caps are placed. The reduction maneuver is reversed and used to disengage the extenders from the screws; the extenders are then removed (Fig. 27.15). In this manner minimally invasive instrumentation is placed posteriorly (Fig. 27.16). It should be noted that a single midline incision could be made with the fascia being kept intact and opened only for screw placement if cosmesis is required. Additionally, for thoracolumbar fractures or thoracic fractures, it may be possible to drop a rod through the proximal screw extender without a second incision.

Fig. 27.12 A rod (on a rod holder) is passed using free-hand technique. Lateral fluoroscopy helps direct placement

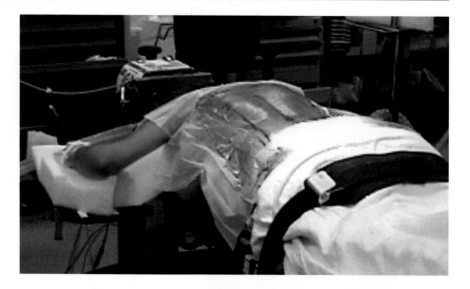

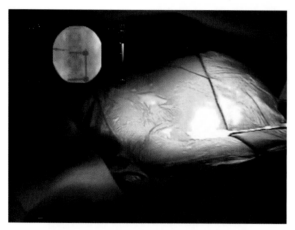

Fig. 27.13 A rod tester confirms the presence of the rod in the screw extender. Note the *green line*, which confirms that the tester cannot seat in the screw head as the rod is in the extender (*arrow*)

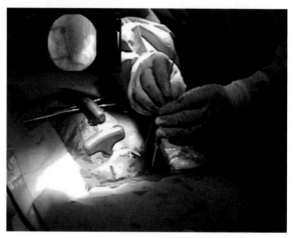

Fig. 27.15 The reduction device is reversed and the screw extenders are removed after caps are finally tightened

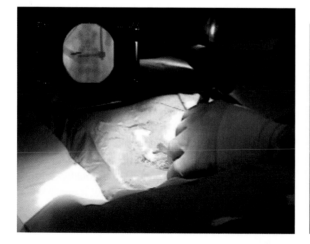

Fig. 27.14 A reduction device is used to reduce the rod. This is confirmed with lateral fluoroscopy

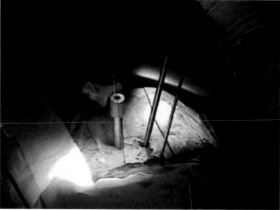

Fig. 27.16 Final construct AP and lateral fluoroscopic images

27.5.2 Technical Peals and Pitfalls

We prefer to cannulate all our pedicles using the AP projection, and only after our pedicles are cannulated are guide wires placed and advanced using the lateral projection. This method saves considerable time and reduces the amount of radiation used. Additionally, operating room lights are dimmed in order to maximize visualization on the fluoroscopy unit screen. If there is a problem with a screw extender or screw head, one can always extend the minimally invasive style incision and open up the fascia and dissect down to the level of the rod. In this manner open persuasion can be performed or open seating of a rod can be performed of the screw head. Open surgery always remains a bail out if there is a problem.

Should a posterior fusion also need to be performed, the simplest posterior fusion can be performed by simply extending the incision about the screw heads and exposing the facet. A high-speed burr is then used to decorticate the facet, and local bone autograft, allograft, or biologics can be used to obtain a facet fusion.

27.5.3 Postoperative Considerations

The first two authors typically brace these patients for three months after surgery, while the last author never braces after these procedures. Alternatively, patients may opt to undergo minimally invasive fixation instead of bracing for stable burst fractures. In the setting of fusion, however, we recommend postoperative bracing. Providing there was no significant neurologic deficit before surgery, we ambulate patients as early as possible. Additionally, deep venous thrombosis prophylaxis is used starting on postoperative day 1.

Potential complications of minimally invasive spinal fusion or minimally invasive fixation include instrumentation misplacement, infection, bleeding, pseudoarthrosis, and adjacent segment degeneration. It is especially vital to monitor the position of the guide wires at all times to avoid inadvertent advancement anteriorly. Complications of MIS posterior fixation reported in two series included screw misplacement requiring revision, neurological injury, radicular pain, instrumentation prominence (in a series where the rod was placed suprafascially), and wound infection [10, 15]. If there is any concern for the quality of imaging of the spine, especially with regard to AP fluoroscopy, we recommended open surgery. Any theoretical benefit of minimally invasive spine surgery is lost if screw placement is not accurate. Inaccurate screw placement can result in serious neurologic or vascular, viscus, or pulmonary injury. If there is any difficulty of the placement of minimally invasive instrumentation specifically, also with regard to seating the rod, consideration should be made for extending the procedure to an open one. In order to avoid instrumentation failure in the future, the decision to perform a short segment fusion vs. a longer fusion is based on the principles of McCormack et al. [6]. Additionally, we recommend patients be placed on a Jackson table in order to maintain lordosis. Effort should also be made to avoid violating the supraadjacent facet.

27.5.4 Conclusion

Minimally invasive fixation represents a less tissue-injuring alternative to open posterior fixation or open posterior fixation and fusion in the setting of spinal trauma. Current-generation systems allow multisegment fixation with significantly less difficulties than earlier-generation instrumentation. Long-term outcomes regarding MIS posterior fixation for trauma (compared with open procedures) are currently being reported. As these data become available, we believe there will be increased use of MIS in the treatment of spinal fractures.

References

1. Anand N, Baron EM, Dekutoski MB (2009) Minimally invasive posterior stabilization techniques (single and multiple segment) percutaneous exposure in trauma. In: Vaccaro AR, Fehlings MG, Dvorak M (eds) Management of spine and spinal cord trauma: an evidence based analysis. Medtronic, Memphis
2. Baron EM, Zeiller SC, Vaccaro AR, Hilibrand AS (2005) Surgical management of thoracolumbar fractures. Contemp Spine Surg 6(12):1–9
3. Kawaguchi Y, Matsui H, Tsuji H (1994) Back muscle injury after posterior lumbar spine surgery. Part 2: histologic and histochemical analyses in humans. Spine 19(22):2598–2602
4. Kawaguchi Y, Yabuki S, Styf J et al (1996) Back muscle injury after posterior lumbar spine surgery. Topographic evaluation of intramuscular pressure and blood flow in the porcine back muscle during surgery. Spine 21(22):2683–2688

5. Lu K, Liang CL, Cho CL et al (2002) Oxidative stress and heat shock protein response in human paraspinal muscles during retraction. J Neurosurg 97(1 suppl):75–81

6. McCormack T, Karaikovic E, Gaines RW (1994) The load sharing classification of spine fractures. Spine 19(15):1741–1744

7. Potter BK, Lenke LG, Kuklo TR (2004) Prevention and management of iatrogenic flat back deformity. J Bone Joint Surg Am 86-A(8):1793–1808

8. Rampersaud YR, Annand N, Dekutoski MB (2006) Use of minimally invasive surgical techniques in the management of trauma: current concepts. Spine 31(11 suppl):S96–S102; discussion S104

9. Rechtine GR, Bono PL, Cahill D, Bolesta MJ, Chrin AM (2001) Postoperative wound infection after instrumentation of thoracic and lumbar fractures. J Orthop Trauma 15(8):566–569

10. Ringel F, Stoffel M, Stuer C, Meyer B (2006) Minimally invasive transmuscular pedicle screw fixation of the thoracic and lumbar spine. Neurosurgery 59(4 suppl 2):ONS361–ONS366; discussion ONS366–ONS367

11. Spoonamore M (2008) Pedicle-targeting techniques for minimally invasive lumbar fusions. In: Lewandrowski K, Yeung C, Spoonamore M, McLain RF (eds) Minimally invasive spinal fusion techniques. Summit Communications, Armonk

12. Suwa H, Hanakita J, Ohshita N, Gotoh K, Matsuoka N, Morizane A (2000) Postoperative changes in paraspinal muscle thickness after various lumbar back surgery procedures. Neurol Med Chir (Tokyo) 40(3):151-154; discussion 154-155

13. Verlaan JJ, Diekerhof CH, Buskens E et al (2004) Surgical treatment of traumatic fractures of the thoracic and lumbar spine: a systematic review of the literature on techniques, complications, and outcome. Spine 29(7):803–814

14. Weber BR, Grob D, Dvorak J, Muntener M (1997) Posterior surgical approach to the lumbar spine and its effect on the multifidus muscle. Spine 22(15):1765–1772

15. Wild MH, Glees M, Plieschnegger C, Wenda K (2007) Five-year follow-up examination after purely minimally invasive posterior stabilization of thoracolumbar fractures: a comparison of minimally invasive percutaneously and conventionally open treated patients. Arch Orthop Trauma Surg 127(5): 335–343

16. Zeiller SC, Baron EM, Hilibrand AS, Anand N, Vaccaro AR (2007) Thoracolumbar fractures: classification and management. In: Jallo JI, Loftus CM, Vaccaro AR (eds) Neurosurgical trauma and critical care. Thieme, New York

Surgical Stabilization Options for Fractures and Fracture-Dislocations at the Lumbosacral Junction and for Posterior Pelvic Ring Reconstruction

28

Thomas A. Schildhauer, Carlo Bellabarba, M.L. Chip Routt, and Jens R. Chapman

28.1 Indications

The pelvic ring and lumbar spinal transition zone provide our trunk and lower extremities with a sound structural foundation and conduit for neurovascular structures, as well as a floor to our intestines and urogenital structures. Injuries to this area are typically the result of high-energy injuries, neoplastic disease, or insufficiency fractures in the presence of impaired bone substance. Due to its unique reliance on a combination of firm bony structures encased by strong ligamentous support structures, the pelvic ring and lumbosacral juncture are exposed to a wide variety of possible injury constellations in terms of musculoskeletal injuries and associated organ system injuries. Ultimately, preservation or restoration of the three-dimensional alignment of this region with a solidly healed injury zone is desirable (Fig. 28.1). The goals of surgical treatment of pelvic ring and lumbosacral zone injuries are providing an environment to allow for best possible regeneration of neural injury and facilitating the recovery process through early pain-free mobilization without interfering with the care of other injured organ systems.

While there has to be some room for individualized treatment given the multiple-injury patient and injury manifestations, there is little doubt that a number of generally acceptable treatment algorithms have prevailed over the last 2 decades.

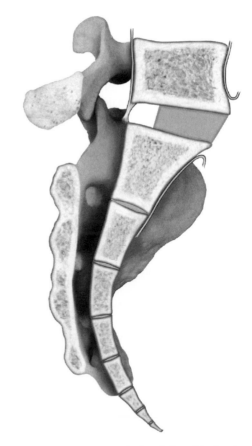

Fig. 28.1 The sacrum forms the foundation of the Lumbar spine and heavily influences its alignment. Together with strong ligaments it provides the foundation for the posterior pelvic ring. It also serves as a protective conduit for the lumbo-sacral plexus and the iliac vessels

T.A. Schildhauer
Chirurgische Klinik und Poliklinik, BG-Universitätskliniken 'Bergmannsheil', Ruhr-Universität, Buerkle-de-la-Camp-Platz 1, 44797 Bochum, Germany

C. Bellabarba, M.L.C. Routt and J.R. Chapman (⊠)
Department of Orthopaedic Surgery, Harborview Medical Center, 325 Ninth Avenue, Seattle, WA 98104, USA
e-mail: jenschap@u.washington.edu

V.V. Patel et al. (eds.), *Spine Trauma*,
DOI: 10.1007/978-3-642-03694-1_28, © Springer-Verlag Berlin Heidelberg 2010

In principle, patients who have mainly ligamentous injuries or major structural disruption of their posterior lumbosacral region can be expected to have more favorable outcomes with appropriate surgical reconstruction compared with nonoperative treatment results for the same indications. Similarly, polytraumatized patients and patients with regional neurologic injuries will generally benefit from well-performed and timely surgical reconstruction. Beyond that, there are a large number of specific circumstances, which may make surgical intervention preferable to other treatment forms.

28.2 Contraindications

As in any patients with open fractures or in injuries with severe soft-tissue trauma (i.e., degloving injuries, contusions), open reduction and extensive hardware fixation have to be used with caution due to an increased potential for impaired soft-tissue healing. For patients with peripelvic injuries, occult open fractures may be present in case of perforation of the vaginal or rectal vaults, or in the presence of major dorsal deglovement injuries (Morel-Lavallee) (Fig. 28.2). On the other hand, mechanical bony stability has been identified as the only beneficial variable for patients with infection following open pelvic injuries.

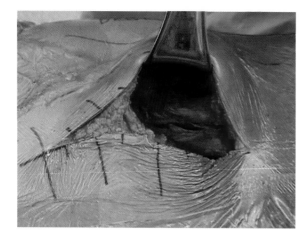

Fig. 28.2 A Morel-Lavalle lesion represents a deglovement injury of the dorsal integument from the lumbo-dorsal fascia. It can extend from the lower ribcage to the gluteal region and can considerably affect decision making about the type of posterior fixation of posterior pelvic ring trauma

Nondisplaced fractures, especially in situations without neurological symptoms, very rarely present as indications for surgical stabilization.

28.3 Techniques

Surgical treatment of the sacral fracture and posterior pelvic ring trauma is performed at the earliest point after emergent surgical needs of other organ systems have been adequately addressed and the patient has been deemed physiologically stable for sacral surgery, ideally less than 2 weeks after injury. Emergent operative intervention is recommended only in patients with: (1) open fractures, (2) lumbodorsal, presacral soft-tissue compromise caused by displaced fracture fragments, and (3) a deteriorating neurologic examination.

For patients with open fractures, appropriate wound debridement should be performed as soon as the patients' hemodynamic condition is stable. Rectal involvement requires early loop colostomy, preferably of the transverse colon, followed by a distal colonic wash out. Soft-tissue contusions and Morel-Lavallee lesions have to be addressed; nonviable tissues require early and sometimes repetitive debridement. Degloved soft-tissue pockets require thorough debridement and the use of meticulous dead space closure and drainage techniques.

Most commonly, the presence of a clinically relevant anterior pelvic ring disruption should be surgically reconstructed as anatomically as possible, as it may aid in the indirect reduction of the posterior pelvic ring and provide partial pelvic stability. Anterior pelvic stabilization may involve plating of the symphysis or antegrade and retrograde superior pubic ramus screw fixation. Upon the completion of this part of the pelvic ring reconstruction, the posterior pelvic ring and lumbosacral junction injury can be addressed as needed with the patient either in supine or even prone position as necessary.

28.4 Treatment Options and Decision-Making

In patients with nondisplaced fractures and good bone quality, as well as in polytraumatized or elderly polymorbid patients, a nonoperative approach for treatment may be indicated. Nonoperative care can range from simple activity limitations to brace wear with hip spica using uni- or bilateral hip extension attachments. Prolonged recumbent skeletal lower extremity traction followed by mobilization with brace wear has been historically used for more unstable injuries. Time periods recommended for nonoperative care vary from a few weeks to 3 or more months. Concerns surrounding nonoperative care center around the potential for posterior skin breakdown and pressure ulcers, thromboembolic events, pulmonary emboli and pulmonary decompensation, secondary deformity, increased pain, and secondary neurologic deterioration.

Surgical treatments can be differentiated into neural decompression surgery and stabilization efforts. Neural decompression procedures vary from limited or extensile neural element decompression in the form of selective foraminotomy to comprehensive laminectomy with or without ventral spinal canal disimpaction. Surgical stabilization efforts include percutaneous internal or external fixation or formal open reduction and internal fixation. Of course, there are a number of conceivable combinations of surgical stabilization in response to the multiple variations of injuries that patients present with. It has to be kept in mind, however, that many of these fixation techniques typically do not stabilize the lumbosacral junction itself, but offer a limited stabilization of the posterior pelvic ring in the horizontal plane. Also, these techniques preclude early full weight-bearing activities postoperatively due to their inherent biomechanical limitations and high forces with ambulation. If there are structural concerns regarding the integrity of the lumbosacral junction or if secondary symptoms at the lumbosacral junction emerge, inclusion of this critical transition zone with adequate instrumentation surgery should be considered.

28.4.1 External Fixation

This technique has maintained a role in emergency management of unstable pelvic ring fractures and for adjuvant stabilization of posterior pelvic ring disruptions. The most common insertion sites, by far, are the anterior iliac spinous processes with the pins engaging the iliac crest bilaterally. An alternative or supplemental anterior fixation site consists of the abductor tubercle on the superior and lateral aspect of the iliac crest.

Although there have been descriptions of external fixator pin placements into the posterior iliac crest and application of posteriorly based or circumferential external fixateur frames, these devices are not practical in everyday life. Anterior frames represent the majority of routinely applied external fixation devices for the distinct purpose of closing down a splayed anterior pelvic ring and reducing the volume of a disrupted pelvic ring as an adjunct resuscitation aid. Predictably, these devices have a very limited biomechanical effect on the posterior pelvic ring. There is also a strong trend toward pin tract infections and pin loosening in anterior external fixateurs kept in place for 2 weeks or more. Due to these factors, anterior pelvic external fixateurs have largely maintained a supplemental treatment role.

28.4.2 Transiliac Sacral Bars

This early form of internal splinting offered restoration of a posterior pelvic ring tension band by means of placing one or two threaded rods through the posterior superior iliac spinous processes on either side bridging across the posterior sacral elements. The option of achieving some compressive effect across the posterior pelvic ring was affected by placing nuts and washers over the rods to the medial and lateral aspects of the posterior iliac crests on either side. While the concept and implant cost of the device were simple and "low-tech," actual clinical applications were hampered by the needs to perform a relatively extensile dorsal exposure through two parallel parasagittal incisions with an increased potential for wound healing complications and a potential for difficult in vivo implant handling. Fixation strength was directly related to integrity, size, and bone quality of the posterior iliac crests on both sides of the pelvis. Over time, the popularity of this device has waned due to its inherent limitations.

28.4.3 Transverse Transiliac Plating

Restoration of the posterior pelvic tension band function can be provided by a large fragment plate that is placed transversely across the posterior iliac crests in a way that the plate ends overlap the posterior superior iliac spinous processes and allow for placement of screws through the plate holes to cross back into the sacrum. Compared to the posterior transiliac bars, this device application holds theoretical biomechanical advantages due to a greater bone fixation strength by virtue of multidirectionally directed large fragment screws, instead of unidimensional threaded bars with some compressive effect. The clear disadvantages of this instrumentation technique are the need for an extensile dorsal exposure using either two longitudinal parasagittal incisions or a transverse incision. Both exposure techniques rely on less than desirable soft-tissue stripping techniques for adequate fracture reduction and would likely lead to an undesirable rate of wound healing complication, infection, and buttock incision.

28.5 Open Reduction and Internal Fixation with Small Fragment Plate and Screw Devices

The concept of performing an open reduction and internal fixation through a posterior midline exposure dates back to the beginning of the use of plates and screws for fracture care. Due to the relatively small nature of the sacrum and its relatively shallow soft-tissue coverage, small plate fixation is usually preferred. Roy-Camille suggested small fragment posterior plate and screw fixation along the posterior ala lateral to the posterior neuroforamina for the treatment of transverse sacral fractures. Screw purchase relies on anterior alar cortical engagement in the region just adjacent to the sacroiliac joint. There are many possible further variations of hardware placement across the multitude of fracture configurations in which posterior pelvic ring disruptions can be present. Extensile exposure may also be necessary to achieve comprehensive fixation of the various fracture segments of the more complex fracture variants that may present in this region. This further limits the applicability of this fixation philosophy (Fig. 28.3).

Overall, fracture fixation stability, however, is very much contingent upon bone quality and fracture comminution. In reality, most posterior pelvic and sacral fractures present with less than straightforward fracture patterns, limiting the practicality of rigid fracture fixation with this technique.

28.5.1 Iliosacral Screws

Advances of intraoperative image intensification and the increasing availability of these devices have made the percutaneous application of screws placed through

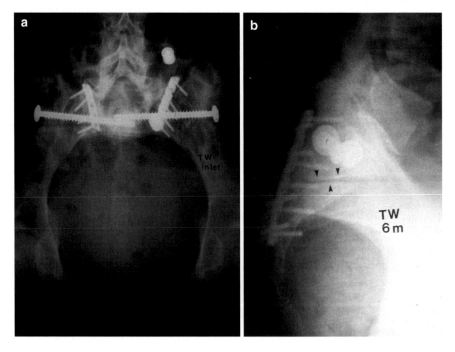

Fig. 28.3 (**a, b**) Open reduction and internal fixation of unstable posterior pelvic ring fractures with plates and screws has become largely obsolete due to its improvisational nature and lack of effective biomechanical stability

the ilium into the bodies of the first and/or second sacral segment an increasingly popular treatment. Refinements of this basic treatment concept have been plenty and range from improvement of closed reduction techniques with percutaneous implant placement and increased understanding of anatomy and timing of intervention to cannulated screw systems of various dimensions and thread lengths. With these varied screw systems, it is possible to achieve compression or "pull-effects" of fractured segments by deliberate placement of partially threaded devices or achieve a "holding" or buttress function by placing fully threaded devices in nonorthogonal angles. Screw washers are used to minimize the risk of screw pullthrough. For osteoporotic patients, screws may have to be placed across the midline to minimize toggle-loosening or cantilevering. While the

use of CT-scans for screw placement has been suggested by some, this technology application has not become a mainstay of posterior pelvic reduction due to spatial access limitations and dissociation of fracture care from the operating room or the emergency room. Undoubtedly, the utilization of percutaneous SI screws has provided a dramatic improvement for the treatment of patients with posterior pelvic ring disruption. Intricate knowledge of posterior lumbopelvic anatomy and recognition of normal-variants are important prerequisites prior to engaging in surgery. Timing of surgery within 48 h may facilitate closed reduction due to less fracture hematoma congealment and lower radiographic interference from posttraumatic ileus formation. Limitations of this technique mainly lie in its biomechanical performance in patients with impaired bone quality or vertically displaced posterior ring fractures, as well as difficulties in safe device placement for patients with anatomic segmentation anomalies and upper sacral fracture displacement (Fig. 28.4).

28.5.2 Segmental Lumbopelvic Fixation

Lumbopelvic fixation is indicated in injuries to the lumbosacral junction with multidirectional instabilities. These occur primarily under two circumstances. In the first circumstance, a vertical sacral fracture, which constitutes the posterior pelvic ring injury, extends rostrally into or medial to the S1 superior facet, thereby disarticulating the L5-S1 facet from the stable sacral fracture fragment. In the second, a multiplanar sacral fracture comprises bilateral longitudinal fractures and a transverse fracture component separates the upper central sacrum and remainder of the spine from the peripheral sacrum and attached pelvis. The result of this fracture pattern and its variants is the dissociation of the lumbar spine from the pelvic ring and functional lumbosacral instability. These injuries are frequently associated with neurologic deficits ranging from lower extremity monoradiculopathies to complete cauda equina deficits. Attempts at surgical decompression of compromised neural elements, however, would lead to further instability of the lumbosacral junction.

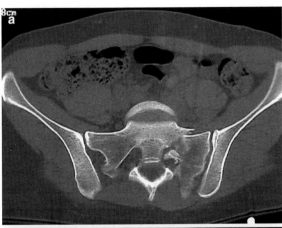

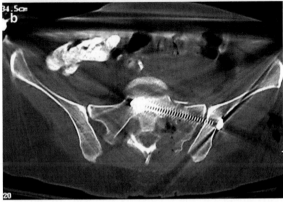

Fig. 28.4 Sacroiliac screw fixation allows for restoration of bony continuity and provides some posterior pelvic ring stability through a percutaneous approach. Keys to success with this technique are appropriate case selection, timing, surgical expertise and suitable surgical resources. In this patient a small laminotomy was added to a percutaneous SI-screw fixation to remove a bone fragment which was impinged in the S1 foramen

Other indications for lumbopelvic fixation are posterior pelvic ring injuries in severe osteoporosis or bony comminution or in sacral fractures with concomitant posterior ilium fractures, which may preclude any other standard posterior pelvic ring osteosynthesis technique, such as iliosacral screw or transiliac plate osteosynthesis. Secondary fracture dislocation after standard osteosynthesis techniques of the posterior pelvic ring, pseudarthrosis, and bony defects after tumor and infection may be other reasons for considering lumbopelvic fixation as a salvage procedure to stabilize the lumbosacral junction and posterior pelvic ring. The advantage of lumbopelvic fixation with a long iliac screw in these situations is that the anchor screw in the ilium bypasses any posterior pelvic pathology, since it gains its bony anchor in two iliac constrictions at 3 and 8 cm anterior to the posterior superior iliac spine (PSIS).

Lumbopelvic fixation comprises variants of a bridging osteosynthesis for injuries to the lumbosacral junction. This osteosynthesis technique transfers axial loads from the upper body and trunk directly to the ilium, thereby bypassing any lumbosacral junction injury itself. It anchors in the pedicles of the lower lumbar spine and connects distally to long ilium screws positioned between the PSIS and the anterior inferior iliac spine (AIIS). Since a two-point fixation with only one anchor screw cranially and caudally to the injury may allow splaying, this bridging stabilization has to be combined either with an additional horizontal fixation, such as an iliosacral screw or a transiliac plate osteosynthesis, or has to be extended vertically by additional level pedicle and/or iliac screws. In bilateral sacral injuries or complex lumbopelvic fracture-dislocations with spino-pelvic dissociation, a bilateral lumbopelvic fixation includes horizontal transconnectors between the two vertical connecting rods. These compensate any other horizontal fixation.

28.6 Results

The variability of injury type and injury magnitude, the lack of consistently applied injury and outcome classification systems, and a relatively low incidence of these injuries have precluded comparative studies to evaluate various treatment algorithms. In our experience, the majority of surgical decompression and lumbopelvic fixation for sacral fracture-dislocations with spino-pelvic dissociation and cauda equina deficits (Roy-Camille type 2–4) presented fracture healing in all patients without secondary loss of reduction. Average sacral kyphosis improved from 43 to 21°. Eighty-three percent had

full or partial recovery of bowel and bladder deficits. Wound infection occurred in 16% of patients, two thirds of whom originally had been diagnosed with traumatic closed soft-tissue degloving lesions. Eleven percent of patients required surgical reexploration because of seroma/pseudomeningocele formation. Nevertheless, in both patients concurrent traumatic dural tears or sacral root avulsions were identified. At the latest follow-up examination, 31% of patients had at least one broken longitudinal rod between the lowest lumbar and most rostral iliac screw. Because of the lack of a sacro-iliac joint arthrodesis and the resulting likelihood of eventual fatigue failure of the rods between the iliac and lumbar screws, this was interpreted as an incidental finding in the absence of referable clinical symptoms, such as pain with weight bearing or external hip rotation, and in absence of radiographic signs of loss of fracture reduction. Conversely, in all patients with absent rod failure, bridging callus of the posterolateral arthrodesis mass to the ilium could be identified on follow-up radiographs.

28.6.1 Exposure

After preoperative bowel preparation, patients are positioned prone on a Jackson operating table under somatosensory evoked potentials and electromyogram monitoring along with C-arm visualization in the lateral plane. Posterior midline surgical dissection is carried from the L4 to the S4 segment, with subperiosteal lateral dissection to the lumbar transverse processes, sacral ala and PSIS bilaterally (Fig. 28.5).

28.6.2 Neural Decompression, Fracture Reduction, Lumbopelvic Fixation

In sacral fracture-dislocations with spino-pelvic instability, bilateral lumbar pedicle screw fixation is initially applied to the L5 and S1 segment. We prefer a low-profile side opening system (e.g., Universal Spine System, Synthes, Paoli, PA). If comminution of the S1 segment precludes screw placement at this level, supplemental screw placement into the L4 segment is performed to provide a "4-point" fixation of the lumbar component of the fracture.

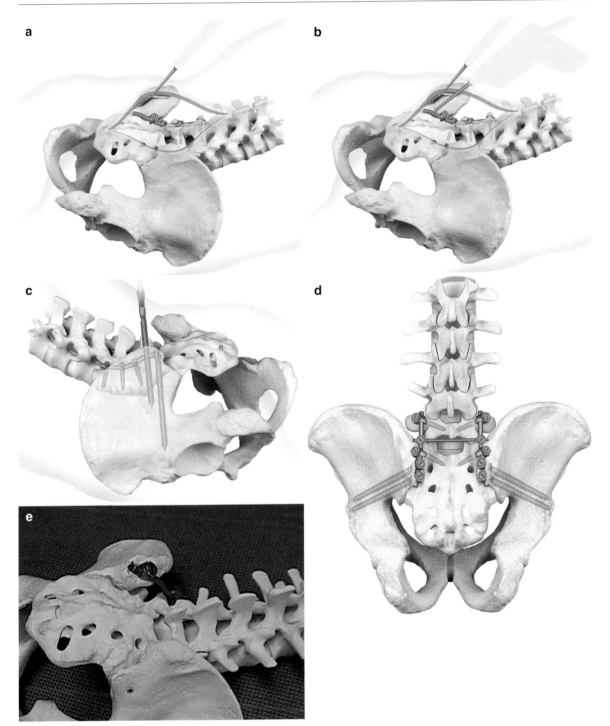

Fig. 28.5 (**a–e**) Sequence of segmental lumbo-pelvic stabilization. (**a**) Following posterior midline exposure and dissection of the posterior iliac crests bilaterally necessary neural element decompressions and direct fracture reduction are carried out. (**b**) Following placement of pedicle screws into the L5 and if needed L4 segments, rods are contoured to fit into the groove between posterior iliac crest and sacrum. (**c, d**) Tangential to the caudal ends of the rods drilling of the posterior iliac crest commences just medial to the posterior superior iliac spinous process aiming for the anterior inferior iliac spinous process. This is usually done under lateral C-arm guidance to avoid penetration of the iliac notch. (**e**) Final screw anchoring is accomplished in a low profile fashion to avoid soft tissue irritation or breakdown

Decompression of neural elements can be accomplished by several techniques. Indirect fracture reduction may relieve nerve root compression, but it is most effective if performed prior to fracture hematoma consolidation. Direct neural decompression can be performed through anterior or posterior approaches. The anterior approach is rarely indicated due to the difficult access resulting from sacral inclination, visceral structures, and the presence of an extensive venous plexus overlying the sacrum. Nevertheless, if fragments of the anterior sacral ala impinge on the L5 nerve root, direct access for fracture reduction and decompression of the nerve root can only be gained by an anterior approach through the Olerud window. Otherwise, neural decompression is performed through the posterior above-mentioned approach. Single bony fragments that encroach on a nerve root and require selective ventral foraminal decompression are removed by focal laminectomy, which allows the involved sacral root to be followed and decompressed through its anterior neuroforaminal exit. In complex sacral fractures involving extensive areas of the sacral spinal canal, a comprehensive sacral laminectomy is necessary. While performing a sacral laminectomy, it is usually advantageous to identify the more cranial sacral roots and then to follow them to their respective ventral foramen. Ventral canal decompression can be accomplished by freeing the sacral roots in the injury zone from their epidural venous cuff and then proceeding with ventral disimpaction or direct removal of protruding bone fragments. Ventral disimpaction may be facilitated by placing an elevator into the fracture as a lever or using an impactor to directly push the dorsal wall of the injured sacral vertebral bodies and thus correct the posterior displacement. It is helpful to perform the sacral decompression surgery under lateral C-arm control for orientation purposes and help to assess sacral alignment and associated decompression of the spinal canal.

Traumatic dural tears are relatively common. When possible, suture repair is undertaken with 6-0 Prolene®. Otherwise, patching or sealing techniques may be used, including the use of dural allograft, dural graft matrix, or one of various biologic sealants. Containment of cerebrospinal fluid is ascertained with a Valsalva maneuver held to 30-cm H_2O for 10 s (see Chap. 33).

For overall fracture reduction in lumbosacral fracture-dislocations with spino-pelvic dissociation, the angulated upper sacral body segment can be secured with a Schanz screw placed between the S1 and S2 roots, allowing for disimpaction and direct manipulative reduction of this fragment. To achieve this goal, sacral length is reestablished to prevent the caudal sacral fragment from impeding reduction, using bifemoral skeletal traction or unilateral versus bilateral use of an AO femoral distractor between a pedicle screw or Schanz screw in the L5 pedicle and another in the ilium. Alignment is occasionally maintained by the interdigitation and partial intussusception of the upper sacrum on the lower sacrum. When possible, iliosacral screws are used to provide initial fixation; however, because of typically occurring comminution of the sacral ala in these fractures, the iliosacral screws are positioned as transfixation screws, rather than compression screws, to decrease the potential for neuroforaminal overcompression (Fig. 28.6).

The cephalad fracture component consisting of the lumbar spine and central upper sacral segment is then secured to the caudal fracture fragment consisting of the pelvis and lower/peripheral sacral segments by connecting the lumbosacral pedicle screws to iliac screws. Before placing these iliac screws, longitudinal rods are secured to the lumbosacral pedicle screws after having been contoured in a manner that positions their caudal segment just medial to the PSIS and, therefore, adjacent to the intended starting point of the iliac screws. The iliac screws can then be placed adjacent to the prepositioned rod. Placement of the iliac screws adjacent to the precontoured, prepositioned rod eliminates the more difficult rod-contouring required when pedicle screws and iliac screws are placed independently, before rod application. A true lateral view of the pelvis with precise overlap of the sciatic notches is vital to the safe placement of iliac screws. If these radiographic landmarks cannot be confidently visualized, the sciatic notch can also be directly palpated to guide safe screw placement by dissecting the gluteus muscles off the outer table of the ilium. A 3.2 mm channel is drilled through the bone corridor between the PSIS and the AIIS. The combination obturator-outlet oblique view, which projects the column of bone along the intended screw trajectory as a teardrop shape, is useful to confirm the correct starting point and final screw position. The longest possible screws are used, typically with a maximum length of 140 mm. This allows for maximum thread contact with the cortical bone of the inner and outer tables along the narrower midportion of the ilium, a best grip of the screws within the two cortical constrictions within the bony canal, and a better 3-point fixation due to the iliac curvature. Images that are

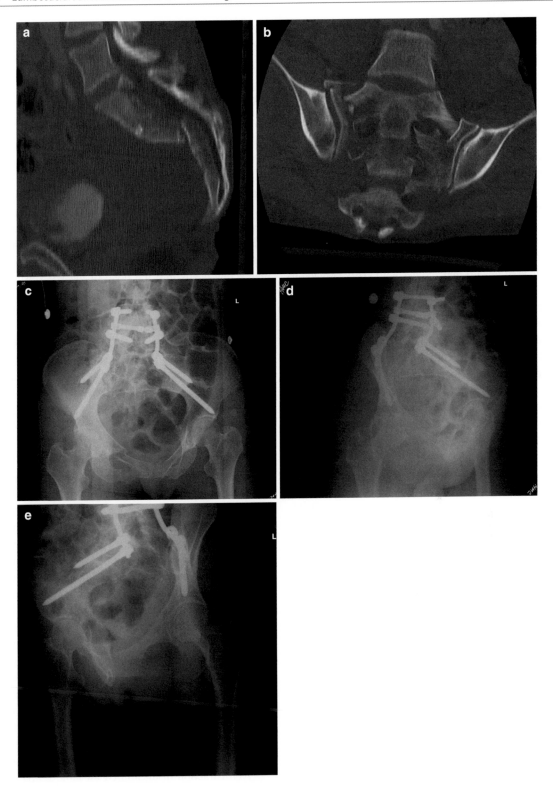

Fig. 28.6 In this series a 28 year old male with Denis Zone 3, Roy-Camille Type 2 injury is shown with incomplete cauda equina injury (**a**, **b**). (**c**) Demonstrates the use of segmental lumbo-pelvic fixation on a pelvic antero-posterior radiograph, while left and right iliac oblique images demonstrates co-axial intertable iliac screw placement bilaterally (**d**, **e**). In presence of neural continuity comprehensive neural element decompression and stabilization within anatomic parameters has been shown to consistently improve neurologic outcomes

essential to confirm acceptable screw position are the orthogonal obturator-outlet and obturator-inlet views, which confirm that screws are contained within the ilium without medial or lateral penetration, and the lateral and iliac oblique views, which confirm appropriate screw length and the absence of sciatic notch or acetabular penetration. In highly unstable situations at the lumbopelvic junction or in severe osteoporotic bone, a second iliac screw placement is recommended. The second iliac screw is placed either along the same trajectory, adjacent to the first iliac screw, or is started at a point cephalad to the optimal PSIS-AIIS path and aimed from the iliac tubercle to the AIIS to allow better triangulation, increased pull-out strength, and rotational stability. The longitudinal connecting rods are then compressed toward one another with cross-connectors or transverse bars as needed to reestablish physiologic posterior pelvic ring alignment.

In unilateral sacral fractures with rostral extension into and medial to the L5/S1 facet, the so-called triangular osteosynthesis, consisting of lumbopelvic fixation between the pedicle of L5 and the ilium associated with ipsilateral iliosacral screw fixation, has been shown to result in stable fracture fixation allowing early full weight bearing.

After thorough wound irrigation, local bone graft from the sacral laminectomy is applied to the decorticated posterolateral elements from the most rostral instrumented lumbar vertebra to the sacral ala. The pelvis and posterior ilium, however, are not included in the arthrodesis. Therefore, the iliosacral joints are not formally fused.

28.7 Postoperative Management

Postoperatively, patients are mobilized immediately and allowed to fully weight bear and ambulate as tolerated, unless precluded by other injuries. Since the iliosacral joints are not formally fused, micromotion at the iliosacral joints, which are bridged by the lumbopelvic fixation, may result in failure of the longitudinal connection rods between the pedicle and iliac screws. This hardware failure is not a result of a pseudarthrosis at the fracture site, but a result of constant cyclic loading. Early hardware removal of the lumbopelvic fixation after fracture healing (after 6–12 months) can prevent this hardware breakage. Another alternative is to simply allow the hardware breakage to occur and proceed with removal only if clinically indicated.

28.8 Avoiding Pitfalls and Complications

Painful hardware, especially at the insertion site of the iliac screw, is always a concern in lumbopelvic fixation. Also, prominent iliac screws may have an influence on wound healing complications or may result in pressure ulcers, especially in postoperatively immobilized patients and posttraumatic soft-tissue compromise (e.g., degloving, contusion). Recessing of the iliac screw heads into the bone of the PSIS using an osteotome is, therefore, recommended.

Some pedicle and iliac screw hardware systems provide only partially threaded iliac screws with limited length and diameter. It has to be kept in mind that pull-out strength is directly related to screw-cortical bone interface, as well as screw length and width. Therefore, surgeons should strive for optimal implants for maximum iliac screw fixation to avoid iliac screw loosening and "windshield-wiper-effect," which is known from the Galveston technique.

In highly unstable pelvic ring injuries with lumbopelvic instability, postoperative secondary vertical displacement may be prevented by lumbopelvic fixation. However, flexion deformity may result if the anterior pelvic ring injury is not stabilized and if the iliac screws are not having a strong purchase within the cancellous bone of the ilium (e.g., in osteoporosis or when having only short and thin iliac anchor screws available). In these situations it is of importance to initially stabilize the anterior pelvic ring injury with a "dynamic" osteosynthesis, such as a superior pubic ramus screw, and then to perform posterior sacral fracture reduction and fixation. If the posterior reduction and triangular osteosynthesis is performed first without having a perfect anterior ring reduction, a secondary anterior pelvic ring reduction and osteosynthesis is immediately working against the much stronger posterior ring fixation. This may result in early loosening and failure of the anterior pelvic ring fixation.

Overdistraction of an injured unstable L5/S1 facet joint is always a concern while performing lumbopelvic fixation techniques, especially performing a distraction maneuver on an injured L5/S1 joint for sacral fracture reduction. Therefore, while applying the lumbopelvic fixation and reduction maneuver along a vertical connecting rod, the surgeon should be aware of such an injury to the L5/S1 facet and actively search for it preoperatively on the computerized tomography scans. If such an injury is present and if distraction forces are applied along the longitudinal connecting rod of the lumbopelvic fixation for vertical reduction of the sacral fracture, this reduction maneuver should be followed by horizontal fixation with an SI-screw. Then, the distraction force over the injured L5/S1 facet should be released, the appropriate position and reduction of the L5/S1 junction should be reassessed, and only then should the final fixation of the lumbopelvic implants at the screw-rod interface be performed. Lumbopelvic fixation has to be understood as a bridging osteosynthesis stabilizing a reduced fracture, and not as a "distracting" osteosynthesis. Overdistraction at the lumbopelvic junction can occur as well when the bony facet is intact but the joint capsule is transected, which may happen iatrogenically when L5 pedicle screws are positioned. Tilting at the L5/S1 junction due to overdistraction should be differentiated from tilting due to insufficient reduction of the injured hemipelvis in the vertical direction. In that case, the sacral ala may engage on an uninjured or nondisplaced L5 transverse process.

Distraction along a longitudinal connecting rod of the lumbopelvic fixation may result in displacement of the fracture laterally and posteriorly along the vector of the rod, if it is bent only in one plane. We prebend the longitudinal rod in an s-shape in the frontal as well as in the sagittal plane. Rotating the rod within the L5 pedicle screw and the iliac screw during reduction maneuvers may then help to close down the fracture site. The lumbopelvic fixation should never be finalized before performing the horizontal fixation with the SI-screw. It should rather be a concomitant procedure, using the longitudinal connecting rod for vertical reduction, followed by horizontal final fixation and then finalization of the lumbopelvic fixation with correction of any distraction at the L5/S1 junction.

Further Reading

1. Alexander RH, Proctor HJ (eds) (1993) Advanced trauma life support for physicians: ATLS instructor manual, 5th edn. American College of Surgeons, Chicago
2. Archdeacon MT, Hiratzka J (2006) The trochanteric c-clamp for provisional pelvic stability. J Orthop Trauma 20(1):47–51
3. Bellabarba C, Stewart JD, Ricci WM, DiPasquale TG, Bolhofner BR (2003) Midline sagittal sacral fractures in anterior-posterior compression pelvic ring injuries. J Orthop Trauma 17(1):32–37
4. Bellabarba C, Schildhauer TA, Vaccaro AR, Chapman JR (2006) Complications associated with surgical stabilization of high-grade sacral fracture-dislocations with spino-pelvic instability. Spine 31(11S):S80–S88
5. Ben-Menachem Y, Coldwell DM, Young JW, Burgess AR (1991) Hemorrhage associated with pelvic fractures: causes, diagnosis, and emergent management. AJR Am J Roentgenol 157(5):1005–1014
6. Blake SP, Connors AM (2004) Sacral insufficiency fracture. Br J Radiol 77(922):891–896
7. Bonnin JG (1945) Sacral fractures and injuries to the cauda equina. J Bone Joint Surg Am 27:113–127
8. Browner BD, Cole JD, GRaham JM, Bondurant FJ, Nunchuck-Burns SK, Colter HB (1987) Delayed posterior internal fixation of unstable pelvic fractures. J Trauma 27:998–1006
9. Carter SR (1994) Occult sacral fractures in osteopenic patients. J Bone Joint Surg Am 76(9):1434
10. Chiu FY, Chuang TY, Lo WH (2004) Treatment of unstable pelvic fractures: use of a transiliac sacral rod for posterior lesions and an external fixator for anterior lesions. J Trauma 57(1):141–145
11. Dasgupta B, Shah N, Brown H, Gordon TE, Tanqueray AB, Mellor JA (1998) Sacral insurrficiency fractus: an unsuspected cause of low back pain. BR J Rheumatol 37:789–793
12. Denis F, Davis S, Comfort T (1988) Sacral fractures: an important problem. Retrospective analysis of 236 cases. Clin Orthop Relat Res 227:67–81
13. Esses SI, Botsford DJ, Huler RJ, Rauschning W (1991) Surgical anatomy of the sacrum. A guide for rational screw fixation. Spine 16(6 Suppl):S283–S288
14. Fisher RG (1988) Sacral fracture with compression of cauda equina: surgical treatment. J Trauma 28(12):1678–1680
15. Fountain SS, Hamilton RD, Jameson RM (1977) Transverse fractures of the sacrum. A report of six cases. J Bone Joint Surg Am 59(4):486–489
16. Fujii M, Abe K, Hayashi K, Kosuda S, Yano F, Watanabe S, Katagiri S, Ka WJ, Tominaga S (2005) Honda sign and variants in patients suspected of having a sacral insufficiency fracture. Clin Nucl Med 30(3):165–169
17. Gotis-Graham I, McGuigan L, Diamond T, Portek I, Quinn R, Sturgess A, Tulloch R (1994) Sacral insufficiency fractures in the elderly. J Bone Joint Surg Br 76(6):882–886
18. Griffin DR, Starr AJ, Reinert CM, Jones AL, Whitlock S (2003) Vertically unstable pelvic fractures fixed with percutaneous iliosacral crews: does posterior injury pattern predict fixation failure? J Orthop Trauma 17:399–405
19. Hak DJ, Olson SA, Matta JM (1997) Diagnosis and management of closed internal degloving injuries associated with pelvic and acetabular fractures: the Morel-Lavallee lesion. J Trauma 42(6):1046–1051
20. Harma A, Inan M (2005) Surgical management of transforaminal sacral fractures. Int Orthop 29(5):333–337
21. Henderson RC (1989) The long term results of nonoperatively treated major pelvic disruptions. J Orthop Trauma 3:41–47

22. Incagnoli P, Viggiano M, Carli P (2000) Priorities in the management of severe pelvic trauma. Curr Opin Crit Care 6(6):401–407

23. Isler B (1990) Lumbosacral lesions associated with pelvic ring injuries. J Orthop Trauma 4(1):1–6

24. Kabak S, Halici M, Tuncel M, Avsarogullar L, Baktir A, Basturk M (2003) Functional outcome of open reduction and internal fixation for completely unstable pelvic ring fractures (type C): a report of 40 cases. J Orthop Trauma 17(8):555–562

25. Käch K, Trentz O (1994) Distraction spondylodesis of the sacrum in vertical shear lesions of the pelvis. Unfallchirurg 97:28–38

26. Kellam JF, McMurtry RY, Paley D, Tile M (1987) The unstable pelvic fracture. Operative treatment. Orthop Clin North Am 18(1):25–41

27. Kellam JF (1998) Long-term functional prognosis of posterior injuries in high-energy pelvic disruption. J Orthop Trauma 12(3):150–151

28. Klineberg E, McHenry T, Bellabarba C, Wagner T, Chapman JR (2008) Sacral insufficiency fractures caudal to instrumented posterior lumbosacral arthrodesis. Spine 33(16):1806–1811

29. Korovessis PG, Magnissalis EA, Deligianni D (2006) Biomechanical evaluation of conventional internal contemporary spinal fixation techniques used for stabilization of complete sacroiliac joint separation: a 3-dimensional unilaterally isolated experimental stiffness study. Spine 31(25): E941–E951

30. Kuklo TR, Potter BK, Ludwig SC, Anderson PA, Lindsey RW, Vaccaro AR (2006) Radiographic measurement techniques for sacral fractures consensus statement of the spine trauma study group. Spine 31(9):1047–1055

31. Krappinger D, Larndorfer R, Struve P, Rosenberger R, Arora R, Blauth M (2007) Minimally invasive transiliac plate osteosynthesis for type C injuries of the pelvic ring: a clinical and radiological follow-up. J Orthop Trauma 21(9):595–602

32. Latenser BA, Gentilello LM, Tarver AA, Thalgott JS, Batdorf JW (1991) Improved outcome with early fixation of skeletally unstable pelvic fractures. J Trauma 31(1):28–31

33. Lindahl J, Hirvensalo E, Bostman O, Santavirta S (1999) Failure of reduction with an external fixator in the management of injuries of the pelvic ring: long-term evaluation of 110 patients. J Bone Joint Surg Br 81-B(6):955–962

34. Moed BR, Geer BL (2006) S2 iliosacral screw fixation for disruptions of the posterior pelvic ring: a report of 49 cases. J Orthop Trauma 20(6):378–383

35. Nork SE, Jones CB, Harding SP, Mirza SK, Routt ML Jr (2001) Percutaneous stabilization of U-shaped sacral fractures using iliosacral screws: technique and early results. J Orthop Trauma 15(4):238–246

36. Nothofer W, Thonke N, Neugebauer R (2004) Die therapie instabiler sakrumfracturen bei beckenringbrüchen mit dorsaler sakrumdistanzosteosynthese. Unfallchirurg 107:118–127

37. Olson SA, Pollak AN (1996) Assessment of pelvic ring stability after injury: indications for surgical stabilization. Clin Orthop Relat Res 329:15–27

38. Pohlemann T, Angst M, Schneider E, Ganz R, Tscherne H (1993) Fixation of transforaminal sacrum fractures: a biomechanical study. J Orthop Trauma 7(2):107–117

39. Routt ML Jr, Nork SE, Mills WJ (2000) Percutaneous fixation of pelvic ring disruptions. Clin Orthop Relat Res (375):15–29

40. Routt ML Jr, Simonian PT, Agnew SG, Mann FA (1996) Radiographic recognition of the sacral alar slope for optimal placement of iliosacral screws: a cadaveric and clinical study. J Orthop Trauma 10(3):171–177

41. Routt ML Jr, Simonian PT, Swiontkowski MF (1997) Stabilization of pelvic ring disruptions. Orthop Clin North Am 28(3):369–388

42. Routt ML Jr, Simonian PT, Mills WJ (1997) Iliosacral screw fixation: early complications of the percutaneous technique. J Orthop Trauma 11(8):584–589

43. Roy-Camille R, Saillant G, Gagna G, Mazel C (1985) Transverse fracture of the upper sacrum. Suicidal jumper's fracture. Spine 10(9):838–845

44. Schildhauer TA, Ledoux WR, Chapman JR et al (2003) Triangular osteosynthesis and iliosacral screw fixation in unstable sacrum fractures. A cadaveric and biomechanical evaluation under cyclic loads. J Orthop Trauma 17(1):22–31

45. Schildhauer TA, Josten C, Muhr G (1998) The triangular osteosynthesis of vertically unstable sacrum fractures: a new concept allowing early weight-bearing. J Orthop Trauma 12(5):307–314

46. Schildhauer TA, McCullough P, Chapman JR, Mann FA (2002) Anatomic and radiographic considerations for placement of transilial screws in lumbopelvic fixations. J Spinal Dis Tech 15(3):199–205

47. Schildhauer TA, Bellabarba C, Nork SE, Barei DP et al (2006) Decompression and lumbopelvic fixation for sacral fracture-dislocations with spino-pelvic dissociation. J Orthop Trauma 20(7):447–484

48. Simonian PT, Routt ML Jr (1997) Biomechanics of pelvic fixation. Orthop Clin North Am 28(3):351–367

49. Simonian PT, Chip Routt ML Jr, Harrington RM, Tencer AF (1996) Internal fixation for the transforaminal sacral fracture. Clin Orthop Relat Res 323:202–209

50. Simpson T, Krieg JC, Heuer F, Bottlang M (2002) Stabilization of pelvic ring disruptions with a circumferential sheet. J Trauma 52(1):158–161

51. Templeman D, Goulet J, Duwelius PJ, Olson S, Davidson M (1996) Internal fixation of displaced fractures of the sacrum. Clin Orthop Relat Res 329:180–185

52. Tiemann AH, Schmidt C, Josten C (2003) Triangular vertebropelvine stabilisation of unstable posterior pelvic ring fractures. Zentralbl Chir 128:202–208

53. Tile M (1995) Pelvic ring fractures: should they be fixed? J Bone Joint Surg Br 70:1–12

54. Tile M (1999) The management of the unstable pelvic ring fractures. J Bone Joint Surg Br 81-B(6):941–943

55. Tseng S (2006) Tornetta P III:Percutaneous management of Morel Lavalee lesions. J Bone Joint Surg Am 88:92–96

56. van Zwienen CM, van den Bosch EW, Snijders CJ, Kleinrensink GJ, van Vugt AB (2004) Biomechanical comparison of sacroiliac screw techniques for unstable pelvic ring fractures. J Orthop Trauma 18(9):589–595

57. Waites MD, Mears SC, Mathis J, Belkoff SM (2007) The strength of the osteoporotic sacrum. Spine 32(23):E652–E655

58. Weber M, Hasler P, Gerber H (1993) Insufficiency fractures of the sacrum. Twenty cases and review of the literature. Spine 18(16):2507–2512
59. Wood KB, Geissele AE, Ogilvie JW (1996) Pelvic fractures after long lumbosacral spine fusions. Spine 21(11): 1357–1362
60. Zelle BA, Gruen GS, Hunt T, Speth SR (2004) Sacral fractures with neurological injury: is early decompression beneficial? Int Orthop 28(4):244–251
61. Chapman JR, Harrington RM, Lee KM et al (1996) Factors affecting the pull-out strength of cancellous bone screws. J Biomech Eng 118:391–398

Sacral Screw Fixation

29

Todd McCall, Daniel Fassett, and Andrew Dailey

29.1 Introduction

Historically, the lumbosacral junction has been the area in the spine where it is most difficult to achieve an arthrodesis. Pseudarthrosis and hardware failure have been reported to occur at alarmingly high rates in long fusions including the sacrum [6]. For example, Camp et al. [4] noted a 44% rate of sacral screw failure with Cotrel-Dubousset instrumentation. Several factors contribute to the high pseudarthrosis rate. First, the lumbosacral facet joints are oriented coronally and thus allow more rotation than the lumbar facet joints [10]. Second, the sacrum does not contain pedicles defined by a ring of bone into which screws can obtain a firm purchase as is seen with the lumbar or thoracic spine [24]. Third, long spine fusion constructs can function as a cantilever arm through which the cephalad end of the construct generates excessive forces on the sacral screws.

Because of the challenge of obtaining strong sacral fixation, the optimization of sacral fixation has received specific attention in the literature. In general, the two principal methods that have been advocated for obtaining strong sacral fixation are the anteromedial [11, 26] and anterolateral [18] trajectories for screw placement into the first vertebra of the sacrum. In the anteromedial approach, the screw passes through the pedicle into the centrum or promontory, whereas in the anterolateral

T. McCall (✉) and D. Fassett
Illinois Neurological Institute, University of Illinois
College of Medicine–Peoria, Peoria, 61656, USA
e-mail: todd.mcall@gmail.com

A. Dailey
Department of Neurosurgery, University of Utah,
Salt Lake City, UT, USA

approach the screw is seated into the sacral ala. A third, but less frequently utilized approach involves placing screws into the second sacral vertebra.

In this chapter, we will first review the relevant sacral anatomy that should be considered when placing sacral instrumentation. The different techniques will then be compared with regard to important factors that influence the biomechanical strength of sacral screw fixation, including bone density, cortical fixation, and screw length. Finally, standard screw entry sites and trajectories that maximize safety and screw fixation will be described. Although fixation into the ilium (discussed elsewhere) has become much more common in recent years, techniques for sacral fixation still play an important role in the treatment of traumatic and degenerative conditions of the lumbosacral spine .

29.2 Relevant Anatomy

The sacrum (Fig. 29.1) consists of five vertebrae in a kyphotic configuration that functions as a keystone, transferring force from the spine through the sacroiliac joints into the pelvis. Superiorly, the first two vertebrae are comparable in size to lumbar vertebrae while the lower three vertebrae are progressively smaller. The sacral promontory is the ventral and cephalad aspect of the S1 body that protrudes into the pelvis. The S1 vertebra articulates with the fifth lumbar vertebra by two zygapophyseal (facet) joints and an intervertebral disc. Contiguous transverse processes laterally form the sacral ala, or wings, which articulate with the pelvis and form the sacroiliac joints. Four paired neuroforamina on both the dorsal and ventral surfaces allow passage of the corresponding rami. The dorsal surface of the sacrum has a

V.V. Patel et al. (eds.), *Spine Trauma*,
DOI: 10.1007/978-3-642-03694-1_29, © Springer-Verlag Berlin Heidelberg 2010

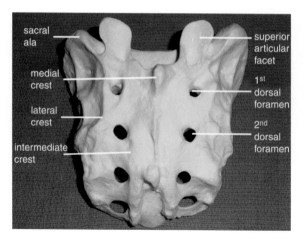

Fig. 29.1 Photograph of the dorsum of the sacrum showing standard bony landmarks often used for the placement of sacral screws

median crest from the remnant spinous processes, and the fused articular processes form a pair of intermediate crests between the median crest and foramina.

Critical anatomic structures lie directly on the ventral surface of the sacrum and can be at risk of injury when screws penetrate the anterior cortex. Anterior to L5, S1, and S2 are the common iliac arteries and veins, internal iliac arteries and veins, elements of the lumbosacral plexus, and retrosigmoid colon [21]. Other structures on the ventral surface of the sacrum include the sympathetic trunk and middle sacral artery and vein [8].

29.3 Bone Mineral Density

Bone quality is one of the most critical factors for obtaining strong screw fixation [30]. Bone mineral density (BMD) in the sacrum measured by quantitative computed tomography (CT) directly correlates with screw insertional torque [25, 28]. Increased sacral BMD also correlates with increased maximal load tolerated by screws and reduced compliance (increased stiffness) [25].

The authors of several studies have carefully evaluated the BMD of the sacrum and consistently found that the sacral ala has a diminished density compared with other portions of the sacrum. In a CT and microscopic evaluation of the sacrum, Peretz et al. [23] found that trabecular bone was densest near the endplates and lacking in the ala, which they termed an "alar void." Zheng et al. [28] found

that the mean BMD of the sacrum measured by quantitative CT in a young population (mean age of 31 years) was 382 mg/cm^3 in the sacral body, which was 32% higher than in the ala. The superior sacral endplate had the highest BMD. Likewise, Smith et al. [25] measured the BMD of the sacrum by quantitative CT in an older population (mean age of 74 years) and found the centrum (130 mg/cm^3) to be 60% more dense than the ala. The substantial diminution of BMD in an older population (382 mg/cm^3– 130 mg/cm^3) is noteworthy.

29.4 Cortical Fixation

It is generally accepted that increased cortical purchase improves screw fixation [9, 20, 21, 24, 29]. Screws placed deep enough to engage both the posterior and anterior cortex of a vertebral body have significantly greater pull-out force than screws that penetrate the posterior cortex alone [29]. In the sacrum, the need for bicortical cortical screw purchase may be of particular importance because the sacral pedicle is formed by a confluence of cancellous bone, and thus, there is not a true cortical ring for a screw to engage as in thoracic and lumbar pedicles [24]. The value of additional cortical bone–screw interface was demonstrated by Lehman et al. [16], who described a tricortical technique via an anteromedial trajectory, in which screws directed at the apex of the sacral promontory were able to penetrate the cortex of the superior endplate of S1 along with the posterior and anterior cortex. Tricortical screws were found to have 99% greater insertional torque than standard bicortical screws that parallel the superior endplate.

Unicortical screw placement appears to be less biomechanically robust but has the advantage of not placing critical structures at risk. The concept of safe zones on the ventral surface of the sacrum, where the risk of injury to adjacent structures is minimized, has been advocated by several authors [9, 17, 21]. The medial safe zone, where bicortical anterolateral screws protrude through the anterior cortex of the sacrum, is larger than the lateral safe zone associated with anterolateral screw placement. As such, anteromedial screws are considered safer.

Anatomic cadaver studies have shown that the use of bicortical anteromedial screws is most likely to place the middle sacral artery and vein, sympathetic trunk, and common iliac vein at risk [8, 17]. Anterolateral screws place the lumbosacral trunk and internal iliac vein at risk of injury [17, 21]. Bicortical anterolateral screws placed parallel to the S1 endplate and 30° laterally do not touch structures on the ventral surface of the sacrum 53% of the time, whereas screws placed 45° laterally avoid contact only 27% of the time [21]. Thus, although a more lateral trajectory increases the potential length of the screw insertion (see below), the risk of complication when the anterior cortex is perforated likely increases as well. S2 pedicle screws also have the potential to injure neurovascular structures including the middle sacral artery and vein, sacral sympathetic trunk, and lateral sacral vein [21].

29.5 Screw Length

The concept that longer screw length corresponds with stronger screw fixation is both intuitive and borne out by biomechanical studies. In a study using fresh human lumbosacral vertebrae, Zindrick et al. [30] demonstrated that screws inserted all the way to the anterior cortex required 91% more loading cycles in the medial–lateral direction prior to loosening than screws placed to only 50% depth. The number of loading cycles increased over 1,000% when loading of the deeper screws was performed in a cephalad–caudad direction. Screws that were inserted though the anterior cortex had an additional 194% increase in cyclical loading strength. Similarly, Krag et al. [14] found that vertebral screw fixation was significantly improved when screws were inserted to 80% of the available depth compared with 50% depth for both "cut-out"/twisting and "cut-up"/extension loads.

These findings pertain to sacral screws because an anteromedial path through the pedicle traverses a mean length of 49.7 mm (in male patients), whereas an anterolateral course into the ala with the screw at a 25° lateral angle traverses only 38.3 mm [3]. Further increasing the lateral angle of an anterolateral screw can increase the length it traverses. For example, the mean length of a bicortical alar screw placed at a 30° lateral trajectory (38 mm) was 6 mm shorter than the mean length of a screw placed at a 45° trajectory (44 mm) [21]. The lengths of the typical S2 transpedicular and lateral mass screws are only 25.2 mm and 32.8 mm, respectively [7].

29.6 Biomechanical Comparisons

Given the advantages of an anteromedial trajectory for sacral screw placement over an anterolateral trajectory with respect to BMD and screw length, anteromedially placed screws would be expected to be biomechanically superior, and this has generally been corroborated by studies. In load-to-failure tests comparing anteromedially and anterolaterally placed screws in the sacrum, anterolateral screws withstood 23% [5] and 24% [25] less force than their anteromedial counterparts, which were statistically significant differences. Anteromedial placement also appears to decrease compliance (improve stiffness) [25].

Not all authors have concluded that anteromedial screw placement is superior to anterolateral screw placement, though. Zindrick et al. [30] compared the pull-out force of screws placed with a 45° lateral trajectory into the ala, a straight trajectory into the ala, a medial trajectory through the S1 pedicle, or a medial trajectory through the S2 pedicle. The mean pull-out force for the 45° alar screws (1007 N) was highest, followed by that of the S1 pedicle screws (870 N), straight alar screws (668 N), and S2 pedicle screws (185). The S2 pedicle screws were significantly inferior to all of the others. The difference between the 45° alar and S1 pedicle screws was not reported to be significantly different. The clinical relevance of these results by Zindrick et al. [30] has been called into question, however, since the pull-out test was done with tension loading along the screw axis whereas in vivo loading occurs perpendicular to the screw axis [5].

29.7 Technique of Screw Placement

29.7.1 Anteromedial (Pedicle) S1 Screw

Most techniques for placing screws in the first sacral vertebra anteromedially through the pedicle describe the starting point in relation to the inferior aspect of the superior S1 facet. Usually, the posterior cortex is penetrated lateral to the inferior aspect of the facet, with a more lateral entry point necessitating a more medial trajectory. Smith et al. [25] and Carlson et al. [5] described the same technique, starting at a point 2 mm lateral to the inferior aspect of the facet and then

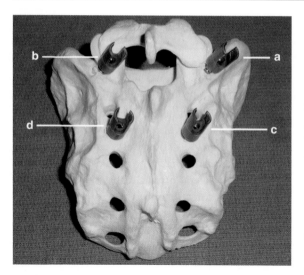

Fig. 29.2 Photograph demonstrating the dorsal entry points for sacral screws. (**a**) S1 anteromedial screw started 2 mm lateral to the base of the superior articular facet. (**b**) S1 anterolateral screw started at the base of the superior articular facet. This entry point may be moved inferiorly and slightly medially for an even longer screw trajectory. (**c**) S2 pedicle screw started midway between the first and second sacral foramina. (**d**) S2 pedicle screws also started midway between the first and second sacral foramina

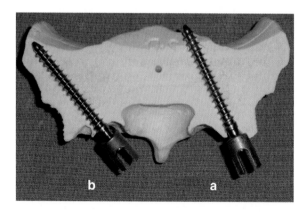

Fig. 29.3 Photograph demonstrating axial trajectories of S1 screws. (**a**) S1 anteromedial screw angled 30° medially. (**b**) S1 anterolateral screw angled 40° laterally

angling the screw 30° anteromedially along the axial plane and about 20° anterocaudally along the sagittal plane to parallel the endplate (Figs. 29.2a and 29.3a).

There are many variations to this standard technique. As previously noted, Lehman et al. [16] proposed a trajectory in the sagittal plane directly toward the apex of the sacral promontory to obtain tricortical screw fixation, which resulted in a 99% increase in insertional torque. Luk et al. [19] described an even

more cephalad trajectory in the sagittal plane, with the screw piercing the superior endplate of S1. This technique has the biomechanical advantages of traversing the thicker trabecular bone adjacent to the S1 endplate and achieving bicortical fixation while minimizing the risk to neurovascular structure anterior to the sacrum. According to the authors [19], in vitro mean pull-out force and cyclic loading were significantly improved with this technique compared with screws placed in a standard fashion parallel to the superior S1 endplate.

29.7.2 Anterolateral (Alar) S1 Screw

Even more variations exist for placing sacral alar screws. The starting point can be the same as for a pedicle screw, at the base of the facet, or even inferiorly and medially to the facet joint (Fig. 29.2b) [5, 13, 21, 25]. As with pedicle screws, the trajectory should be oriented cranially toward the S1 endplate. The lateral angulation in the axial plane can vary greatly, ranging somewhere between 25° and 45°, with 30° being common (Fig. 29.3b) [3, 5, 12, 21, 25]. A more medial or inferior starting point should be complemented with a more angulated trajectory. When placing alar screws, the anterior cortex of the sacrum should be engaged with the tip of the screw to provide bicortical fixation and improve pull-out strength.

29.7.3 S2 Screws

Screws placed into the second sacral vertebrae are started between the first and second dorsal foramina, either at the midpoint or slightly rostral (Fig. 29.2c, d) [7, 8, 21]. A transpedicular approach can be attained by simply choosing a trajectory perpendicular to the dorsal sacral surface [8] or directing the screw medially up to 30°, in which case a mean screw length of 25.2 mm can be used (Fig. 29.4a) [7]. A lateral mass screw can be placed with a lateral trajectory of 22°, allowing a mean screw length of up to 32.8 mm (Fig. 29.4b) [7]. Because of the variability in dimensions of the second sacral vertebra, preoperative measurements to determine proper screw lengths should be considered. Because of the relatively short length of screws placed in S2 and the substantially lower pull-out

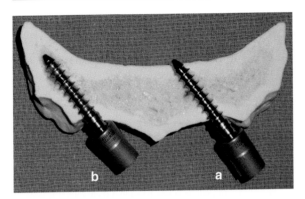

Fig. 29.4 Photograph demonstrating axial trajectories of S2 screws. (**a**) S2 pedicle screws can be placed perpendicular to the dorsal surface of the sacrum or angled medially up to 30° on average. (**b**) Lateral mass screws are placed with a mean lateral angulation of 22°. The angulation of S2 screws can vary greatly because of anatomical variability

strength, S2 screws alone are not deemed adequate for sacral fixation.

29.8 Choice of Technique

Anteromedial screw placement into the first sacral vertebra has become the preferred method by most spine surgeons given the relative ease, safety, and biomechanical superiority of the technique. However, in some clinical situations a surgeon may still rely on anterolateral screws into the ala for sacral fixation. Various pathologic processes, such as discitis or metastasis, may compromise the integrity of the sacral promontory and centrum, rendering an anteromedial trajectory insufficient (Fig. 29.5). In this circumstance, alar screws provide an alternative.

The question of whether to place screws through the anterior cortex to achieve stronger fixation at the risk of neurovascular injury needs to be addressed on a case-by-case basis. If a patient has osteopenic bone or if a longer fusion is being performed, then the added risk assumed with additional cortical purchase is justified. While stand-alone S2 screws are generally not considered an adequate alterative to S1 screws given their short length and poor biomechanical strength, they can be used to supplement S1 screws and further protect the S1 screws from pulling out of the sacrum [20].

Iliac screw fixation has evolved from the Galveston technique [1, 2] of inserting contoured rods directly into the ilium as an alternative to sacral screw fixation because of the high failure rate of sacral screws [4]. Low pseudarthrosis rates have been reported with the use of iliac fixation for long fusions to the sacrum [15]. However, a retrospective study comparing sacral-only fixation and iliac fixation for long fusion constructs from S1 to at least T10 found no difference in pseudarthrosis rates between the two groups at a minimum of 5-year follow-up [27]. Iliac implants have additional comorbidity because of the extensive exposure required, leading to a potential increase of blood loss or infection [22]. Iliac implants can also be quite prominent and cause discomfort, leading to removal in 26% of cases in one series [27]. The technique for iliac fixation and the indications for its use are discussed elsewhere in this textbook.

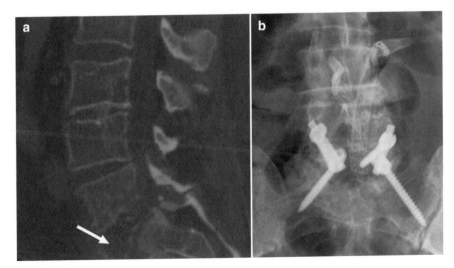

Fig. 29.5 Sagittal computed tomography (CT) image demonstrating sacral promontory destruction (*arrow*) in a case of discitis (**a**) requiring alar screw fixation (**b**) for lumbosacral arthrodesis

29.9 Conclusions

Successful sacral screw fixation has proven to be difficult because of the high biomechanical demands placed on the instrumentation and the challenging anatomy of the sacrum. The quality of bone, purchase of cortical bone, and screw length all influence the strength of a construct. The added fixation afforded with bicortical placement of screws must be balanced with the added risk of neurovascular injury. Anteromedial (pedicle) S1 screws are generally the best option because of their relative safety and strength, as determined by load-to-failure studies; however, anterolateral (alar) S1 screws offer a viable alternative when S1 pedicle screws are not feasible. S2 screws are usually insufficient by themselves but can be used to supplement S1 screws when additional fixation is deemed necessary.

References

1. Allen BL Jr, Ferguson RL (1988) A 1988 perspective on the Galveston technique of pelvic fixation. Orthop Clin North Am 19:409–418
2. Allen BL Jr, Ferguson RL (1988) The Galveston experience with L-rod instrumentation for adolescent idiopathic scoliosis. Clin Orthop Relat Res 229:59–69
3. Asher MA, Strippgen WE (1986) Anthropometric studies of the human sacrum relating to dorsal transsacral implant designs. Clin Orthop Relat Res 203:58–62
4. Camp JF, Caudle R, Ashmun RD et al (1990) Immediate complications of Cotrel-Dubousset instrumentation to the sacro-pelvis. A clinical and biomechanical study. Spine 15:932–941
5. Carlson GD, Abitbol JJ, Anderson DR et al (1992) Screw fixation in the human sacrum. An in vitro study of the biomechanics of fixation. Spine 17:S196–S203
6. Devlin VJ, Boachie-Adjei O, Bradford DS et al (1991) Treatment of adult spinal deformity with fusion to the sacrum using CD instrumentation. J Spinal Disord 4:1–14
7. Ebraheim NA, Lu J, Yang H et al (1997) Anatomic considerations of the second sacral vertebra and dorsal screw placement. Surg Radiol Anat 19:353–357
8. Ergur I, Akcali O, Kiray A et al (2007) Neurovascular risks of sacral screws with bicortical purchase: an anatomical study. Eur Spine J 16:1519–1523
9. Esses SI, Botsford DJ, Huler RJ et al (1991) Surgical anatomy of the sacrum. A guide for rational screw fixation. Spine 16:S283–S288
10. Grobler LJ, Frymoyer JW, Robertson PA et al (1993) Biomechanics of the lumbar spine. Semin Spine Surg 5:59–72
11. Harrington PR, Dickson JH (1976) Spinal instrumentation in the treatment of severe progressive spondylolisthesis. Clin Orthop Relat Res 117:157–163
12. Kostuik JP, Errico TJ, Gleason TF (1986) Techniques of internal fixation for degenerative conditions of the lumbar spine. Clin Orthop Relat Res 203:219–231
13. Kostuik JP, Hall BB (1983) Spinal fusions to the sacrum in adults with scoliosis. Spine 8:489–500
14. Krag MH, Beynnon BD, Pope MH et al (1988) Depth of insertion of transpedicular vertebral screws into human vertebrae: effect upon screw-vertebra interface strength. J Spinal Disord 1:287–294
15. Kuklo TR, Bridwell KH, Lewis SJ et al (2001) Minimum 2-year analysis of sacropelvic fixation and L5-S1 fusion using S1 and iliac screws. Spine 26:1976–1983
16. Lehman RA Jr, Kuklo TR, Belmont PJ Jr et al (2002) Advantage of pedicle screw fixation directed into the apex of the sacral promontory over bicortical fixation: a biomechanical analysis. Spine 27:806–811
17. Licht NJ, Rowe DE, Ross LM (1992) Pitfalls of pedicle screw fixation in the sacrum. A cadaver model. Spine 17:892–896
18. Louis R (1986) Fusion of the lumbar and sacral spine by internal fixation with screw plates. Clin Orthop Relat Res 203:18–33
19. Luk KD, Chen L, Lu WW (2005) A stronger bicortical sacral pedicle screw fixation through the s1 endplate: an in vitro cyclic loading and pull-out force evaluation. Spine 30:525–529
20. McCord DH, Cunningham BW, Shono Y et al (1992) Biomechanical analysis of lumbosacral fixation. Spine 17: S235–S243
21. Mirkovic S, Abitbol JJ, Steinman J et al (1991) Anatomic consideration for sacral screw placement. Spine 16:S289–S294
22. Moshirfar A, Rand FF, Sponseller PD et al (2005) Pelvic fixation in spine surgery. Historical overview, indications, biomechanical relevance, and current techniques. J Bone Joint Surg Am 87(suppl 2):89–106
23. Peretz AM, Hipp JA, Heggeness MH (1998) The internal bony architecture of the sacrum. Spine 23:971–974
24. Robertson PA, Plank LD (1999) Pedicle screw placement at the sacrum: anatomical characterization and limitations at S1. J Spinal Disord 12:227–233
25. Smith SA, Abitbol JJ, Carlson GD et al (1993) The effects of depth of penetration, screw orientation, and bone density on sacral screw fixation. Spine 18:1006–1010
26. Steffee AD, Biscup RS, Sitkowski DJ (1986) Segmental spine plates with pedicle screw fixation. A new internal fixation device for disorders of the lumbar and thoracolumbar spine. Clin Orthop Relat Res (203):45–53
27. Weistroffer JK, Perra JH, Lonstein JE et al (2008) Complications in long fusions to the sacrum for adult scoliosis: minimum five-year analysis of fifty patients. Spine 33:1478–1483
28. Zheng Y, Lu WW, Zhu Q et al (2000) Variation in bone mineral density of the sacrum in young adults and its significance for sacral fixation. Spine 25:353–357
29. Zindrick MR, Wiltse LL, Doornik A et al (1987) Analysis of the morphometric characteristics of the thoracic and lumbar pedicles. Spine 12:160–166
30. Zindrick MR, Wiltse LL, Widell EH et al (1986) A biomechanical study of intrapeduncular screw fixation in the lumbosacral spine. Clin Orthop Relat Res 203:99–112

Percutaneous Placement of Iliosacral Screws

30

John C. France

30.1 Case Example

This is the case of a 46-year-old male who fell 20 ft from a roof while putting up Christmas lights and landed on the driveway, partially striking a car on the way. He suffered numerous injuries including a pelvic "U" fracture or spinopelvic dissociation. The fracture involved the pedicle on the right at L5 as the plane of injury extended up from the sacral ala and into the spine creating a combined lumbar spine and pelvic fracture (Fig. 30.1). This typical pattern benefits from a combined posterior approach to address the spinal and pelvic components. The spine is fixed to the pelvis with lumbosacral fixation (this construct included L4 to span the right pedicle fracture at L5) including iliac wing screws and the fixation between the iliac wings and the sacral vertebrae is reinforced with iliosacral screws placed percutaneously (Fig. 30.2).

30.2 Background

The use of iliosacral screws originated and has traditionally fallen within the realm of the musculoskeletal trauma surgeon. Because sacroiliac joint pain is often in the differential of causes of low back pain, the spine surgeon usually sees these groups of patients. Although

the debate about the true incidence and contribution of the sacroiliac joint to back pain roars on, there is enough evidence to believe that it plays a role in some patients. In the patient recalcitrant to nonoperative measures a computed tomography (CT)-guided injection can be used therapeutically and diagnostically by combining a corticosteroid with a long-acting analgesic such as bupivacaine. This author prefers CT guidance to fluoroscopic to maximize the accuracy of needle placement and verify exact location. It is most important to be certain that the needle was in the exact location in patients who fail to benefit. In those patients who experience 100% relief temporarily but no lasting benefit on two separate occasions, one can have reasonable confidence that the pain source has been identified and consider a sacroiliac fusion. Thus, the spine surgeon plays an integral role in evaluation and is often the one to perform the fusion if warranted and needs to be familiar with the technique of iliosacral screws as a means of fixation.

In addition, more complex pelvis fractures can extend through the L5–S1 facet and include a facet dislocation. The pelvic H-fracture or spondylopelvic dissociation is another example of combined spine and pelvic pathology where the lumbar spine and upper sacrum are essentially torn free from the pelvic ring (Fig. 30.3). Under these circumstances, the spine may require stabilization in conjunction with the pelvis. This type of procedure may fall solely under the realm of the spine surgeon or be performed in conjunction with the trauma surgeon depending on the circumstances such as training and level of comfort with the necessary techniques such as iliosacral screw fixation.

J.C. France
Department of Orthopaedic Surgery, West Virginia University,
P.O. Box 9196, Morgantown, WV 26542, USA
e-mail: jfrance@hsc.wvu.edu

V.V. Patel et al. (eds.), *Spine Trauma*,
DOI: 10.1007/978-3-642-03694-1_30, © Springer-Verlag Berlin Heidelberg 2010

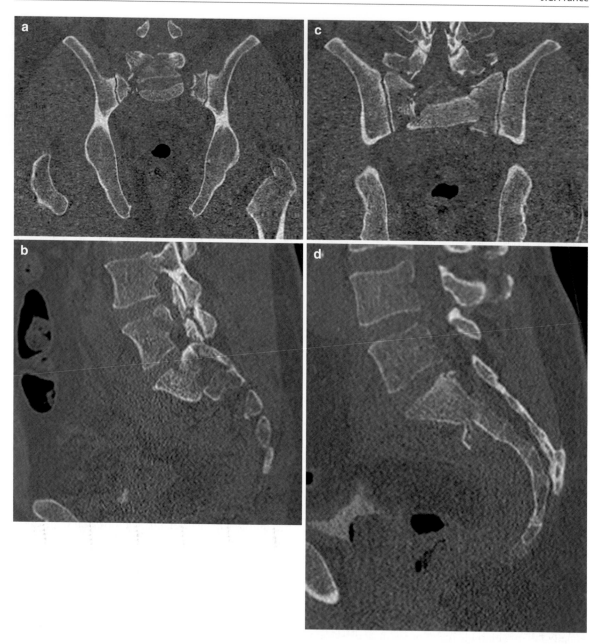

Fig. 30.1 (**a**) Computed tomography (CT) coronal reconstruction showing the right L5 pedicle fracture at the base and one can see how this plane of injury extends up from the sacral ala fracture, and in (**b**) a sagittal reconstruction of the same injury. The coronal in (**c**) demonstrates the bilateral sacral fractures in zone 2 on the *right* and zone 1 on the *left*, and (**d**) is a sagittal of the transverse sacral component through zone 3. The two parallel vertical fracture and one transverse sacral fracture combine into the "U" fracture pattern allowing the spine to separate from the pelvic ring and displace anteriorly

30.3 Indications and Advantages for Procedure Contraindications and Disadvantages for Procedure

Iliosacral screws are generally utilized in the setting of pelvic fractures to address the posterior component.

This can be a sacroiliac dislocation or involve fracture through the sacrum. Some fractures through the sacrum extend into the L5–S1 facet and may be associated with a facet dislocation (Fig. 30.4). In these instances the hemipelvis is typically translated posterior and superiorly, and the reduction can be achieved with the patient prone and via a midline posterior spine

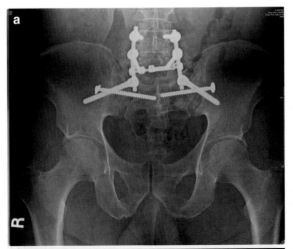

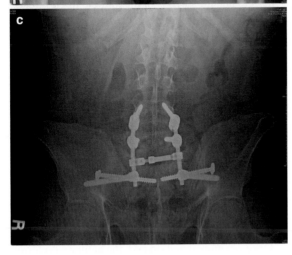

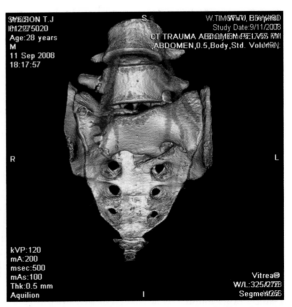

Fig. 30.3 A three-dimensional reconstruction of a lumbosacral spine showing a "U" type fracture of the sacrum with right sacral ala fracture extending transversely across the sacral vertebral bodies and into the left sacroiliac joint essentially breaking the spine free from the pelvic ring

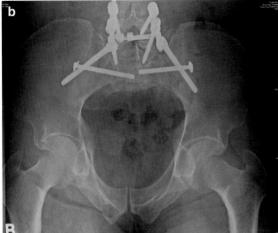

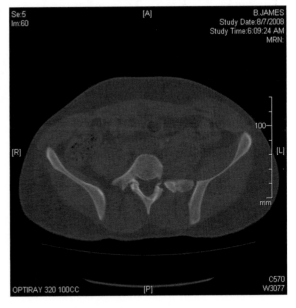

Fig. 30.4 An axial CT of the pelvis at the lumbosacral junction demonstrating a dislocation of the left L5–S1 joint as part of a hemipelvis fracture. The pattern is best handled posteriorly to aid in reduction and fixation can then extend into the lumbar spine to fix both the spine and pelvic components

Fig. 30.2 The postoperative fixation with screws at L4 and L5 connecting to iliac wing screws and bilateral percutaneous iliosacral screws is shown in an AP (**a**), inlet (**b**), and outlet (**c**) views

approach, which may involve the spine surgeon. One effective fixation technique utilizes lumbar pedicle screws and iliac wing screws. The fixation can be supplemented with percutaneous iliosacral screws as in the above case example. These are typically very unstable pelvic fractures and adding iliosacral screws offers another direction of fixation improving the stability without having to reposition or redrape the patient. If an adequate reduction cannot be accomplished then iliosacral screws are relatively contraindicated because the distorted anatomy potentially puts the neural elements into the path of the screw.

Sacroiliac fusion can also be accomplished using iliosacral screws. This can be done easily with the patient prone to allow access for direct exposure of the joint and percutaneous screw placement. Compression across the joint helps to create stability and aids in gaining bony union.

30.4 Procedure

30.4.1 Equipment Needed

If one is treating a sacroiliac fracture that extends through the L5–S1 junction as in the case example, then standard spine instrumentation is needed. For the iliosacral screw insertion, large cannulated screws are used, typically 7.0 or 7.3 mm in diameter. If compression is desired then partially threaded screws are used. If compression is to be avoided then a fully threaded screw is used. This is covered in more detail later in the technique.

30.4.2 Anesthetic and Neuromonitoring Considerations

If reduction of the hemipelvis is necessary then muscle relaxation is beneficial. Because the pelvis has a complex three-dimensional anatomy and air or stool in the colon can impede visualization, the surrounding neural elements are at risk. A bowel prep can be considered especially in the trauma setting where they may received a CT scan with bowel contrast that would markedly impair visualization. Also during reduction the roots can become entrapped. Thus,

neuromonitoring specifically to assess L5, S1, and lower sacral root function is prudent. A Foley catheter is used to drain the bladder to improve imaging.

30.4.3 Patient Positioning and Room Setup

The patient can be positioned either prone or supine. This can be based on surgeon preference or may be dictated by the circumstances that warrant the placement of an iliosacral screw. For example, if the patient has a pelvic fracture and an external fixator frame is being used then it would be easier to position the patient supine. If the patient has a sacroiliac fracture dislocation and associated L5–S1 facet dislocation then prone positioning would allow the surgeon to address the spine component and the sacroiliac screw simultaneously.

Prone: C-arm excursion is important and requires enough room under the table to tilt the arm into inlet and outlet views so the operating room table must be radiolucent over a wide area. The Jackson frame is ideal for C-arm access and the spine positioning pads work well. The prep should include the buttock and anteriorly as far as the hip/thigh pads will allow.

Supine: A folded blanket or towel can be placed under the patient's pelvis in the midline to elevate the patient off the table, which improves the access to the lateral aspect of the buttock. The prep should be done as posterior as the table will allow to assure inclusion of the starting point. Criteria for C-arm access are similar to prone positioning and the Jackson flat top again is ideal.

30.4.4 Surgical Approach, Reduction Technique, and Fixation Technique

Step 1: Lateral C-arm

Once positioned and draped, the author's preferred starting position is with the C-arm in lateral. The first step is to manipulate the fluoroscopy unit into a "true" lateral image (Fig. 30.5). The true lateral is determined by aligning the sciatic notches and hip joints in perfect parallel. This finding gives a lateral image of the sacrum. Because the sacrum is aligned obliquely to the floor, one can easily get confused on the anterior–posterior and caudal–cephalad planes, which makes it difficult to direct the guide pin and screw. The anterior–posterior (Fig. 30.6b) and cephalad–caudal (Fig. 30.6a) planes of the sacrum can be marked on the exterior of the patient to be used as a reference

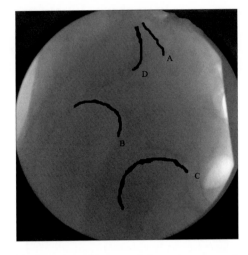

Fig. 30.5 A true lateral fluoroscopic image is necessary to accurately assess the anatomic landmarks. *Line A* is the superior S1 endplate and should be perpendicular to the image beam. *Line B* is the sciatic notches perfectly overlapped and *line C* is the acetabulum perfectly overlapped. Lastly, *line D* shows the sacral ala, which is important to identify in order to avoid the L5 nerve root

throughout the remainder of the procedure (Fig. 30.6c). Lastly, the anterior edge of the sacral ala should be noted.

While the C-arm is in the lateral position the starting point can be identified (Fig. 30.7a). The anticipated direction in the axial plane runs from posterior to anterior; thus, the starting point on the lateral image appears to be in the central canal and can be planned from the preoperative CT scan of the pelvis (Fig. 30.7b). The guide pin is inserted through a small stab down to contact with the bone. The insertion stab can be widened around the guide pin to accommodate the working cannulas after the site has been radiographically verified as the proper site. By doing this, the insertion site can easily be revised without creating a large incision.

Step 2: Inlet and outlet images

Once the guide pin is positioned on the lateral image, it is held firmly against the bone and the C-arm is rotated into the inlet and outlet views. The starting point can be reviewed and then the direction of insertion can be completed. The *inlet view* (Fig. 30.8) is obtained by tilting the C-arm approximately in line with the cephalad–caudal line drawn on the patient and is used to direct the anterior–posterior direction of the guide pin. A clear picture of the anterior border of the S1 vertebral body, the spinal canal, and the anterior edge of the sacral ala housing the L5 root must be

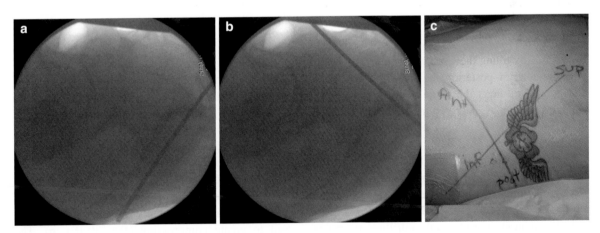

Fig. 30.6 The lateral image can be used to set up the C-arm angles for the inlet and outlet views and to help the surgeon understand the anterior–posterior and cephalad–caudal directions while working under the image. (**a**) Lateral sacral view with a Steinmann pin oriented along the cephalad–caudal direction of the sacrum, this line can translated onto the skin (**c**). Movement along that line guides cephalad–caudal adjustments and when the image beam is parallel to the same line it is in the inlet view. (**b**) The Steinmann pin oriented in the anterior–posterior direction to guide adjustments (**c** this line translated onto the skin) and when the beam of the image is parallel to this line it is in the outlet view

Fig. 30.7 The starting point on the lateral image should appear posterior in the canal (**a**) since the direction of the screw should run posterior to anterior as can be seen on the uninjured side of the pelvis in axial CT scan in (**b**)

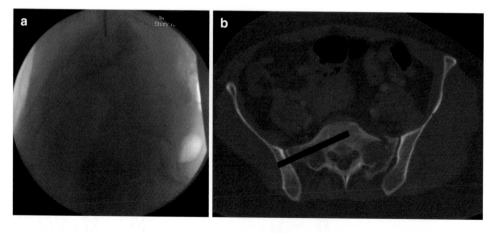

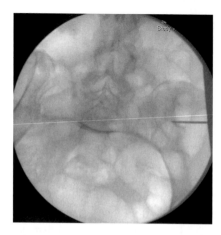

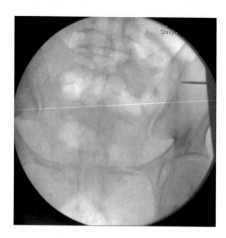

Fig. 30.8 The inlet view should provide a good view of the S1 vertebral body and anterior border of the sacral ala, to avoid the canal posteriorly and the L5 root anteriorly

Fig. 30.9 The outlet view should provide a tangential view across the superior endplate of S1 and the S1 neuroforamin should be well seen to avoid the corresponding nerve root

obtained to minimize risk. The *outlet view* (Fig. 30.9) is obtained by tilting the C-arm approximately in line with the anterior–posterior line drawn on the patient and is used to direct the guide pin in the cephalad–caudal direction. A clear picture of the S1 foramina and L5–S1 disc must be obtained to minimize risk of injuries in this view.

By working back and forth between the inlet and outlet views the guide pin can be gradually passed through the ilium, across the sacroiliac joint, and into the body of the S1 vertebrae. The type of screw selected will determine if the path requires drilling or tapping, or is a self-drilling or self-tapping screw.

Step 3: The screw

The author prefers a cannulated 7.3 mm screw that is self-drilling and self-tapping to eliminate steps,

others use a 7.0 mm screw that requires drilling and tapping with a noncutting screw tip, but the latter has a smaller diameter guide wire that is more challenging to direct. If there is a fracture through the sacral foramina then one must avoid compression across the fracture that may close the foramina and injure the sacral roots. Similarly, compression should be avoided in a comminuted alar fracture that would contribute to shortening the alar wing. When the prior two circumstances are present a fully threaded screw should be used, otherwise a partially threaded screw can be used to create compression (Fig. 30.10a, b). The author prefers to use a washer to prevent the screw head from penetrating the outer cortex of the iliac wing and to aid the compression force. In addition, as the screw is nearing full insertion the C-arm can be rotated more in-line with the iliac wing to better

Fig. 30.10 (**a**) Shows the inlet view with a fully threaded screw. (**b**) Shows an outlet view

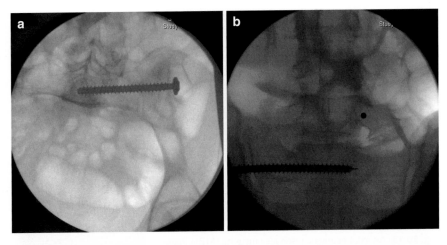

Fig. 30.11 The view can be used to verify that the screw is fully seated with the washer against the lateral ilium. It is an inlet/obturator oblique view (rotate the C-arm about 45° off AP, while in the inlet position). (**a**) Shows the screw short of being seated with the washer loose. (**b**) Shows the screw fully seated with the washer tight against the lateral cortex of the iliac wing

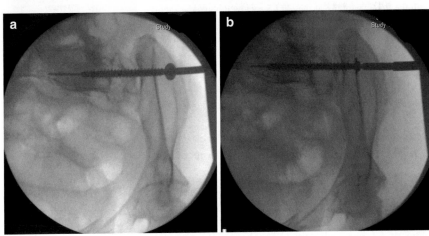

visualize the outer cortex of the iliac wing and the surgeon will see the washer touch the cortex and realign itself flat against the cortex as it is tightened (Fig. 30.11a, b). This appearance resembles an obturator oblique view.

If additional stability is needed a second screw can be inserted. This can sometimes be done at the S1 body level but at times is done at the S2 body level (Fig. 30.12).

30.5 Complications and Postoperative Considerations

The most common significant complication associated with this technique is neurological injury. The L5 nerve is most vulnerable if a screw is directed too anterior since it lays on the anterior surface of the sacral ala (Fig. 30.13). In patients with typical anatomy the

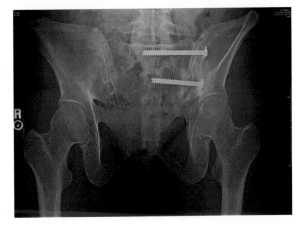

Fig. 30.12 An outlet view of two iliosacral screws, one at S1 and the other at S2

anterior surface of the ala can be well visualized on the inlet view (also the lateral can be useful), but there are many anatomic variants that include sacralization of

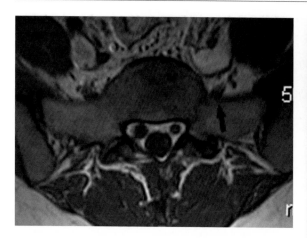

Fig. 30.13 An axial magnetic resonance imaging (MRI) image with the *arrow* pointing at the *left* L5 root as it abuts the sacral ala making it vulnerable to injury if an iliosacral screw is inadvertently directed too anterior

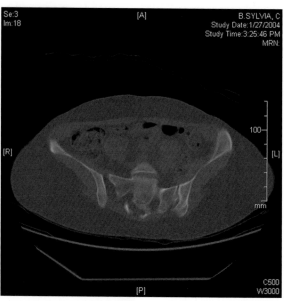

Fig. 30.14 An axial CT of an anomalous sacrum with the anterior surface of the *left* ala more posterior than the anterior surface of the *right* ala. This can be difficult to appreciate on intraoperative fluoroscopy and creates a shallow "safe zone" for passage of the screw

the L5 vertebrae and lumbarization of the S1 vertebrae. Additionally some people have a deeper groove for the ala that narrows the "safe zone" (Fig. 30.14) for screw insertion. Careful inspection of the preoperative CT images can allow the surgeon to recognize these anomalies and minimize risk. The S1 root is vulnerable within the anterior foramen. The outlet view is used to define the S1 foramen. Typically, the C-arm is tilted on the outlet view to make the superior endplate of S1 perpendicular to the beam. But, the S1 foramen may run anterior–inferior to posterior–superior relative to that end plate so it is useful to adjust the tilt into slightly more "outlet" to get a more tangential view through the S1 foramen. The more caudal sacral roots can be injured if the screw is directed too posterior and enters the central canal. The L5, S1, and lower sacral roots are not only vulnerable to screw misdirection but can be injured during reduction when entrapped within an alar fracture and if the fracture extends through the sacral foramen or central canal. When these circumstances are present, a fully threaded screw would be utilized to prevent compression. Because intraoperative fluoroscopy has limited visualization, it is a good idea to obtain a postoperative CT scan to accurately evaluate the screw positions. Once recognized, the offending screw can be removed and replaced or redirected if the degree of neurological compromise warrants.

The potential for bowel or vascular injury is rare but exists if a screw is directed too anterior or if the guide

wire is inadvertently advanced while passing the drill, tap, or screw. Thus, frequent fluoroscopic images should be obtained during these steps to recognize this problem and the postoperative CT scan will identify any screw that is excessively long. Some injury could go unrecognized so one must remain vigilant and aware of potential intra-operative while the patient convalesces.

In more severely displaced fractures loss of fixation can occur as the posterior pelvis rotates around the screw or is angulated. This can be minimized with the addition of a second posterior screw and other means to control the anterior pelvis such as plating and external fixation (Fig. 30.15).

Over time many sacroiliac joints will autofuse if the injury is through the joint. When fusion fails to occur, screw loosening or breakage can occur over time. This does not typically pose a problem since the pelvis has usually become stable prior to breakage. In circumstances where sacroiliac fusion is the primary purpose of the procedure the cleaning the cartilage and fibrous tissue from the joint, then packing bone graft is important to avoid a nonunion and screw breakage or loosening (Fig. 30.16).

There is no need for external bracing. The weight-bearing status is more dependent on the pathology

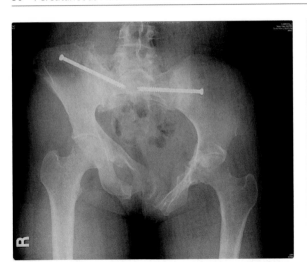

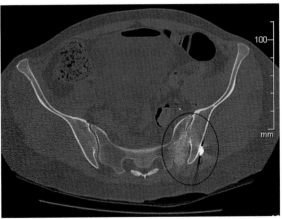

Fig. 30.16 An axial CT with a circle around the bone graft impacted into the sacroiliac joint for fusion

Fig. 30.15 This is an AP pelvis of a 25-year-old female who initially had an unstable pelvic fracture treated with bilateral iliosacral screws and an anterior external fixator frame. Her injury was further complicated by the fact that she had delivered a baby 6 weeks earlier and had lax ligamentous support for her pelvis. Despite an anatomic reduction, initially her hemipelvis continued to rotate and displace. A second iliosacral screw may have better controlled these rotational forces

being treated. For a highly unstable pelvic fracture, touch down weight bearing for 6–12 weeks is recommended. For intrinsically stable condition such as sacroiliac fusion for arthrosis, which will maintain that stability postoperatively, weight bearing as tolerated is used, often with ambulatory aids for 6 weeks as a reminder to the patient to minimize the rotational and axial loads across the joint. The healing across the sacroiliac joint can be followed with specific sacroiliac views (essentially an obturator oblique view) to look directly through the joint, and the overall pelvic alignment is evaluated with Antero Posterior (AP), inlet, and outlet pelvic radiographs. If a better view of the actual fusion integrity is required after 6 months then CT scanning is the modality of choice.

Iliac Fixation in Trauma

31

Robert Morgan

31.1 Introduction

Iliac fixation for spinal constructs has been utilized since the initial description of the Galveston technique by Allen and Ferguson in 1982 [2]. Utilization in trauma constructs has also been well described for a variety of injury patterns including lumbopelvic dislocations and fracture dislocations [7], sacral fractures [8], and low lumbar burst fractures [9]. The key indication for placement of an iliac screw for trauma is the identification of the need for an additional point of fixation in order to assure postoperative stability. This may necessitate two screws placed ipsilaterally for rotational stability as one screw, particularly if smaller in diameter, may toggle and loosen during early weight bearing [1]. Complications of iliac screw placement for trauma involve late pain from implant prominence and wound complications related to the dissection [3].

31.2 Technique

31.2.1 Exposure

The iliac crest may be approached in several ways. If a canal exploration or decompression is necessary, a standard midline approach may be used with placement of pedicle screws at indicated spinal levels as needed. This may then be extended laterally elevating the erector spinae out to the ilium. This may be difficult in the

young trauma patient. Another option is to make a separate fascial incision directly overlying the posterior superior iliac spine. The fascia is then elevated off of the PSIS both medial and laterally so that a portion of the PSIS may be resected in order to recess the screw head. Only the portion necessary for screw head recession should be removed to minimize postoperative pain. Once the PSIS is exposed and prepared, actual placement of the screw can be performed.

31.2.2 Screw Placement

The key part of placing a single iliac screw is identification of the column of bone passing between the posterior and anterior inferior iliac spines just superior to the acetabulum. This trajectory may be approximated without fluoroscopy in a nontraumatized patient, but in the patient with pelvic disruption image guidance will maximize fixation (Figs. 31.1–31.3).

A typical image for the screw trajectory is presented in Fig. 31.4. This image is obtained with the patient in the prone position and the C-arm positioned in a combined Judet and outlet views of the pelvis. Because of anatomic variability, an approximate C-arm setting is 30° caudal, 45° coronal. This is similar to the image obtained for anterior supra-acetabular external fixator pin placement as described by Haidukewych et al. with the important caveat that the addition of caudal angulation allows the pin to pass above the greater sciatic notch, which is critical for safe screw placement [4].

Following identification of an appropriate starting point, depending on whether one or two screws is planned (see Figs. 31.4 and 31.5), a 3.2 mm pilot hole may be drilled following the trajectory of the C-arm. Repeat imaging demonstrating the drill bit remaining

R. Morgan
University of Minnesota, 640 Jackson Street,
Saint Paul, MN, USA
e-mail: robert.a.morgan@healthpartners.com

V.V. Patel et al. (eds.), *Spine Trauma*,
DOI: 10.1007/978-3-642-03694-1_31, © Springer-Verlag Berlin Heidelberg 2010

Fig. 31.1 (**a**) and (**b**) Sagittal computed tomography (CT) scan and magnetic resonance imaging (MRI) demonstrating complex lumbosacral dislocation with CSF leak dorsal and ventral. Iliac screw placement strategies must factor in the need for duraplasty and postoperative cerebrospinal fluid drainage

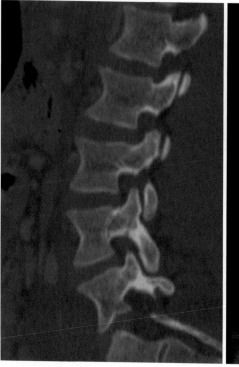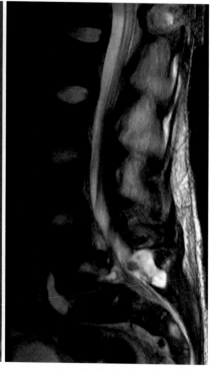

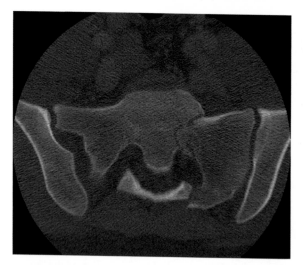

Fig. 31.2 Axial CT scan demonstrating sacral fracture involving comminution of the S1 body and pedicle precluding pedicle screw placement on the involved side. Iliac screw placement strategies will require additional torsional stability, possibly warranting stacked (double) ipsilateral iliac screws

centered on the image will ensure the trajectory is within the column of bone. A blunt pedicle probe may also be used if the cancellous bone is soft enough. A straight probe is recommended but a curved probe can also be used. In this case, the probe is advanced along the inner table until resistance is increased, then the probe is rotated 180° toward the outer table and again advanced until resistance is increased. A lateral image may be useful for ensuring the sufficiency of screw length to extend beyond the greater sciatic notch but is not usually necessary (see Fig. 31.6). Note that the lateral image can be deceiving, particularly in the trauma patient, because the sciatic notches may not perfectly line up due to pelvic ring disruptions. A perfect lateral image should demonstrate the screw trajectory to be superior to both the sciatic notch and the dome of the acetabulum [10].

Unlike osteopenic patients, the typical trauma patient has dense cancellous bone in this region. An 8.5 mm diameter screw will give significant torsional resistance to insertion at typical screw lengths around 100 mm so tapping is often necessary. The torsional resistance for a 7.5 mm tap may be significant and sequential tapping may be useful. "Line-to-line" tapping may be useful if two screws are placed ipsilaterally to prevent iatrogenic fracture (Figs. 31.7 and 31.8).

31.2.3 Connecting the Construct

Depending on the nature of the fracture being treated and the system being used, a variety of strategies may

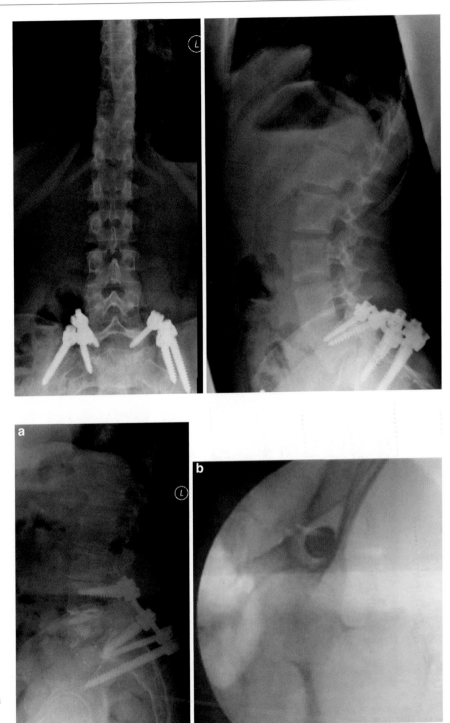

Fig. 31.3 AP and lateral standing radiographs demonstrating posterior stabilization of sacral facet and comminuted pedicle fracture. Note the unilateral pedicle screw on the *right*, double 7.5 mm diameter iliac screws on the *left*

Fig. 31.4 (**a**) Sacral insufficiency fracture below a prior fusion. Iliac extension of instrumentation allowed immediate weight bearing [5, 6]. (**b**) Screw trajectory on C-arm. The screw depicted is 8.5 mm × 100 mm

be used to connect the iliac screw to the rest of the construct. Several considerations at this stage of the procedure are

1. Will I need a cross-link? The close proximity of implants at L5, S1, and the ilium will often preclude a cross-link unless the construct is extended to L4 or the system being used allows for a cross-link to be applied directly to the screw head. Another option is to use an offset connector from the iliac screw to the rest of the construct, which will allow a more traditional cross-link to be placed.

Fig. 31.5 Screw trajectory anatomic landmarks. Placement of two screws would necessitate a more eccentric starting point

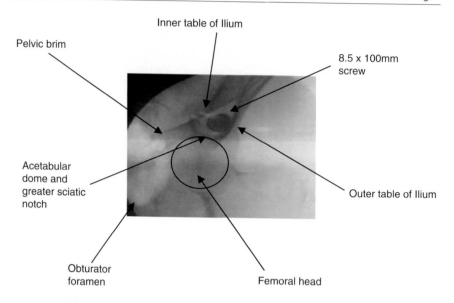

Inner table of Ilium

Pelvic brim

8.5 x 100mm screw

Acetabular dome and greater sciatic notch

Outer table of Ilium

Obturator foramen

Femoral head

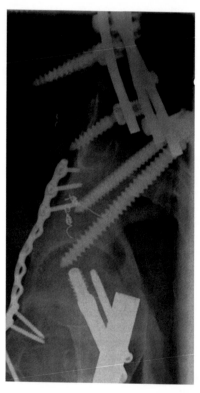

Fig. 31.6 Complex polytrauma patient with apparent iliac screw in hip joint. Note asymmetric sciatic notches. This is due to mal-reduction of the pelvis and changing the screw trajectory would result in violation of the inner table of the pelvis

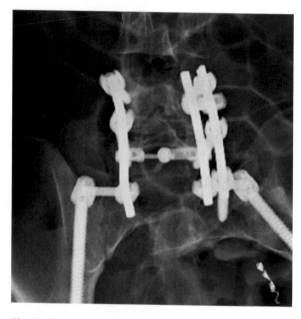

Fig. 31.7 Late lumbopelvic fracture dislocation demonstrating offset connectors combined with cross-links

2. Will I use offset connectors? Contouring of the rod is simplified if these connectors are used, particularly if a construct involving the S1 pedicles is being

used. These can be easily tunneled under the extensor musculature so that there is little implant prominence when the iliac screw is properly recessed into the ilium. They also can facilitate reduction of fractures and dislocations by providing a point for compression/distraction/and rotation prior to final tightening. It is important that the system characteristics be understood prior to rod placement as the strategy for final rod placement will differ depending on whether the connector is open or closed.

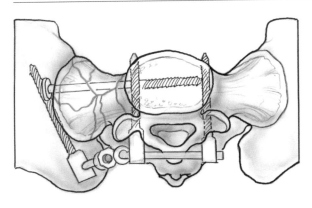

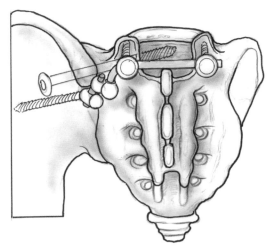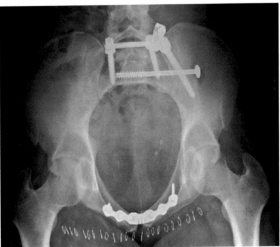

Fig. 31.8 Contoured rods and cross-link used in place of offset connector for comminuted Zone II sacral fracture requiring open reduction and anterior pelvic ring plating. Construct allowed immediate weight bearing [6]

31.2.4 Closure

It is important to close the fascia overlying the iliac screw if a separate fascial incision was made for screw placement. This will help to reduce late symptomatic implants but a prominent implant may erode through even intact overlying fascia resulting in either late pain or wound problems.

31.3 Conclusion

Placement of iliac screws is a safe and effective means of obtaining distal fixation in low lumbar and sacral trauma. Careful attention to operative technique and implant selection will allow for construct stability and often early

patient mobilization. Wound problems and late implant-related pain are reported complications despite meticulous attention to detail and may be unavoidable sequelae of the often devastating injuries that result in the indication for iliac fixation.

References

1. Akesen B, Wu C, Mehbod AA, Sokolowski M, Transfeldt EE (2008) Revision of loosened iliac screws: a biomechanical study of longer and bigger screws. Spine 33(13):1423–1428
2. Allen BL Jr, Ferguson RL (1982) The Galveston technique for L rod instrumentation of the scoliotic spine. Spine 7(3):276–284
3. Bellabarba C, Schildhauer TA, Vaccaro AR, Chapman JR (2006) Complications associated with surgical stabilization of high-grade sacral fracture dislocations with spino-pelvic instability. Spine 31(11 Suppl):S80–S88, discussion S104

4. Haidukewych GJ, Kumar S, Prpa B (2003) Placement of half-pins for supra-acetabular external fixation: an anatomic study. Clin Orthop Relat Res (411):269–273

5. Korovessis PG, Magnissalis EA, Deligianni D (2006) Biomechanical evaluation of conventional internal contemporary spinal fixation techniques used for stabilization of complete sacroiliac joint separation: a 3-dimensional unilaterally isolated experimental stiffness study. Spine 31(25):E941–E951

6. Mouhsine E, Wettstein M, Schizas C, Borens O, Blanc CH, Leyvraz PF et al (2006) Modified triangular posterior osteosynthesis of unstable sacrum fracture. Eur Spine J 15(6): 857–863

7. Schildhauer TA, Bellabarba C, Nork SE, Barei DP, Routt ML Jr, Chapman JR (2006) Decompression and lumbopelvic fixation for sacral fracture-dislocations with spino-pelvic dissociation. J Orthop Trauma 20(7):447–457

8. Schildhauer TA, Ledoux WR, Chapman JR, Henley MB, Tencer AF, Routt ML Jr (2003) Triangular osteosynthesis and iliosacral screw fixation for unstable sacral fractures: a cadaveric and biomechanical evaluation under cyclic loads. J Orthop Trauma 17(1):22–31

9. Wang MY, Ludwig SC, Anderson DG, Mummaneni PV (2008) Percutaneous iliac screw placement: description of a new minimally invasive technique. Neurosurg Focus 25(2):E17

10. Ziran BH, Wasan AD, Marks DM, Olson SA, Chapman MW (2007) Fluoroscopic imaging guides of the posterior pelvis pertaining to iliosacral screw placement. J Trauma 62(2):347–356, discussion 356

Minimally Invasive Treatment for Ankylosing Spondylitis and DISH Thoracolumbar Fractures

32

Neel Anand, Eli M. Baron, Rebecca Rosemann, and Mark Dekutoski

32.1 Case Example

Fifty-nine-year old male with a history of ankylosing spondylitis (AS) suffered a slip and fall injury with axial back pain. He was seen in the Emergency Department, diagnosed with compression fracture, and discharged home in TLSO brace without further evaluation. His pain persisted for 3 months with progressive kyphotic deformity. He presented to spine clinic with continued pain for further evaluation (Fig. 32.1).

Given his AS history, an MRI was ordered to rule out ligamentous injury and evaluate healing potential. MRI showed three-column disruption and gross instability (Fig. 32.2).

He was treated with multisegment percutaneous pedicle screw and rod instrumentation without fusion. He tolerated the procedure well and was discharged home in stable condition on postoperative day 1. Pain improved significantly and he returned to many of his normal activities postoperatively (Fig. 32.3).

32.2 Background

Spinal trauma can be particularly devastating in patients with AS and diffuse idiopathic skeletal hyperostosis (DISH) [3]. These patients have an autofusion of the spine, commonly known as the "bamboo spine," and as a result, fractures in this population are more similar to long bone fractures. Many are three-column injuries and often have extensive ligamentous injuries with increased instability patterns and dislocation. Because of this, surgical stabilization is often required in this patient population and has historically required long constructs with multiple points of fixation. Focus must be on ensuring support of the anterior column.

Segmental fixation, specifically with pedicle screws and rods, has become the primary technique for fixation of thoracolumbar fractures [2]. Traditionally, this has been performed with or without fusion via open surgical technique. Nevertheless, open surgical technique is associated with high morbidity, high infection rates, and mean blood loss of greater than 1,000 cc [14]. Rechtine reported an infection rate as high as 10% [10]. Given the muscle damage associated with paraspinal muscle stripping procedures [4–6, 13, 15], minimally invasive techniques have been developed. They are associated with theoretically lower blood loss, less muscle damage, and overall reduced morbidity [17].

32.3 Advantages

Advantages of the minimally invasive surgical technique include reduced blood loss, reduced morbidity, and possibly reduced infection rates, given the

N. Anand (✉), E.M. Baron and R. Rosemann
Department of Surgery, Cedars Sinai Institute for Spinal Disorders, Cedars Sinai Medical Center, Los Angeles, CA 90048, USA
e-mail: neel.anand@cshs.org

M. Dekutoski
Department of Orthopedic Surgery, Mayo Clinic Graduate School of Medicine, Gonda 14, 200 First Street SW, Rochester, MN, USA

V.V. Patel et al. (eds.), *Spine Trauma*,
DOI: 10.1007/978-3-642-03694-1_32, © Springer-Verlag Berlin Heidelberg 2010

Fig. 32.1 Preoperative radiographs showing T12 compression fracture

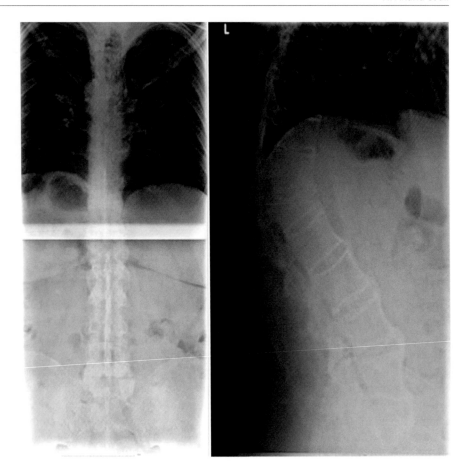

reduction in tissue trauma [9]. Nevertheless, an open approach may be technically more feasible, especially if a decompression or open reduction technique is considered (e.g., transpedicular vertebrectomy and cage placement). Additionally, minimally invasive pedicle screw placement is highly fluoroscopy dependent, theoretically increasing operating room staff, surgeon, and patient radiation exposure. Nevertheless, as image guidance becomes more available, this disadvantage may disappear.

32.4 Procedure

The technique for minimally invasive instrumentation and correction for fractures in this population is very similar to that described in Chapter 27. Please find further tips specific to this population below.

32.5 Technical Perils and Pitfalls

Because of the deformed position and kyphosis of the spine, positioning becomes critical. The regular Jackson table may not be appropriate for these patients. Radiolucent tables with logrolls and extra chest and pelvic padding may be required. At times, a table that breaks into kyphosis may be necessary.

In patients with intact neurology, we feel it is best to fix the fracture in its original deformed position and not make valiant attempts to correct existing deformity. Hence, the existing kyphosis is realigned and instrumentation extended at least 3–4 segments above and below the fracture. In patients with complete neurological deficit, an attempt could be made to correct the deformity at the fracture site so as to better align the spine. A pedicle subtraction osteotomy or Smith–Peterson osteotomy may need to be added to correct the deformity in select cases.

Fig. 32.2 MRI demonstrating ligamentous and bony disruption in all three columns with compression fracture

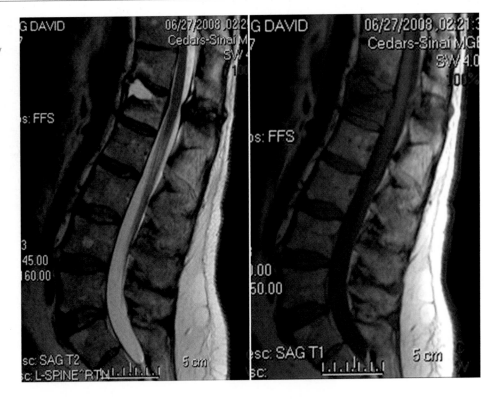

Occasionally, extreme kyphosis can prevent safe prone positioning and fracture reduction, and instrumentation may have to be done with the patient in the lateral position.

We prefer to cannulate all our pedicles using the AP projection, and once our pedicles are cannulated, guide wires are placed and advanced using the lateral projection. This method saves considerable time and reduces the amount of radiation used. Additionally, operating room lights are dimmed in order to maximize visualization on the fluoroscopy unit screen. If there is a problem with a screw extender or screw head, one can always extend the minimally invasive-style incision and open up the fascia and dissect down to the level of the rod. In this manner open persuasion can be performed or open seating of a rod can be performed of the screw head. Open surgery always remains a bail out if there is a problem.

In our experience in through bone flexion distraction injuries (chance fractures), posterior fusion is usually not required as the instrumentation serves as an internal brace allowing the fracture to heal naturally. In ligamentous hyperextension injuries, focal fusion at the fractured segment is recommended.

32.6 Postoperative Considerations

We brace patients minimally for 3–6 months after surgery. Pulmonary toilet, personal hygiene, and early ambulation are important goals in the acute postoperative period. Wound healing may be an issue secondary to the kyphosis and possible chronic steroids used to control systemic disease. Additionally, for deep venous thrombosis, prophylaxis is used starting on postoperative day 1.

In addition to the known complications of MIS fixation for thoracolumbar fractures, AS and DISH patients can have significant osteoporosis making visualization and targeting of percutaneous screws extremely demanding.

32.7 Results

We conducted a retrospective review of AS and DISH fractures treated at three major centers between 1994 and 2007. Open surgical techniques were used during 1994–2002, and from 2002 to 2007, constrained and unconstrained percutaneous instrumentation was used [3].

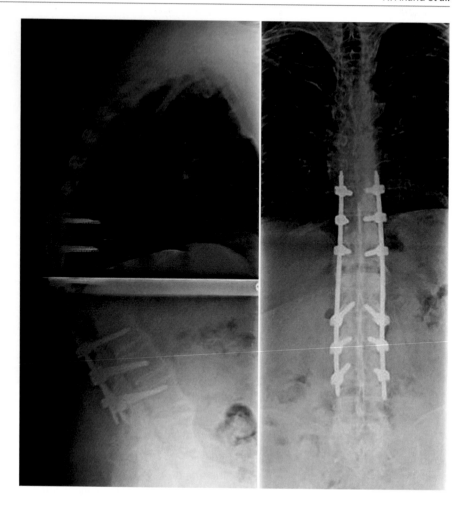

There were 18 open, 8 constrained (CP), and 9 unconstrained percutaneous (UP) procedures, the outcomes of which were as below

- Ninety day perioperative deaths occurred in three patients (2 open, 1 CP, 0 UP).
- Wound complications occurred in five (4 open, 1 CP, 0 UP), which included four persistent drainage/infections in the open group. The one wound breakdown in a constrained percutaneous patient wherein the curved rod prominence contributed to a wound dehiscence.
- Reoperation for instrumentation-related complications occurred in three patients (2 open, 1 CP, 0 UP).
- EBL, hospitalization, and ICU stay were significantly reduced in the CP and UP groups.

32.8 Conclusions

Our results would suggest that open techniques result in significantly greater perioperative morbidity and mortality than percutaneous (constrained and unconstrained) techniques [3].

Unconstrained techniques reduced instrumentation and wound complications by lower rod profile and greater flexibility with segmental fixation placement and reduced implant prominence [3].

Minimally invasive fixation represents a less tissue-injuring alternative to open posterior fixation or open posterior fixation and fusion in the setting of spinal trauma in patients with AS and DISH. Current-generation systems such as the Medtronic CD-Horizon Longitude system allow multisegment fixation with significantly less difficulties than earlier-generation instrumentation. As more data become available, we believe there will be increased use of MIS in the treatment of spinal fractures.

References

1. Anand N, Baron EM, Dekutoski MB (2009) Minimally invasive posterior stabilization techniques (single and multiple segment) percutaneous exposure in trauma. In: Vaccaro AR, Fehlings MG, Dvorak M (eds) Management of spine and spinal cord trauma: an evidence based analysis. Medtronic, Memphis

2. Baron EM, Zeiller SC, Vaccaro AR, Hilibrand AS (2005) Surgical management of thoracolumbar fractures. Contemp Spine Surg 6(12):1–9

3. Dekutoski M, Huddleston P, Anand N, Riina J, Isaacs R, Gahr R (2009) Thoracolumbar fracture management with selective fusion and instrumentation removal. Spine J 9(10): 83S–84S

4. Kawaguchi Y, Matsui H, Tsuji H (1994) Back muscle injury after posterior lumbar spine surgery. Part 2: Histologic and histochemical analyses in humans. Spine 19(22):2598–2602

5. Kawaguchi Y, Yabuki S, Styf J et al (1996) Back muscle injury after posterior lumbar spine surgery. Topographic evaluation of intramuscular pressure and blood flow in the porcine back muscle during surgery. Spine 21(22):2683–2688

6. Lu K, Liang CL, Cho CL et al (2002) Oxidative stress and heat shock protein response in human paraspinal muscles during retraction. J Neurosurg 97(1 suppl):75–81

7. McCormack T, Karaikovic E, Gaines RW (1994) The load sharing classification of spine fractures. Spine 19(15):1741–1744

8. Potter BK, Lenke LG, Kuklo TR (2004) Prevention and management of iatrogenic flatback deformity. J Bone Joint Surg Am 86-A(8):1793–1808

9. Rampersaud YR, Annand N, Dekutoski MB (2006) Use of minimally invasive surgical techniques in the management of trauma: current concepts. Spine 31(11 suppl):S96–S102, discussion S104

10. Rechtine GR, Bono PL, Cahill D, Bolesta MJ, Chrin AM (2001) Postoperative wound infection after instrumentation of thoracic and lumbar fractures. J Orthop Trauma 15(8):566–569

11. Ringel F, Stoffel M, Stuer C, Meyer B (2006) Minimally invasive transmuscular pedicle screw fixation of the thoracic and lumbar spine. Neurosurgery 59(4 suppl 2):ONS361–ONS366, discussion ONS366–367

12. Spoonamore M (2008) Pedicle-targeting techniques for minimally invasive lumbar fusions. In: Lewandrowski K, Yeung C, Spoonamore M, McLain RF (eds) Minimally invasive spinal fusion techniques. Summit Communications, Armonk

13. Suwa H, Hanakita J, Ohshita N, Gotoh K, Matsuoka N, Morizane A (2000) Postoperative changes in paraspinal muscle thickness after various lumbar back surgery procedures. Neurol Med Chir (Tokyo) 40(3):151–154, discussion 154–155

14. Verlaan JJ, Diekerhof CH, Buskens E et al (2004) Surgical treatment of traumatic fractures of the thoracic and lumbar spine: a systematic review of the literature on techniques, complications, and outcome. Spine 29(7):803–814

15. Weber BR, Grob D, Dvorak J, Muntener M (1997) Posterior surgical approach to the lumbar spine and its effect on the multifidus muscle. Spine 22(15):1765–1772

16. Wild MH, Glees M, Plieschnegger C, Wenda K (2007) Five-year follow-up examination after purely minimally invasive posterior stabilization of thoracolumbar fractures: a comparison of minimally invasive percutaneously and conventionally open treated patients. Arch Orthop Trauma Surg 127(5):335–343

17. Zeiller SC, Baron EM, Hilibrand AS, Anand N, Vaccaro AR (2007) Thoracolumbar fractures: classification and management. In: Jallo JI, Loftus CM, Vaccaro AR (eds) Neurosurgical trauma and critical care. Thieme, New York

Surgical Treatment of Thoracic or Thoracolumbar Fractures of Ankylosing Spondylitis (AS) or Diffuse Idiopathic Skeletal Hyperostosis (DISH)

Courtney W. Brown

33.1 Case Report

This 73-year-old male was working on his roof at 10 o'clock at night and fell, landing on his back, hyperextending it over a fence. He was brought in a level I emergency room and found to have a ruptured aorta, as well as a T 11–12 fracture-dislocation of a preexisting diffuse idiopathic skeletal hyperostosis (DISH) spine (Fig. 33.1). He was taken immediately to the operating room for the aortic repair. However, his postoperative clinical status was so poor that he was not returned to the operating room for stabilization of his spine for 10 days.

In addition, because of his comatose state, neurological status was variable to undetermined. At surgery, posterior instrumentation, three above and three below, was performed, returning the patient to his preoperative contour (Fig. 33.2). The length of stabilization above and below the fracture dislocation was done to control the long lever arms of the DISH spine. After approximately 6 weeks, the patient became alert and was found to be neurologically intact. After long-term rehabilitation, the patient is now totally recovered, both physically and mentally.

33.2 Introduction

Ankylosing spondylitis and DISH patients have similar pathological spinal problems, that of spontaneous

C.W. Brown
Department of Orthopaedics, University of Colorado
Health Science Center, Panorama Orhopedics & Spine Center,
660 Golden Ridge Road, Suite 250, Golden,
CO 80401-9522, USA
e-mail: cbrown@panoramaortho.com

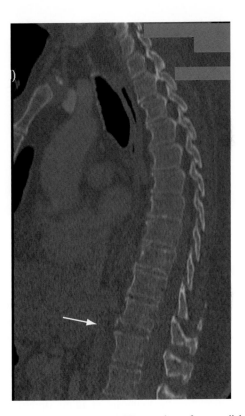

Fig. 33.1 Preoperative sagittal CT scan shows fracture dislocation at T 11–12 that has spontaneously reduced

ligamentous stiffening and fusing of the spine. If fractured in the thoracic or thoracolumbar regions, two long bone levers are created, producing extreme spinal instability that risks the spinal cord and the anterior vascular structures. Because of these risks, surgical stabilization of the spine is absolutely necessary. Usually, this will require longer instrumentation than is commonly needed for a similar fracture in the spines with normal anatomy. Three or more levels above and below the fractured level need to be included in the instrumentation.

V.V. Patel et al. (eds.), *Spine Trauma*,
DOI: 10.1007/978-3-642-03694-1_33, © Springer-Verlag Berlin Heidelberg 2010

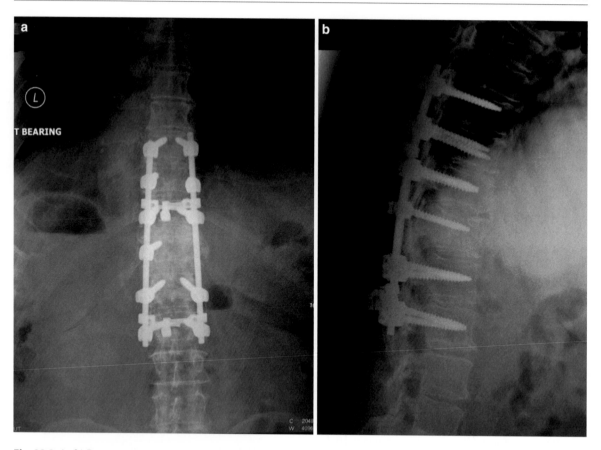

Fig. 33.2 (**a**, **b**) Postoperative erect AP and lateral X-ray 11 months after injury and surgeries

33.3 Equipment

A radiolucent operating table that can be adjusted to match the preinjury spinal alignment is necessary. In most cases of ankylosing spondylitis, reestablishing the preexisting anatomical alignment is indicated, especially if there is evidence of spinal cord injury. Trying to perform a corrective osteotomy through the fractured spine, correcting the kyphosis, is, in my opinion, contraindicated if there is a spinal cord injury. This may be detrimental toward potential spinal cord recovery. DISH patients usually have relatively normal global balance prior to injury, and therefore, any spinal deformity correction is usually unnecessary.

A general anesthetic with IV antibiotics is required. Neuromonitoring is appropriate, including both motor and sensory, even if the patient has a spinal cord injury, as it may be incomplete.

Most spinal instrumentation systems are adequate for this type of surgery but must include both pedicle screws and hooks. I prefer titanium, and if the bone

is osteoporotic, commercially pure rods (vs. alloy rods) are preferred, The hooks need to be available because the vertebral bodies and pedicles in severe ankylosing spondylitis patients can sometimes be totally void of any cancellous bone. The posterior elements, including the lamina and the facets, are the strongest bone structures available for fixation. If these are the only stable structures available, hook fixation may be necessary.

It should be noted that ligamentum flavum in ankylosing spondylitis is sometimes completely calcified. Therefore, the ligamentum flavum must be carefully dissected and removed prior to any insertion of laminal hooks. Hook instrumentation should be of a claw construct above and below the fracture, such that there is adequate length to the instrumentation to control the long bone character of the pathology. This commonly will require three levels of instrumentation, both proximally and distally. Occasionally, cement augmentation into the pedicles and vertebral bodies will give adequate fixation for screws, but this is not always possible, thus forcing the use of hooks.

33.4 Patient Positioning

If the patient is neurologically intact, two options are available. First, the patient should be placed on a flexed table repositioning the spine in its normal preinjury alignment. In ankylosing spondylitis, this will usually require a kyphotic position similar to the patient's preoperative status. In ankylosing spondylitis, a corrective osteotomy utilizing the fracture level in the neurologically intact patient is possible, but is of a high risk and needs to be performed with the patient's consent and full understanding of the risks. A second position option in ankylosing spondylitis with extreme kyphosis is to place the patient on his side in the flexed position corresponding to his preoperative status. Care must be taken to avoid translation of the fracture in either anterior/posterior or lateral alignment. Multiple biplane X-rays need to be obtained while positioning the patient. Various types of padding or pillows may facilitate positioning and avoid displacement. In DISH, normal pre-operative alignment is usually adequate.

33.5 Procedure

After the patient is adequately positioned, a routine posterior exposure is performed exposing the ankylosed and autofused spine above and below the level of instability for a minimum of three levels in both directions. However, if there is mobility between the second and third instrumented distal levels in the lower lumbar spine, that level may not need to be incorporated. Once the exposure is obtained, pedicle screw fixation should be performed under X-ray control. Three levels above and three levels below, and perhaps even four, may be necessary. Once that is obtained, the chosen rods should be bent to contour so that the fractured spine is immobilized in its relatively normal preinjury position. Cross-links should be applied above and below. The fracture level should be decorticated with a burr to avoid any loosening of the instrumentation. Bone grafting is then performed (Fig. 33.2).

Preoperative MRI imaging will show whether a neurologically significant epidural hematoma exists. If so, decompressive laminectomy should be performed proximally or distally as indicated. If a large amount of lamina is removed, hooks will not be possible and pedicle cement augmentation may be necessary.

Postoperatively, these patients are usually maintained in a Jewett brace with a gibbus pad over the incision, thus eliminating irritation to the incision. They should be mobilized as soon as the next day to facilitate pulmonary status and avoid DVTs. Adequate blood support is necessary.

33.6 Complications

Infection is always a concern and one reason titanium is most appropriate in these spinal cases. Titanium is more resistant to bacterial infection than stainless steel. If there is infection, do not remove the metal until the fracture has completely healed by CT scan.

Nonunion is rare as most of these patients will autofuse anteriorly even if there is an opening anterior wedge. Metal cutout is rare.

References

1. Kubiak EN, Moskovich R, Errico TJ, Di Cesare PE (2005) Orthopaedic management of ankylosing spondylitis. J Am Acad Orthop Surg 13(4):267–278
2. Sapkas G, Kateros K, Papadakis SA, Galanakos S, Brilakis E, Machairas G, Katonis P (2009) Surgical outcome after spinal fractures in patients with ankylosing spondylitis. BMC Musculoskelet Disord 10:96
3. Taljanovic MS, Hunter TB, Wisneski RJ, Seeger JF, Friend CJ, Schwartz SA, Rogers LF (2009) Imaging characteristics of diffuse idiopathic skeletal hyperostosis with an emphasis on acute spinal fractures: review. AJR Am J Roentgenol 193 (3 suppl):S10–S19; Quiz S20–S24
4. Thumbikat P, Hariharan RP, Ravichandran G, McClelland MR, Mathew KM (2007) Spinal cord injury in patients with ankylosing spondylitis: a 10-year review. Spine (Phila Pa 1976) 32(26):2989–2995
5. Westerveld LA, Verlaan JJ, Oner FC (2009) Spinal fractures in patients with ankylosing spinal disorders: a systematic review of the literature on treatment, neurological status and complications. Eur Spine J 18(2):145–156
6. Whang PG, Goldberg G, Lawrence JP, Hong J, Harrop JS, Anderson DG, Albert TJ, Vaccaro AR (2009) The management of spinal injuries in patients with ankylosing spondylitis or diffuse idiopathic skeletal hyperostosis: a comparison of treatment methods and clinical outcomes. J Spinal Disord Tech 22(2):77–85

Traumatic Dural Tears

34

Amgad S. Hanna, Ahmad Nassr, and James S. Harrop

34.1 Case Example

An 18-year-old male was involved in a motocross bike
collision where he fell backwards and landed on his
buttocks resulting in flexion and axial load of his spine.
Immediately after the injury, he had complete loss of
sensory and motor function in the lower extremities,
which improved minimally en route to the hospital.
On examination, he had weakness of the left lower
extremity: proximally (iliopsoas and quadriceps) 1/5,
and distally 2/5. The right lower extremity strength was
minimally weak (4+/5). Sensation was normal, but rectal examination showed decreased tone and volition.
Computerized tomography (CT) revealed L1 burst fracture with retropulsion and 75% canal compromise, as
well as laminar fracture (Fig. 34.1). Magnetic resonance
imaging (MRI) revealed, in addition, T2 signal changes
in the conus medullaris (Fig. 34.2a) and possibly an
avulsed nerve root on the right side (Fig. 34.2b).

The patient underwent a posterior decompression with
instrumented fusion. After the laminectomy, spontaneous
cerebrospinal fluid (CSF) was noted in two different locations; one was a small midline tear, the other was at the
origin of an avulsed right L1 nerve root. These were both

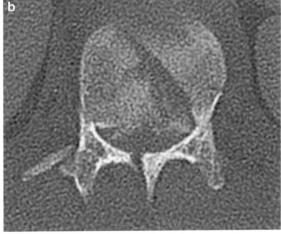

Fig. 34.1 Sagittal (**a**) and axial (**b**) CT showing L1 burst fracture with a retropulsed fragment and canal compromise, as well
as laminar fracture

A.S. Hanna (✉)
Department of Neurosurgery, University of Wisconsin,
600 Highland Avenue, Madison, WI 53792, USA
e-mail: ah2904@yahoo.com

A. Nassr
Department of Orthopedics, Mayo Clinic, 200 First Street SW,
Rochester, MN 55905, USA,

J.S. Harrop
Department of Neurosurgery, Thomas Jefferson University
Hospital, 909 Walnut Street, Philadelphia, PA 19107, USA

V.V. Patel et al. (eds.), *Spine Trauma*,
DOI: 10.1007/978-3-642-03694-1_34, © Springer-Verlag Berlin Heidelberg 2010

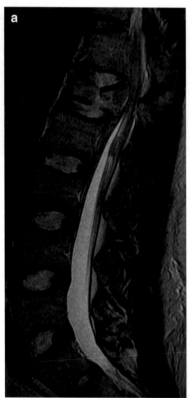

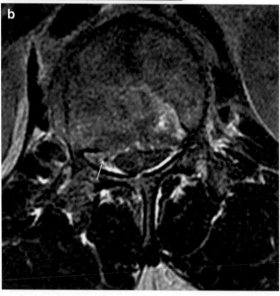

Fig. 34.2 Sagittal (**a**) T2-weighted MRI showing L1 burst fracture and edema of the conus medullaris. Axial (**b**) MRI shows the burst fracture and a possibly avulsed nerve root on the right (*arrow*)

corpectomy and bone grafting due to limited anterior column support as a result of the fracture. After the corpectomy, CSF leak was noted through an anterior dural tear, which was not amenable to direct repair. A piece of DuraGen was cut and placed on top of the dura as an onlay graft, which was covered by DuraSeal. Postoperatively, the wounds remained dry, with no evidence of CSF leak; this was consistent after the drains were removed and the patient was mobilized out of bed. The patient also made a good functional recovery.

34.2 Background

The incidence of traumatic dural tears has been reported to range from 7.5 to 19% of spinal fractures [3, 6, 11]. The highest incidence is noted with thoracolumbar burst fractures, particularly those associated with laminar fractures. Further, the presence of a neurological deficit is highly predictive of dural tears. One possible explanation is when the flexion/axial load force is applied, the retropulsed fragment pushes the neural elements and dura through the laminar defect. After the dissipation of the axial load, the dura +/− the nerve roots are entrapped within the fractured lamina [3].

Persistent CSF leak can be a considerable cause of morbidity including infections and poor wound healing.

34.3 Indications and Advantages for Procedure

The decision to operate is based on the need to stabilize the spine and/or decompress the spinal cord or cauda equina. Chronic contained dural tears, i.e., pseudomeningoceles, should only be treated when symptomatic, e.g., intractable headaches or spinal cord compression.

34.4 Contraindications and Disadvantages for Procedure

There are no contraindications to surgical treatment of traumatic dural tears identified intraoperatively. However, a suspected contained dural tear (pseudomeningocele) may not be an indication for immediate exploration.

primarily sutured using 5-0 PROLENE figure-of-eight stitch. Two Davol drains were placed subfascially, then the fascia was tightly closed using No. 1 Vicryl. Three days later, the patient was taken back for an anterior

34.5 Procedure

34.5.1 Suture Material

Small diameter nonabsorbable suture is typically utilized to close the dura, including 4-0 NUROLON (ETHICON, Inc., a Johnson & Johnson company, Cincinnati, OH), SILK (ETHICON), 5-0 PROLENE (ETHICON), and 6-0 GORE-TEX (WL Gore & Associates, Inc., Flagstaff, AZ). NUROLON is composed of nonabsorbable braided nylon, dyed black. PROLENE is monofilament nonabsorbable polypropylene, dyed blue. GORE-TEX is nonabsorbable monofilament manufactured from expanded polytetrafluoroethylene (ePTFE), undyed. We are presently using 6-0 GORE-TEX for dural repairs, since the needle hole is smaller than the suture size (Fig. 34.3) and the GORE-TEX suture expands to fill the thread hole limiting cerebrospinal fluid leak through the suture line.

34.5.2 Dural Substitutes

Historically, numerous materials have been employed to close dural openings. Rubber and gold foil were used in the late 1800s [1, 5], gelatin products in the mid-1900s, and synthetics such as silicone in the 1980s. However, silastic dural grafts were associated with high incidence of delayed subdural hemorrhage from neovascularization after encapsulation [13]. Cadaveric dura mater grafts have the potential of infectious agent and cases of Creutzfeldt–Jakob disease have been reported [10].

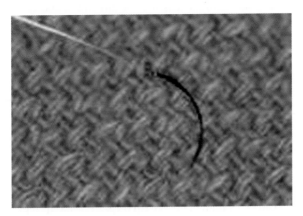

Fig. 34.3 GORE-TEX suture, 6-0. Notice that the needle size is smaller than the suture size

An ideal dural substitute must prevent CSF leaks, induce minimal or no inflammatory and/or immunogenic response, cause little or no adhesion to the neural elements, should not carry an increased risk of infection or bleeding, and be nontoxic, easy to manipulate, and cost-effective [4, 13]. Autologous fascia lata grafts are nonimmunogenic and inexpensive, but can be a cause of donor site morbidity, such as bleeding or infection.

AlloDerm (LifeCell Corp., Branchburg, NJ) is an acellular human dermis allograft. However, being allograft, there is a potential for infection. Therefore, blood samples from each skin donor are tested for hepatitis B and C, HIV types 1 and 2, human T-cell leukemia virus, and syphilis to minimize these risks. AlloDerm completely incorporates by 3 weeks and is characterized by intense fibroblast invasion and organized collagen formation [15]. Two months postimplantation, the trabecular framework of the graft is filled with endogenous collagen [14]. AlloDerm is immunologically inert and needs to be rehydrated for 10 min before use [17].

DuraGen (Integra LifeSciences Corp., Plainsboro, NJ) and DuraMatrix (Stryker, Kalamazoo, MI) are type I collagen matrix graft manufactured from bovine Achilles tendon. They have no detectable infectivity for bovine spongiform encephalopathy and are treated with sodium hydroxide that inactivates several viral strains including human immunodeficiency virus (HIV) [7]. They have an excellent strength and are pliable [13]. They create an initial chemical seal with fibrin and blood products within 4–8 h of application. Fibroblast proliferation begins at 3–4 days and is fully established at 14 days postsurgery [13]. This is followed by repopulation of the collagen matrix with endogenous collagen. Durepair (Medtronic Neurosurgery, Goleta, CA) is another collagen matrix derived from fetal bovine skin. There is one case report of severe allergic reaction to Durepair necessitating surgical removal [9]. Bovine pericardium has also been successfully used [4]. Dura-Guard (Synovis Surgical Innovations, St. Paul, MN) is a glutaraldehyde-processed, chemically cross-linked collagen derived from bovine pericardium; it has to be initially rehydrated in normal saline before application [2]. Zerris compared the three collagen dural substitutes in a canine model and found that the mechanical properties of Durepair and Dura-Guard were similar to native dura and persisted for 6 months. DuraGen was more fragile and did not maintain its structural integrity beyond 1 month. However, the three products were safe and effective in sealing dural defects [18].

34.5.3 Sealants

Several products are available as dural sealants. Before the sealant application, the operative field should be as dry as possible via meticulous hemostasis and repair of CSF leak. It should either cover approximated dural edges, or the interface between a dural substitute and the native dura. Thin-layered application is usually enough; the sealant takes effect by adhering to the dura/dural substitute, and there is no further benefit to adding more layers of sealant.

DuraSeal (Confluent Surgical, Inc., Waltham, MA) has two precursor liquids: one is an amine and the other is a polyethylene glycol (PEG) available in two syringes [16]. Once applied, they cross-link within 1–2 s forming a hydrogel network, which adheres to tissue. Its blue color enhances visualization. The newly available sprayer allows easier application by preventing clogging of the tip of the applicator. It has a 50% postapplication swelling and is absorbed within 4–8 weeks.

Tisseel (Baxter Healthcare Corporation, Deerfield, IL) is mainly used as a hemostatic agent, but can also be used as a sealant. It contains human thrombin, human sealer protein concentrate including fibrinogen, a synthetic fibrinolysis inhibitor solution containing aprotinin, and calcium chloride. Tisseel carries the infection risk of human plasma products and the allergic risk of the protein products including the rare occurrence of anaphylaxis. It begins to breakdown within 1–2 weeks. Tissucol (Immuno AG, Vienna) is another fibrin sealant manufactured with bovine thrombin. Vitagel (Orthovita, Inc., Malvern, PA) is indicated mainly as a hemostatic agent. It uses patient's own blood, mixed with bovine collagen, bovine thrombin, and calcium chloride. It resorbs within 4 weeks.

CoSeal (Baxter) is a PEG product indicated mainly for vascular reconstruction. It swells after application and resorbs within 4 weeks. BioGlue (CryoLife, Inc., Kennesaw, GA) is composed of bovine serum albumin and glutaraldehyde. It polymerizes within 20–30 s of its application and remains in place for more than 2 years. It is mainly used as an adjunct to vascular repair.

34.5.4 Surgical Technique

- Linear tears: Primary repair is typically the most effective method of closing the defect (Fig. 34.4). We typically use a simple running suture where the suture line starts and ends beyond the dural tear (Fig. 34.4a, f). With the GORE-TEX, at least six knots have to be placed to secure the initial stitch (Fig. 34.4b). It is a good practice to take one stitch behind the knot, away from the dural tear (Fig. 34.4c), then proceed to suturing the dural tear itself (Fig. 34.4d). The assistant should use suction in one hand to maintain a dry field for the primary surgeon from CSF and blood, and a Penfield 4 in the other hand to maintain the neural elements intradurally to protect them and allow the primary surgeon to identify the cut dural edges [8]. In larger tears, this can also be assisted by temporarily placing a cottonoid patty under the dural edges; care must be taken not to suture through the cottonoid patty. Before the last stitch, the intradural space can be filled with normal saline (Fig. 34.4e); this ensures no bleeding intradurally, no major CSF leaks, and should help prevent postoperative headache from CSF hypotension. After suturing, the repair is challenged by asking the anesthesia team to perform a Valsalva maneuver twice, and significant leaks are secured by additional suturing, then the sealant is applied (Fig. 34.4g). Alternatively, a locked running or simple interrupted suture could be used [8]. The disadvantage of the interrupted sutures is that it is time consuming and chances of leak in between the stitches are higher. However, sometimes it is ideal to reconstruct complex tears.
- Large tears with loss of dural substance: Patching may be required, using one of the dural substitutes and a suture technique similar to the one described above.
- Complex tears, including anterior tears, may not be amenable to direct repair or patching, and sometimes can only be treated using an onlay graft, then a sealant.
- Chronic leaks may present a diagnostic challenge. The source of the leak may be difficult to find. MRI with or without intrathecal contrast, radioisotope cisternography, or CT-myelography can be used to localize the leak. When symptomatic, they need to be treated. Epidural blood patch or percutaneous fibrin glue injection can help seal the leak, if not surgical exploration may be required.
- Magnification using surgical loupes [8] or operative microscope enhances visualization and improves surgical accuracy. Microinstruments are also preferred (Fig. 34.5a). Micro-pickups are less traumatic to the dural edges than regular pickups. They can be straight or curved tip (Fig. 34.5b). Fine regular needle drivers can be used, but the microneedle drivers give more precision and are less likely to

Fig. 34.4 Illustration of a simple running suture technique. (**a**) Start in a normal dura outside the tear. (**b**) At least 6–8 knots are recommended with the 6-0 GORE-TEX. (**c**) Take the next stitch behind the knot, away from the tear. (**d**) Proceed with the simple running suturing of the tear. Of note, some surgeons prefer a locking running suture. (**e**) The intradural space being filled with saline. (**f**) Completion of the suture line beyond the tear. At this point, a Valsalva maneuver is performed. (**g**) The sealant is then applied as a thin layer to a dry surface

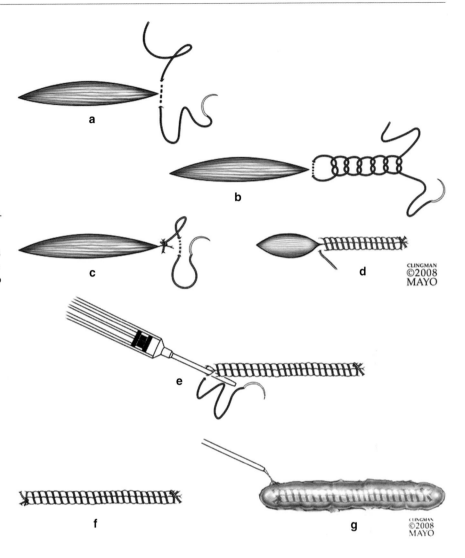

break the smaller needle. They can be straight or curved-tip (Fig. 34.5c), locking (Fig. 34.5d), or nonlocking, according to the surgeon's preference.

- Fascial closure is as important as dural closure. We use a double-layered fascial closure. The first with interrupted No. 1 Vicryl, and the second with a running No. 1 Vicryl. This allows fascia and skin to heal even if the dura does not seal, leading to chronic pseudomeningocele, which is typically asymptomatic.

34.5.5 Surgical Adjuvants

- Lumbar drain: Lumbar drain may be utilized to decrease intradural pressure. When used, we prefer hourly drainage rather than leaving the drain open at a level. We start at 5–10 mL/h, then progressively wean the patient. The drain is removed after a clamping trial for 24 h, if the incision remains dry with the patient sitting up.

- Subfascial drain: The use of subfascial drain is controversial. Some surgeons prefer using a drain to divert CSF and allow the fascia and skin to heal [13]. The drain is placed on low suction or to gravity to prevent CSF hypotension, which can cause headache, mental status change, subdural hematoma, or even herniation. Other surgeons never use subfascial drains in case of CSF leak, to avoid any negative pressure from perpetuating a transdural CSF leak.

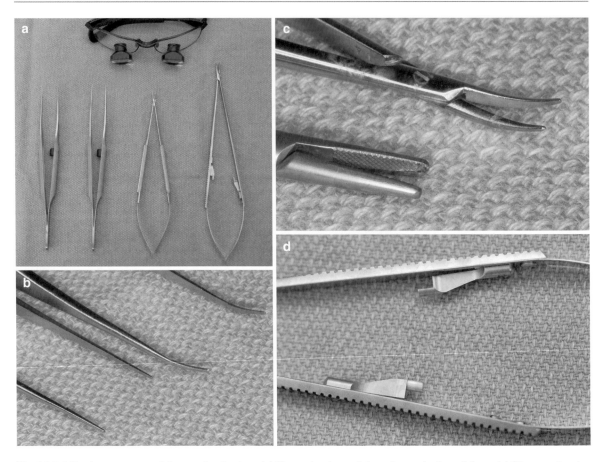

Fig. 34.5 Microinstruments used for suturing the dura. (**a**) *Top*: Loupes used for magnification. From *left* to *right*: Curved micro-pickups, straight micro-pickups, curved nonlocking microneedle driver, straight locking microneedle driver. (**b**) Close-up show-ing the straight and curved micro-pickups. (**c**) Close-up showing the straight and curved microneedle drivers. (**d**) Close-up show-ing the locking mechanism on the needle driver

34.6 Technical Pearls and Pitfalls

- Intraoperative recognition of a dural injury is impor-tant to allow for primary closure. Indirect signs of CSF leak are a collapsed thecal sac or excessive epidural bleeding. Failure to identify a dural tear may cause postoperative CSF leak, delayed wound healing, or infections including meningitis.
- Careful exposure of the lamina is required if a traumatic dural tear is suspected to avoid iatrogenic nerve injury.
- Use of a sealant does not substitute for good surgi-cal technique for dural closure. Most sealants tend to swell after application; extreme care should be taken not to apply a thick layer, which does not add to the sealing power but can cause compression of the neural structures.
- Fascial closure should be watertight. It is the sec-ond line of defense after a watertight dural closure.

- Asymptomatic pseudomeningoceles are common.
- Overdrainage through lumbar drain or subfascial drain can result in serious complications including subdural hematomas [12], herniation, and death. These patients should be carefully monitored while a drain is in place.

34.7 Postoperative Considerations

34.7.1 Activity

The activity is usually dictated by the associated spinal cord injury or spinal instability. Most surgeons prefer a period of flat bed rest after closure of a dural injury. This depends on the ability to close the dura and the location of the injury. Overall, the period of bed rest ranges from none to several days.

34.7.2 Treatment of CSF Hypotension Headache

A reclined position typically eliminates CSF hypotension headaches. Hydration is an important factor, either orally or intravenous. Additionally, intravenous and oral caffeine has been used. Opiate medication seems to have a limited role but may improve symptoms.

34.7.3 Rescue Procedures

A persistent CSF leak or development of a new CSF leak is usually manifested by the egress of CSF from the incision or excessive clear output through a subfascial drain or a chest tube. The incision can be oversewn with a nonabsorbable suture, or DERMABOND (ETHICON) can be added as a sealant. Persistent leak may require placement of a lumbar drain. If the leak persists or reoccurs after clamping or removing the drain, surgical reexploration should be considered. The same techniques discussed above can be employed, in addition to the consideration of mobilizing the paraspinal muscles to close the "dead space" and achieve tight closure of the fascia. Placing a lumbar drain to divert CSF and allowing the wound to heal should be considered as an option if the dura I closure is not water-tight. Finally, with the help of a plastic surgeon, muscular flaps and other vascularized tissue can be mobilized and used as a barrier to CSF leak, especially after complex dural injury with significant dural loss.

34.7.4 Disclosure

None of the authors has any financial interest in any of the products discussed above.

References

1. Abbe R (1895) Rubber tissue for meningeal adhesions. Trans Am Surg Assoc 13:490–491
2. Anson JA, Marchand EP (1996) Bovine pericardium for dural grafts: clinical results in 35 patients. Neurosurgery 39:764–768
3. Aydinli U, Karaeminogullari O, Tiskaya A et al (2001) Dural tears in lumbar burst fractures with greenstick lamina fractures. Spine 26:E410–E415
4. Baharuddin A, Go BT, Firdaus MN et al (2002) Bovine pericardium for dural graft: clinical results in 22 patients. Clin Neurol Neurosurg 104:342–344
5. Beach HHA (1897) Gold foil in cerebral surgery. Boston Med Surg J 136:281–282
6. Cammisa FP Jr, Eismont FJ, Green B (1989) Dural laceration occurring with burst fractures and associated laminar fractures. J Bone Joint Surg Am 71:1044–1052
7. Danish SF, Samdani A, Hanna A et al (2006) Experience with acellular human dura and bovine collagen matrix for duraplasty after posterior fossa decompression for Chiari malformations. J Neurosurg Pediatrics 104:16–20
8. Eismont FJ, Wiesel SW, Rothman RH (1981) Treatment of dural tears associated with spinal surgery. J Bone Joint Surg Am 63:1132–1136
9. Foy AB, Giannini C, Raffel C (2008) Allergic reaction to a bovine dural substitute following spinal cord untethering. J Neurosurg Pediatrics 1:167–169
10. Hoshi K, Yoshino H, Urata J et al (2000) Creutzfeldt-Jakob disease associated with cadaveric dura mater grafts in Japan. Neurology 55:718–721
11. Keenen TL, Antony J, Benson DR (1990) Dural tears associated with lumbar burst fractures. J Orthop Trauma 4:243–245
12. Kuhn J, Hofmann B, Knitelius HO et al (2005) Bilateral subdural hematomata and lumbar pseudomeningocele due to a chronic leakage of liquor cerebrospinalis after a lumbar discectomy with the application of ADCON-L gel. J Neurol Neurosurg Psychiatry 76:1031–1034
13. Narotam PK, Reddy K, Fewer D et al (2007) Collagen matrix duraplasty for cranial and spinal surgery: a clinical and imaging study. J Neurosurg 106:45–51
14. Narotam PK, van Dellen JR, Bhoola KD (1995) A clinicopathological study of collagen sponge as a dural graft in neurosurgery. J Neurosurg 82:406–412
15. Ophof R, Maltha JC, Von den Hoff JW et al (2004) Histologic evaluation of skin-derived and collagen-based substrates implanted in palatal wounds. Wound Repair Regen 12:528–538
16. Preul MC, Campbell PK, Bichard WD et al (2007) ApplicKation of a hydrogel sealant improves watertight closures of duraplasty onlay grafts in a canine craniotomy model. J Neurosurg 107:642–650

Civilian Gunshot Injury to the Spine

35

Zbigniew Gugala and Ronald W. Lindsey

35.1 Introduction

Although recently, the crime rate has steadily declined in the USA, most violent incidents continue to involve firearms. Nonfatal firearm-related crime had plummeted since 1993, before increasing in 2005 (Fig. 35.1). Moreover, the gun availability among civilians is reflected by the rising incidence of assault (57%), self-inflicted (20%), and unintentional (13%) firearm injuries and has culminated in an extremely high prevalence of gunshot injuries in the United States civilian population [10, 27, 66].

Firearm-related injuries have become a public health problem. At present, gunshot injuries constitute the second most common cause of injury-related death in the United States. Nonfatal firearm-related injuries are 3–5 times more common than lethal injuries [2]. Both have a devastating impact on American society causing substantial emotional and financial burden (Table 35.1). A cost analysis of the medical expenses related to gunshot injury in the USA yielded an average cost of $17,000 for every gunshot injury in 1994, which amounted $2.3 billion in lifetime medical expenses for gunshot injury patients [12]. Nearly half of these costs are imposed on US tax payers, creating an enormous burden on the US health system.

Compared to blunt trauma or stabbing injuries, gunshot injuries to the spine are distinct clinical entities (Table 35.2) exhibiting significant differences in injury mechanism, its extent and severity, clinical course, prognosis, and subsequent treatment. The high incidence of

civilian gunshot injuries to the spine demands that all physicians become familiar with the management principles of patients with these injuries. This chapter examines spine injuries secondary to civilian gunshots, including epidemiology, basic wound ballistics, clinical patterns of injury, patient evaluation, and treatment. In the management of spinal gunshot injuries, the authors will address the indications for nonsurgical and surgical therapeutic modalities, as well as emphasize the potential complications pertinent to the penetrating injury.

35.2 Initial Assessment of Patients with Spinal Gunshot Injury

35.2.1 General Evaluation of Patients

Patient evaluation following gunshot injury to the spine begins with a thorough history and initial clinical examination. The pertinent aspects of the history include the type of weapon, shooting distance, bullet type, and its trajectory. These data may be the best early predictors of the spine injury location, severity, and the involvement of the surrounding anatomic structures.

The initial physical examination should determine the location of all entrance and exit wounds, and these wounds should be assessed to establish the extent of local soft-tissue injury and the path of the bullet. Except for excessive bleeding, the wound should not be explored outside of the operating room because of the risk of increased morbidity [26]. As per the Advanced Trauma Life Support (ATLS) guidelines [79], the initial assessment of a patient with spinal gunshot injury includes the patency of airway, breathing, circulation, and neurologic status. A patent airway should be expeditiously identified

Z. Gugala (✉)
R.W. Lindsey
Department of Orthopaedic Surgery and Rehabilitation, University of Texas Medical Branch, 301 University Blvd, Galveston, TX 77555, USA
e-mail: zgugala@utmb.edu

V.V. Patel et al. (eds.), *Spine Trauma*,
DOI: 10.1007/978-3-642-03694-1_35, © Springer-Verlag Berlin Heidelberg 2010

Fig. 35.1 Nonfatal firearm-related crime had plummeted since 1993, before increasing in 2005. Source: [75]

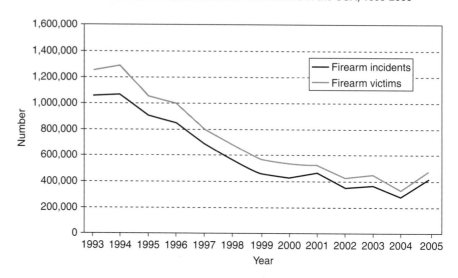

Table 35.1 Medical cost per case for hospitalized patients with nonfatal and fatal gunshot injuries. Hospital discharge data from Maryland 1994–1995

	Nonfatal injuries			Fatal injuries		
	N	Acute care cost [$]	Total care cost [$]	N	Acute care cost [$]	Total care cost [$]
All gunshots	2,394	14,747	36,685	200	11,397	13,191
Assaults	1,470	15,756	41,755	107	13,325	15,410
Unintentional	516	11,897	26,127	21	9,087	10,603
Self-inflicted	50	29,619	47,558	37	8,893	10,245
Intent unknown	357	12,684	29,533	35	9,947	11,033

Total cost is the average of the lifetime cost factors multiplied each case. Adapted from: [12]

Table 35.2 Incidence of cervical spine injury *and/or* cervical spinal cord injury in relation to blunt, stub, and gunshot injury etiology

	Blunt (N=4,390)		Stub (N=7,483)		Gunshot (N=12,573)	
	N	Rate	N	Rate	N	Rate
Spine injury	18	0.41%*	9	0.12%**	165	1.31%
Cord injury	6	0.14%*	8	0.11%*	117	0.94%
Spine *or* cord injury	19	0.43%*	11	0.15%**	168	1.35%
Spine *and* cord injury	5	0.11%*	6	0.08%*	114	0.92%

*$p<0.05$ compared to gunshot injuries; **$p<0.05$ compared to blunt injuries. Adapted from: [58]

or established immediately after the patient's arrival at the hospital. Spontaneous breathing must then be documented or external ventilation initiated. Hemorrhage, the most prevalent cause of deaths after gunshot trauma, must be quickly controlled to ensure hemodynamic stability [79]. The timely diagnosis and treatment of injuries to major vessels has utmost priority and ultimately determines patient survival. Finally, a careful initial neurologic evaluation is performed in accordance with the patient's level of consciousness. Spine gunshot injuries, especially cervical, can be compounded by injuries to the head (Fig. 35.2). Concomitant craniocerebral injuries are particularly devastating. The postresuscitation Glasgow Coma Scale is the most predictive factor

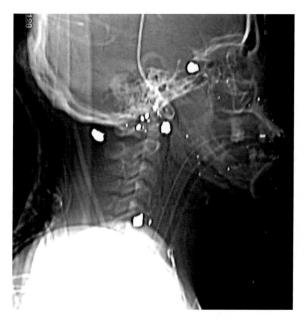

Fig. 35.2 Multiple low-energy gunshot injuries to the neck and head. In the presence of craniocerebral trauma, the postresuscitation Glasgow Coma Scale is the most predictive factor in determining patient survival. Adapted from: [29]

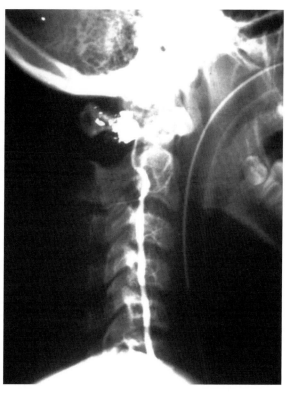

Fig. 35.3 Angiogram depicting cervical (C2) gunshot injury with the vertebral artery damage. The patient developed Wallenberg' syndrome characterized by the decreased blood flow in the posterior inferior cerebellar artery. Clinically, the patient has developed ipsilateral loss of cranial nerves V, IX, X, and XI associated with cerebellar ataxia

in determining patient survival [64]. Subsequently, patients' sensory and motor neurologic status should be documented using the Frankel Scale [25] or the American Spinal Injury Association (ASIA) Impairment Score (ASIA 2002). Most importantly, the clinician must specifically establish the presence of neurologic deficit and designate whether that deficit is complete or incomplete. In gunshot injuries to the spine, it is important to appreciate that the neurologic deficit, if present, may not occur at the level of the wound or bony injury [16]. A thorough neurologic assessment can only be finalized after the resolution of the spinal shock.

The density of vital anatomic structures in the neck makes gunshot injuries in this region extremely susceptible for injuries that are often life threatening [8]. Airway injuries necessitate emergent intubation; carotid and vertebral artery perforations (Fig. 35.3) should be suspected with pulsatile neck bleeding. Immediate restoration of cerebral blood flow is vital and temporary stents can be placed emergently. Pharyngeal and esophageal wounds are often associated with infections and therefore they must also be detected and carefully evaluated. Before multidetector computed tomography (MDCT) can be implemented, endoscopy may be more effective and expeditious for neck gunshot injury assessment and surveillance in the acute setting. The specific indications for

emergent surgery can be further influenced by the location of the neck zone of injury [63] (Fig. 35.4) combined with clinical symptoms at presentation. In particular, zone II injuries deep to platysma frequently require an emergent surgical exploration [32].

Gunshots to the chest are the most prevalent, and yield a high rate of mortality due to fatal cardiac and aortic injuries. Transmediastinal gunshot wounds enter the tight confines of the mediastinum, and therefore, are associated with injuries to vital structures, such as the heart, great vessels, lungs, esophagus, and trachea. Careful chest auscultation can detect asymmetric breath sounds indicating a hemothorax or pneumothorax. Cardiac monitoring, which should include the assessment of distal pulses, can suggest heart perforation, aortic disruption, or tamponade. Also, the incidence of diaphragmatic injuries is extremely high (70–90% for the left lower chest gunshot injuries; 10–20% for abdominal gunshot injuries) and should always be considered.

Fig. 35.4 Neck zone designation is very helpful in determining potential injuries to the neck as a result of penetrating trauma

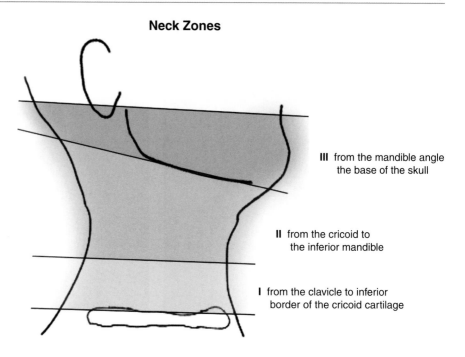

Neck Zones

III from the mandible angle the base of the skull

II from the cricoid to the inferior mandible

I from the clavicle to inferior border of the cricoid cartilage

Similarly, the initial examination of the abdomen is focused on suspected vascular, hollow viscus, and internal organs (kidney, liver, spleen) injuries. In particular, colonic perforations that may occur before the missile traverses through the spine must be recognized, because they are associated with a high rate of spinal infection if appropriate intravenous antibiotics are not promptly administered. In patients with extensive spinal cord deficit, the initial abdominal exam may be unreliable due to the loss of visceral sensation. Diagnostic peritoneal lavage may be indicated even prior to abdominal computed tomography.

In the pelvis, sacral gunshot wounds are most often complicated by hemorrhage. In addition, rectal and genitourinary examination should be done to detect potential injuries to sacral neural structures. For posterior gunshot wounds, sterile packing of the posterior bullet hole using bone wax can be effective in facilitating tamponade. Likewise, emergent angiographic embolization can diminish or halt severe bleeding, but with the risk of possible devascularization of the neural structures.

35.2.2 Spine Injury Evaluation

When the patient has been ventilated and hemodynamically stabilized, spine injury can be evaluated.

The physical examination is similar to that for blunt spinal trauma. Each spinous process must be palpated for tenderness and/or crepitus. An in-depth neurologic examination, which includes motor, sensory reflexes, and anal sphincter tone is mandatory and must be documented precisely. The neurologic examination can be challenging in the intubated or unconscious patient, the neurologic examination can be challenging. However, if paralytic agents have not been administered, deep tendon and bulbocavernosus reflexes may still be elicited.

About 18% of patients with gunshot injury to the neck sustain actual with cervical spine injury [38]. Biomechanically, gunshot injuries to the cervical spine are rarely unstable. Neurologic injuries, however, are highly prevalent, and typically involve the spinal cord and its related structures. The thoracolumbar spine neural structures at risk for gunshot injury include the spinal cord, the conus medullaris, as well as the cauda equina. The neurological findings can range from spinal shock, to upper-, lower- or mixed motor neuron deficits. The precise localization of the level of injury is established by imaging combined with an accurate neurological examination to determine the neural structures involved and the subsequent clinical management and prognosis.

35.2.3 Imaging

Imaging is crucial to the evaluation process, and the minimum study consists of anteroposterior and/or lateral plain radiography spine views (Fig. 35.5). These images can assist in determining the spinal segments involved and the associated structures at risk. Radiographic imaging is not directed toward clearing the cervical spine because most gunshot injuries to this spine are stable.

Hemodynamically stable gunshot injury patients should be promptly evaluated using MDCT to more precisely determine the extent and location of injury (Fig. 35.6). MDCT is especially helpful in accurately visualizing the bullet track and/or the presence of ratained bullet or bone fragments (Fig. 35.7). The ability of MDCT to provide volumetric data during peak vascular contrast enhancement in patients with gunshot injuries permits high-resolution imaging, effective image postprocessing (MPR, MIP mIP), as well as three-dimensional reconstructions. Improved image quality and manipulation of volumetric data allow not only a more accurate diagnosis of injury, detection of injuries secondary to the missile trajectory but also delineates precisely the injuries that have been sustained remotely. MDCT results reliably determine

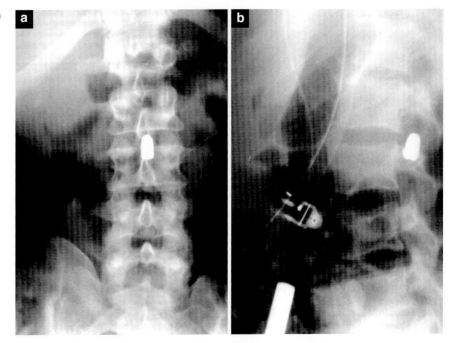

Fig. 35.5 Anteroposterior (**a**) and lateral (**b**) plane radiographs depicting gunshot injury to the lumbar spine with bullet retention in the spinal canal

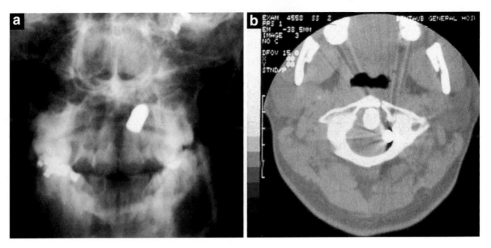

Fig. 35.6 Open-mouth view (**a**) and axial CT scan (**b**) depicting cervical (C1-C2) gunshot injury. The patient was neurologically intact; bony injuries include C1 lateral mass and ring fracture and type II odontoid fracture. The injury rendered the spine unstable and was treated with halo-vest immobilization

Fig. 35.7 Multidetector computed tomography (**a**, coronal; **b**, axial) is the most efficacious imaging modality for spine gunshot injuries in determining bullet trajectory, bullet retention, and also in delineating sustained concomitant injuries

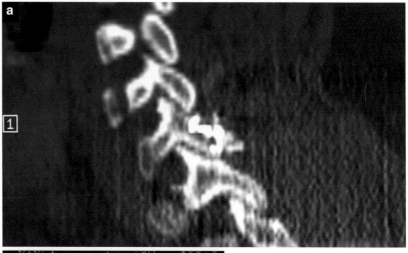

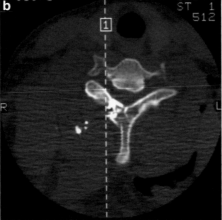

the need for further diagnostic workup and/or clinical intervention (Fig. 35.8).

Magnetic resonance imaging (MRI) of the spine is usually contraindicated in the acute setting even in the presence of neurologic deficit. Ferromagnetism of the missile can produce artifacts and image obscurity as well as induce deflection of the bullet and possibly cause additional injury [74]. Although it has been suggested that MRI better delineates the relation between the retained bullet and the cord than a CT scan [21], the information provided by MRI rarely affects management or outcome. In selected cases of cord injury without retained missile fragments, MRI may complement the CT scan by better characterizing the extent of spinal cord injury [5].

Although spinal stability is often thought to be maintained following gunshot injury to the spine, recent clinical experience suggests otherwise [33]. In the conscious, cooperative, and medically stable patient suspected of late instability, voluntary lateral flexion/extension radiography is reasonable (Fig. 35.9). However, dynamic imaging is rarely indicated in the acute setting.

35.3 Initial Treatment

The treatment of patients with gunshot injury to the spine should adhere to the standard algorithm depicted in Fig. 35.10. The first priority in the treatment of

Fig. 35.8 Voluntary flexion (**a**) and extension (**b**) dynamic radiographs can be useful in ruling out instability in the subacute course of the gunshot injury to the spine with the persistence of symptoms

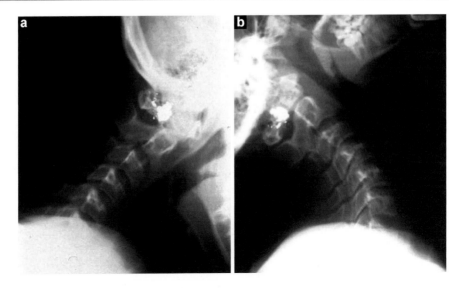

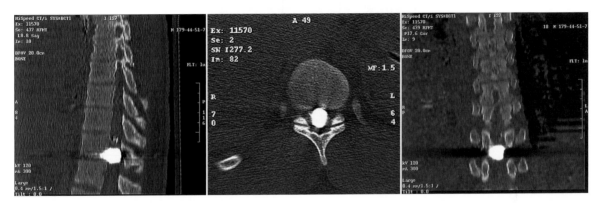

Fig. 35.9 Sagittal (*left*), axial (*middle*) and coronal (*right*) CT projections demonstrating gunshot injury to the thoracic (Th10) spine with bullet lodged in the spinal canal. Patients developed spinal shot and permanent compete spinal cord injury

gunshot injuries to the spine is the general medical condition of the patient [33, 45, 71]. If the patient is medically unstable, it suggests the presence of a visceral or vascular injury, which constitutes an emergency. The visceral injuries associated with spinal gunshot injuries can include hollow viscus and/or major vessel disruption and pulmonary, cardiac, abdominal viscera, and genitourinary lesions. During this phase of treatment, all standard precautions should be employed to protect the spine from additional injury (e.g., back board, sandbags, maintaining the patient in a supine position). At this juncture, apart from an assessment of the patient's neurologic status, all efforts should be focused on stabilizing the patient's potentially life-threatening injuries.

35.4 Pharmacologic Management

35.4.1 Antibiotics

Patients with gunshot injuries to the thoracolumbar spine should be administered high-dose parenteral broad-spectrum antibiotics and tetanus prophylaxis at

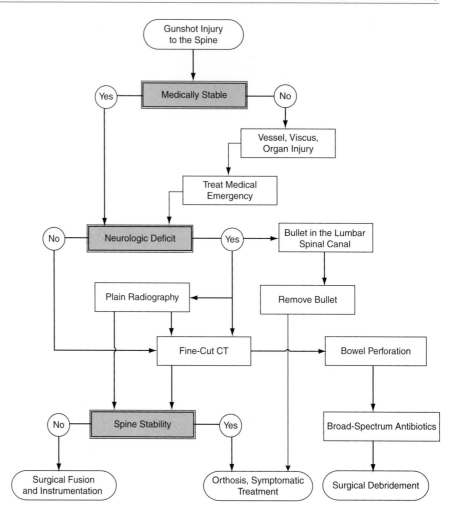

Fig. 35.10 The authors' recommended algorithm for the management of civilian spine gunshot injuries

presentation. Broad-spectrum antibiotic therapy should include coverage for gram-negative and anaerobic organisms, and is especially warranted for high-energy wounds or gunshot injuries in which the bowel is perforated. The antibiotics should be continued through the acute phase of management and/or until the patient has been cleared of associated injury

35.4.2 Steroids

The primary gunshot injury (mechanical) to the spinal cord can be potentiated by the secondary mechanisms (biochemical) that form the premise for the administration of steroids. In blunt spinal cord injury,

it has been demonstrated that all of the damage to the spinal cord does not occur with the initial trauma, but continues with persistent compression [15]. However, the administration of steroids for gunshot spinal cord injury is highly controversial, as presently there are no prospective randomized studies to justify their clinical use. Recent retrospective studies have failed to demonstrate neurologic recovery with steroid administration for ballistic spinal cord injury, and moreover, these studies suggest that steroids in this setting can be extremely hazardous (Table 35.3) [30, 31, 41, 54]. These patients have been shown to be at significantly greater risk for infection or gastrointestinal complications [31]. Therefore, the routine administration of steroids in gunshot spinal cord injury is not recommended.

Table 35.3 Complications of steroid administrations in patients with gunshot injury to the spine [31]

		Spinal infection		Extraspinal infection		Gastrointestinal complication		Pancreatitis	
		%	p value	%	p value	%	p value	%	p value
No steroids	(n = 193)	2.6		16.1		2.6		5.2	
Methylprednisolone	(n = 31)	3.2	0.6	25.8	0.2	0	0.47	16.1	0.04*
Dexamethasone	(n = 30)	10	0.078	20	0.59	13.3	0.021*	0	0.37
Combined steroids	(n = 61)	6.6	0.23	23	0.24	6.6	0.23	8.2	0.36

35.5 Surgical Management

35.5.1 Surgery for Neurologic Deficit

Once the patient is deemed medically stable in the emergency setting, subsequent treatment is determined by the patient's neurologic status. Surgery is not indicated in the presence of a complete neurologic deficit, surgery is not indicated, as the literature, to date, suggests that surgical intervention will not affect the ultimate neurologic outcome. Spine decompression for gunshot-related neurologic deficit has not only proven to be ineffective, but may be detrimental. Stauffer et al. [72] reviewed 185 spine gunshot injury patients with complete neurologic deficits following treatment with surgical decompression. Decompression not only failed to improve the neurologic status of these patients, but also precipitated a multitude of other complications including instability, infection, and spinal fluid fistula [72].

Complete neurologic lesions involving the cauda equina may experience some degree of spontaneous resolution, especially with the typical civilian injury due to a low-energy gunshot wound. Stauffer et al. [72] reported a 94% improvement in patients with cauda equina neurologic deficits treated nonoperatively. Benzel et al. [7] reported improved recovery of nerve root function in all patients with cauda equina gunshot injuries with or without surgery. Isiklar and Lindsey [34] retrospectively studied 37 patients with low-energy gunshot injuries to the spine and further corroborated that neurologic recovery of one or two Frankel grades could be realized in patients with cauda equina injuries.

The presence of a missile fragment in proximity to neural elements may constitute a relative indication for decompression and bullet explantation. A collaborative study was performed by the National Spinal Cord Injury Model Systems, and consisted of serial neurologic examinations of 66 patients with bullet fragments impinging on neural elements. This prospective series concluded that patients with gunshot-related neurologic deficits can experience significant neurologic recovery, if the bullet was removed from the T12-L4 spinal segments [81]. Therefore, the neurologic anatomy of the thoracolumbar region may exhibit a more favorable response to surgical decompression in those patients sustaining low-energy gunshot injuries [13, 81]. The optimal timing for decompression is unclear, but should at least be delayed until spinal shock has resolved. An absolute, but rare, indication for immediate decompression would be a patient's sudden neurologic deterioration in the presence of clear neural element compromise from the gunshot injury.

If the gunshot injury to the thoracic and/or lumbar spine does not present with neurologic deficit, the indication for surgical interventions would be predicated on the risk for complications associated with the retention of the bullet or the presence of spinal instability.

35.5.2 Surgery for Retained Missile Fragments

Bullet removal is rarely indicated following spinal gunshot injuries. Missile fragments that are lodged within the vertebral body, in the posterior elements, or have traversed through the spine and into the surrounding soft tissue are usually not problematic. Relative indications for missile removal would include a missile (or secondary bone fragments) lodged within the spinal canal that may cause late neurologic deficit, the missile that has perforated the alimentary canal prior to entering the spine, or the bullet at risk for causing toxicity. Missile fragments (both bullet and bone) that significantly compromise the spinal canal can threaten the patient's neurologic function, especially when located at the thoracolumbar regions [3, 4, 11]. Early semielective excision of these fragments has been shown to improve motor recovery with conus medullaris and/or cauda equina injuries [37, 60, 81]. When missile fragments do not risk neural compromise, periodic radiographic evaluation is recommended. Retained bullet fragments may migrate and thereby cause late neurologic deficits [4, 36, 40, 50, 73].

35.5.3 Surgery for Debridement

The incidence of infection after spinal civilian gunshot injury is low and usually occurs in patients who have experienced perforation of the alimentary tract before the missile enters the spine. Therefore, for all spinal gunshot injuries with alimentary track involvement, it is crucial to determine not only the wound trajectory but also its direction. The indications for early surgical intervention are especially clear for the spine level when the bullet has perforated the large bowel or hollow viscus. Romanick [62] reported that 7 of 8 patients with spinal gunshot injuries associated with colon perforation developed infections despite receiving prophylactic antibiotics, and concluded that these patients warranted early aggressive surgical debridement. Also Miller et al. [49] advocated surgical intervention with the perforation of the hollow viscus from gunshot wound injuries to the spine, as these contaminated bullets increased the risk of osteomyelitis in associated spinal lesions.

However, the indications for surgical debridement in these patients are also controversial [30]. With the advent of new, potent broad-spectrum antibiotics, a recent trend in the management of low-energy gunshot wounds of the spine traversing the alimentary track has been toward nonoperative treatment and extensive broad-spectrum antibiotic coverage to prevent spinal infection, even when there are bullet fragments lodged in the spinal canal [39, 42, 80, 81]. An initial report by Roffi et al. [61] demonstrated 35 spinal gunshot injury patients with associated alimentary canal perforations, among which 18 were not surgically debrided. Despite the presence of colon perforations in 9 of the 18 nonoperative patients,

none of these patients developed an infection. The authors attributed their results to the sustained use of broad-spectrum intravenous antibiotics for up to 14 days, and recommended the administration of antibiotics for gram-negative and anaerobic organisms for several weeks. In another clinical series [33], only one thoracolumbar spinal gunshot injury became infected; this patient had sustained a colon perforation that was treated only with the antibiotic regimen as recommended by Roffi et al. [61]. More recently, Quigley et al. [56] reviewed 114 patients with low-energy gunshot injuries to the spine, among which 27 (23.7%) sustained a concomitant transgastrointestinal injury. Despite adequate antibiotic coverage, 4 (3.5%) spine and 23 (20.2%) wound infections developed, exhibiting a significantly higher rate ($p=0.001$) in transgastrointestinal spinal gunshot injuries compared to those gunshots that did not traverse the gastrointestinal tract. Three of the five patients (66.6%) with transgastrointestinal gunshot wounds to the spine who underwent spine surgery developed a wound infection, as opposed to 9 of the 22 patients (38.1%) who developed a wound infection without spine surgery. The rate of wound infection with regard to spine surgery was not statistically significant ($p=0.628$).

Although civilian spinal gunshot injuries involving the gastrointestinal tract have raised debate on the merits of surgical debridement in combination with an adequate antibiotic treatment, the authors recommend that strong consideration should be given to the surgical debridement of thoracolumbar spinal gunshot injuries complicated by large bowel perforation.

35.5.4 Bullet Metal Toxicity

Most bullets used in civilian firearms are made from lead. According to the location, the retained lead bullet or its fragments can potentially evolve into lead toxicity, and on this basis preventive early surgical debridement may be indicated. However, this complication is rarely encountered. Lead dissolution typically occurs when the bullet is in contact with the synovial fluid, a pseudocyst, or a disc space [28, 40, 43]. The patient will usually require prolonged exposure to the bullet before experiencing lead poisoning symptoms such as abdominal pain, anemia, headaches, memory loss, and muscle weakness. When this phenomenon occurs, medical treatment consisting of chelation therapy with EDTA (ethylenediaminetetraacetate), D-penicillamine, or dimercaprol may prove effective even prior to the eventual bullet removal [34].

Bullets that contain copper or brass exhibit pronounced toxicity to the spine neural elements when retained in their proximity. In an experimental study [78], implanted copper fragments similar to those contained in bullets induced local neurotoxicity involving as much as 10% of the spinal cord area. Histologically, there was a major destruction of both the axons and the myelin of the dorsal column adjacent to the intradural copper fragments. The results of this study confirmed that copper contained in commercially available bullets can cause varying degrees of neural destruction independent of the mechanical injury, and prophylactic removal may be warranted.

35.5.5 Surgery for Spine Instability

Because low-energy gunshot injuries typically do not render the spine unstable, most spinal gunshot injuries can be treated with an orthosis. Historically, most of the reported cases of instability secondary to spinal gunshot injuries have been iatrogenic as a result of an ill-advised surgical decompression [72]. However, Denis [17] reported a case of lumbar spine instability following gunshot injury, and Isiklar and Lindsey [33] reported a few cases of gunshot-related cervical and lumbar instability despite appropriate external immobilization. These authors concluded that spinal stability following gunshot injuries although common, it is not necessarily guaranteed. This is especially a concern with gunshot injury at the hypermobile cervical region of the spine. Therefore, all patients with spinal gunshot injures should initially be placed in an appropriate orthotic support or brace, and be closely monitored until sufficient spinal stability has been established.

Significant comminution of the entire vertebral body poses a special concern as it increases the risk for late spinal collapse and/or pronounced angular deformity. If surgical intervention to establish stability is warranted, techniques that limit the number of stabilized motion segments are preferred as the extent of instability is usually limited to the traumatized motion segment. Furthermore, extensive decompression of the traumatized segments should be avoided (unless otherwise indicated) as this may only further destabilize the spine. Typically, posterior instrumentation alone will suffice. However, in the case of extensive comminution of both anterior and middle columns of the lumbar region, an anterior procedure may be more appropriate. Surgical techniques which require "front and back" stabilization are rarely indicated.

35.6 Complications

The late complications associated with gunshot injury to the spine are numerous (Table 35.4). Contrary to a blunt spine injury, severe deafferent pain is common in patients with spinal cord injury following gunshot [22]. Symptoms usually consist of a searing, burning sensation that radiates into the paralyzed limbs. Focal pain can occur at the site of injury despite retained stability or bony healing. Pain severity usually subsides with time. Commonly, the pain is not related to the retained missile fragments; therefore, the removal surgery is often ineffective in providing pain relief.

Cerebral spinal fluid leakage with cutaneous fistula formation may occur as a direct sequela of gunshot injury [82], or as a result of surgical intervention [72]. If missile removal is warranted, a 7–10 day delay has been recommended in combination with a tight closure of the dura, paraspinal muscles, and fascia [22].

Late infections occur in approximately 7–12% of spinal gunshot injury patients [80]. The incidence appears to increase with early decompression, or if the bullet has traversed large bowel before entering the spinal column [62]. Infection should always be considered in patients with severe, persistent pain of unknown etiology.

Table 35.4 Complications related to spine gunshot injury [46]

Complication	% of patients (N = 41)
Pain	54
Infection	40
Pneumothorax	24
Fractures (nonspinal)	22
Colon perforation	40
CSF leak	24
Retroperitoneal hematoma	22

35.7 Conclusions

Gunshot injuries to the spine constitute the second most common cause of spinal cord injury in the USA. Therefore, it is imperative for the clinician to be familiar with the distinctions of the penetrating vs. blunt spine injuries. The clinician should appreciate the ballistic principles of missile wounding, and be able to clinically determine gunshot injury severity. At presentation, patients with gunshot injuries to the spine receive parenteral broad-spectrum antibiotics and tetanus prophylaxis. As opposed to blunt spine trauma patients, in penetrating spine trauma with neurologic deficit, steroids are not indicated. Spinal decompression has not proven to be effective for gunshot injuries, and should be reserved for cases in which progressive neurologic deficit or cauda equina injuries exist. Spinal debridement in combination with broad-spectrum antibiotics should be considered in patients with concomitant large bowel perforation. Spinal gunshot injury rarely results in spinal instability; however, the patient warrants careful monitoring until stability has been clearly established.

APPENDIX

Epidemiology of Spinal Civilian Gunshot Injury

There has been a steady increase in the number of patients who are admitted with penetrating injuries to urban trauma centers throughout the United States. Accordingly, there has been a significant rise in the incidence of gunshot injuries to the spine. At present, gunshot injuries to the spine account for 13% of all spinal injuries and rank third only to falls and motor vehicle accidents [81, 83, 84].

In recent years, spinal cord injury as a result of a gunshot almost doubled, from 13% to 25% [91]. Civilian gunshot injuries to the spine in US urban regions constitute the second most common cause of all spinal cord injury following only motor vehicle accidents [9, 46, 82, 90]. Gunshot vs. blunt spinal cord injury patient populations differ epidemiologically, primarily in their ethnicity, socioeconomic status, and injury severity [46] (Table 35.5). Typically,

Table 35.5 Demographic comparison of patients with spinal cord injury secondary to gunshot vs. nonviolent trauma [46]

	GS SCI [%]	NT SCI [%]
Gender		
Male	95.1	79.7
Female	4.9	20.3
Ethnicity		
Caucasian	9.8	51.5
Non-Caucasian	91.2	48.5
Marital status		
Never married	70.7	38.9
Married	19.5	44.3
Not married	9.8	16.8
Employment status		
Employed	41.5	75.4
Unemployed	58.5	24.5
Mean age	27.1	42.2

gunshot spinal cord injury casualties are males, 25–30 years of age [9, 66, 82], and 92% of minority ethnicity [9, 46, 85].

Although gunshot injuries to the thoracic spine are most frequent (50–60%) followed by the lumbar spine, gunshot injuries to the cervical spine are more typically life threatening. Approximately, 80% of spinal gunshot injury patients experience associated injuries to the lungs, heart, hollow viscus, and/or major vessels [9, 35, 46, 90]. Recent advances in trauma care have enhanced the overall survival rate of gunshot injury patients; however, firearm-inflicted injuries to the spine carry a poor prognosis [33] with a considerable inherent risk for permanent complete spinal cord and/or peripheral nerve damage.

Ballistic Principles of a Gunshot Injury

Ballistics is the science of projectile motion and characterizes three phases of missile projection: its passage through the barrel of a firearm (interior ballistics), its subsequent trajectory through the air (external ballistics), and its penetration of the target (terminal ballistics).

Wound ballistics is a part of terminal ballistics that characterizes the motion and interactions of a projectile in living tissues.

All firearms can be classified into three major categories according to their muzzle velocity: low velocity (<350 m/s), medium velocity (350–600 m/s), and high velocity (>600 m/s). Handguns (except for magnums) are low-velocity weapons; shotguns and magnum handguns are of medium velocity; and high-velocity weapons are usually rifles. Gunshot wounds in civilians are typically the result of low- or medium-velocity firearms. Muzzle velocity alone does not determine the wounding potential of a firearm, and therefore, the type of firearm alone is not synonymous with the type of wound created [23, 24, 44]. The type of bullet used can greatly affect wounding, and this is most evident with shotguns. Although shotguns are medium-velocity weapons, the large total mass of their lead pellets dramatically increases their kinetic energy. Depending on the distance to the target and the size of pellets, shotguns can possess the wounding potential of high-velocity firearms or multiple low-velocity weapons.

Wounding Potential

The wounding potential of a projectile reflects its kinematics and physical characteristics while penetrating the target tissue (Table 35.6). The primary determinant of missile wounding potential is the amount of its energy dissipated within the tissue after the impact. Missile deceleration and subsequent energy transfer are functions of the missile entry energy, missile design, (target tissue) characteristics, and missile behavior within the tissue [1].

Impact Energy

Total kinetic energy of the missile at striking the target is the sum of rotational and advancing missile energies, and is proportional to the missile mass and the impact velocity squared ($\sim mv^2$). In general, an impact velocity of approximately 50 m/s is necessary to penetrate the skin, whereas a velocity of 65 m/s is needed to fracture bone [6]. The missile's muzzle and impact energies are not equivalent, because some of the missile energy is

Table 35.6 Missile wounding potential

Impact energy (rotational and advancing kinetic energy)
Type of firearm (handgun, rifle, shotgun)
Muzzle velocity
Distance to the target
Close vs. far range (handguns 45 m; rifles 95 m)
Bullet stability during flight (yawing, precession, nutation)
Missile design
Geometry (bullets, pellets; hollow- and soft-nose; dum-dum)
Mass (birdshot, buckshot shotgun cartridges)
Caliber (standard, magnum)
Material (lead, lead alloys)
Jacket
Target tissue characteristics
Elasticity
Density
Hollow organs
Fluid-filled organs
Target tissue characteristics
Cavitation (permanent, temporary)
Fragmentation
Shock waves

reduced during flight. The magnum shell of a firearm enhances the muzzle velocity of the bullet by 20–60% by increasing the gunpowder charge. The mass of the missile (e.g., shotgun pellets) can be as vital as the muzzle velocity in the determination of the impact energy [67]. It is important to appreciate the amount of energy transferred to the tissue, as this energy constitutes the major wounding potential of a missile. The designation of the wounding potential based on the type of firearm or its muzzle velocity alone is unreliable, since most of the civilian gunshot injuries are inflicted with low- or medium-velocity weapons.

Distance to the Target

The distance between a firearm and the target greatly affects the missile wounding potential. Missile muzzle energy decreases significantly if the distance to the target exceeds 45 m for low- or 90 m for high-velocity firearms. The effect of the distance to the target is best demonstrated with shotguns, where the distance to the target is the basis for classifying shotgun severity [52, 69]. In contrast to typical civilian bullets, which are pointed, round shotgun pellets have poor aerodynamic properties and lose their kinetic energy rapidly during flight. At close range (<5 m), shotgun pellets act essentially as one mass causing massive tissue destruction. The impact energy of a shotgun fired at this distance is similar to that of a high-velocity firearm. Very close proximity of the shotgun to the target (<2 m) results in not only the pellet projection, but also shell fragment and wadding contamination. Pellets projected at a distance of more than 5 m scatter substantially during flight, and their tissue penetration is usually limited to the deep fascia (5–12 m) or superficial skin (>12 m) [69].

Missile Design

The components of missile design such as its geometry, mass, caliber, material, and the presence of a jacket determine the missile interactions with the target tissue. Civilian bullets are typically made of lead and have no jacket. These bullets deform easily on impact, exhibit decreased tissue penetration, and have an increased possibility of bullet retention, thereby dissipating more energy within the tissue. Conversely, military bullets have a copper jacket (Hague Convention 1899) that prevents bullet deformation, increases tissue penetration, and decreases the likelihood of missile retention. The wounding potential of a shotgun is dependent on a "bolus" blast effect which can be reduced by pellet spreading. The wounding potential of buckshot is greater than birdshot, and can be equivalent to multiple low-caliber handgun wounds.

Target Tissue Characteristics

Missile energy dissipation is directly related to the target tissue density and inversely related to the target tissue elasticity. Projectiles striking tissues of low density and high elasticity, such as lungs, result in a small energy dissipation and minor wounding. Organs with very low or no elasticity such as the liver, spleen, blood vessels, and neural structures absorb considerable energy and can be damaged significantly. Fluid-filled organs such as the bladder, heart, great vessels, and bowel can explode because of the pressure waves generated on missile energy transfer. Dense, nonelastic

tissues such as bone are of special concern because of the significant amount of energy that is dissipated, even with little penetration. Secondary missiles caused by bone and/or bullet fragmentation can further compound local tissue damage.

Missile Behavior Within the Target Tissue

Persistent minor deviations of the bullet from its trajectory during flight increase the energy released in the target tissue. Dense tissues increase the tumbling and yawing of the bullet and result in greater energy dissipation. Likewise, bullet fragmentation within the tissue increases the energy transfer. For nonfragmenting missiles, a longer wound track is necessary to impart their full wounding potential.

Clinical Determinants of Gunshot Injury Severity

Clinical severity of a gunshot injury is determined by the amount of projectile energy dissipated within the tissue after the impact and the critical nature of the specific anatomic structures injured [29] (Table 35.7). Primary mechanisms of tissue damage result from the physical consequences of a projectile passing through the tissue, and can include laceration and crushing (permanent cavitation); transient displacement and stretching of the tissue radially outward of the projectile track (temporary cavitation); and shock waves propagated remotely within the tissue (Fig. 35.11). Secondary injuring mechanisms may result from displaced bone fragments, or may occur as a result of the victim's falling after the shot.

Injury Energy

Gunshot wounds are typically designated as low- or high energy, depending on the extent of the kinetic energy of a projectile dissipated within a tissue. Low-energy wounds are typically caused by guns with nonjacketed bullets that create short tracts through less dense and elastic tissues (skin, adipose tissue, muscle, trabecular

Table 35.7 Clinical determinants of gunshot injury severity

Energy dissipated within tissue
    Low-energy injury (handguns)
    High-energy injury (rifles; close-range shotguns)

Vital structure involvement
    Severe (central nervous system; viscera, major vessels)
    Moderate (structural nonvital organ/tissue)
    Mild (transient functional damage)

Gunshot tissue penetration
    Grazing / blast injuries
    Penetrating (no exit wound)
    Perforating (entrance and exit wounds)

Presence of fracture
    Unstable fracture requiring stabilization
    Stable fracture ("drill hole" bone injuries)
    Intraarticular

Degree of wound contamination
    Gross (hollow viscus, large bowel traversing)
    Moderate (clothing debris)
    Relatively clean

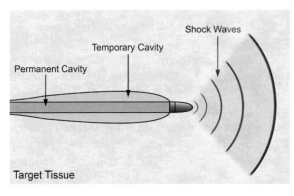

Fig. 35.11 Tissue damage following gunshot results from the physical consequences of a projectile passing through the tissue, and includes laceration and crushing (permanent cavity); transient displacement and stretching of the tissue radially outward of the projectile track (temporary cavity); and shock waves propagated remotely within the tissue

bone). This low-energy trauma is usually localized to the missile track and results in local cutting and/or crushing mechanisms. In rare circumstances, an injury created by a high-velocity missile to low-density tissues may be considered as low energy.

In high-energy transfer gunshot injuries, tissue damage is more significant because of the presence of temporary cavitation. In addition, high-energy missiles can create shock waves that propagate in the target tissue and thereby are capable of inflicting remote injuries. High-mass missiles can result in a high-energy injury, even if inflicted by low- or medium-velocity weapons such as a shotgun [67]. Designation of the energy dissipation within the tissue is done by a thorough clinical assessment of the gunshot wound, since the details of the specific type of firearm and the injury circumstances are rarely available to the clinician.

Anatomic Structure Involvement

In designating the clinical severity of the gunshot injury, apart from the missile energy, it is imperative to determine the involvement of vital anatomic structures and to assess the nature and extent of this damage. In select gunshot injuries, the involvement of vital structures can account for greater clinical severity that could be reflected by the ballistic missile wounding potential. In general, patient injuries following gunshots can be divided into two major categories: wounds to vital structures (central and peripheral neural elements, vessels, and viscera) and those to the musculoskeletal tissues. Life-saving interventions should be performed immediately for injuries that disrupt the airway or compromise breathing or the circulatory system. Gunshot injuries involving musculoskeletal tissues (bone, muscle, joints, ligaments/tendons) can result in morbidity, because of instability, severe functional deficit, infection, or the risk for amputation.

Types of Gunshot Wound

Gunshots can inflict three basic types of wounds that include nonpenetrating, penetrating, and perforating. Nonpenetrating wounds occur without the missile completely entering the target tissue (grazing or blast injury). The depth and area of the tissue involved may vary, but typically, the injury is restricted to the superficial soft-tissue layers. Penetrating wounds consist of a missile entry site but no exit. In this setting, the bullet or its fragments are retained within the tissue and the impact kinetic energy of the missile is dissipated within the tissues entirely. In perforating wounds, missile entry and exit sites are present. Clinical distinctions between the entry and exit sites without knowing the detailed circumstances of the injury can be extremely difficult and misleading [70]. Identification of the bullet entry and exit sites may assist in establishing bullet trajectory.

Distinguishing between the penetrating and perforating types of gunshot wounds is critical in determining missile retention in the tissue and reflects the amount of missile energy transferred [45]. Retained bullet fragments warrant surgical excision if they are present intra-articularly (including disk space) [55, 59], within the spinal canal [81], or have traversed the bowel [62]. Brass- or copper-jacketed bullets lodged in proximity to the central or peripheral neural structures may require surgical removal because of their neurotoxicity [47, 68]. The depth of the wound created by the missile also provides a good indication of the energy dissipated within the tissue. Theoretically, the energy transferred in penetrating injuries equals the entire missile impact energy, whereas the transferred energy in perforating gunshot wounds is the difference between the entry and exit energies. Practically, however, a substantial amount of energy is necessary for complete perforation of the target tissues, and this usually occurs with missiles of high-impact energy. Therefore, perforating gunshot injuries tend to be more severe.

Gunshot Injuries to Bone

Gunshot injuries commonly affect bone and cause fractures. The extent of gunshot injury to bone depends on the missile impact energy and the structural properties of the affected bone. Low-energy gunshot injury to porous, low-density, or cancellous bone can result in a "drilled hole" type of bony defect. These usually occur in the pelvis, distal femur, and spine. Highly comminuted fractures are typically caused by high-energy gunshots. The extent of bone comminution corresponds directly with the amount of the missile energy transferred and also suggests the degree of soft-tissue injury. Occasionally, fractures can be caused or compounded secondarily by the victim's fall after the shot. The severity of bone injury caused by gunshot is determined by the ability to maintain physiologic alignment and stability. Spine fractures due to gunshot rarely result in instability.

Infection Risk Secondary to Gunshot Injury

Missiles projected from firearms are not sterile [77] and some bacteria accumulated before the discharge of the missile can remain at the point of tissue impact [89]. Wound contamination, however, primarily originates from the skin flora, clothing, or any other material encountered in the missile path. Although the risk of infection following typical civilian gunshot is rather low, injuries caused by bullets that traverse grossly contaminated areas such as large bowel carry exceptionally high infection risks. Also high-energy gunshot injuries, in contrast to low-energy counterparts, are extremely prone to infection because of the greater soft-tissue damage and the presence of devitalized tissue debris. The extent of local contamination and the presence of devitalized debris are critical in determining the optimal treatment approach.

Gunshot Injury to the Spine Neural Elements

Injury Pathomechanism

Neural structures of the spine can be injured by a gunshot in the following modes: (1) directly by perforating or penetrating missiles; (2) indirectly by displaced bone fragments; (3) remotely by shock waves generated by high-energy missiles; (4) secondarily, by the disruption of the blood supply to the spinal cord and its structures; and (5) as a consequence of loss of spinal stability and/or alignment. The direct violation of the spinal cord by perforating missiles with tearing of the dura and transection of the cord (total or subtotal) is particularly devastating and typically occurs over several spinal segments. In cases of penetrating missiles, the direct destruction of spinal cord structures is further complicated by the bullet's presence in the spine, which acts as a space-occupying mass [87]. Hematoma and fibrous scarring, precipitated by this mass, may cause subsequent injury [86]. A retained bullet in the canal can also result in late complications due to bullet migration [3, 4, 36, 51, 57], lead poisoning [19, 28], neurotoxicity (copper- or brass-containing bullets) [47], and inflammatory foreign body reaction [14].

Indirect mechanisms inflict damage upon spine neural structures by displacing the bone fragments created by the missile or, less frequently, as a result of spinal instability. These mechanisms usually cause neurologic deficit by cord and/or nerve compression, and more closely resemble the damage typically observed following blunt trauma. Unlike blunt insults, high-energy missiles can remotely cause extensive neurologic damage which extends over a distance above and/or below the level of impact even without making contact with the spinal cord. This was demonstrated in an animal model, in which a high-energy gunshot injury to the spinous process of T12 or L1 consistently produced complete neurologic deficits [18] by pressure shock waves propagated remotely from the missile track. The geometry and material properties of the vertebra can deform and focus pressure waves into localized regions; neural tissue appears to be extremely sensitive to the pressure wave injury mechanism.

The sensitivity of neural elements to direct or indirect insults places the cord and its related structures at extreme risk with both high-energy and low-energy injuries. With direct impact, the cord injury is usually well circumscribed and most severe at the site of the insult. Gross pathology may range from small superficial defects, to localized punctures, or incomplete or total cord transection with varying degrees of cerebral spinal fluid extravasation. When the missile traverses the cervical or thoracic spinal canal, a complete neurologic deficit is almost always assured [82]. Because of the transition of the spinal cord to the cauda equina, gunshot injuries in the lumbar spine may produce only partial neurologic deficits. Owing to indirect mechanisms, remote lesions consisting of edema, necrosis, and/or hemorrhage may still occur in the distal cord. The neurologic injury level tends to be at least one segment higher than the vertebral injury level, while the sensory injury level is usually equal to or below the motor level of injury [82, 85]. The spinal cord is also especially sensitive to ischemic changes; gunshot injuries that disrupt the blood vessels supplying the cord and its neural structures often compound pronounced neurologic deficit.

Patterns of Neurologic Deficit

Depending on the spine level affected by a gunshot, neurologic injury may involve a variety of neural elements, including the spinal cord, nerve roots, conus medullaris, and cauda equina. Spine gunshots predominantly occur in the thoracic vs. the hypermobile cervical or thoracolumbar regions associated with blunt trauma. Furthermore, neurologic deficits due to gunshot injuries differ from blunt spinal trauma in their extent and severity (Table 35.8) [46]. Among spinal gunshot injuries with neurologic deficits, complete neurologic deficits are more common than incomplete [7, 35, 37, 61, 81, 82]: approximately 75% of spinal gunshot injury victims are with a complete neurologic deficit (Frankel Grade A) at presentation. Waters et al. [81] reported that in two-thirds of their patients, this complete neurologic deficit did not change at one year. Among the one-third of patients who did improve by one or two neurologic levels, the injury sustained primarily involved the cauda equina.

Yashon et al. [90] categorized spinal gunshot injury patients into four groups according to their neurologic status: (1) immediate and complete clinical loss of spinal cord function; (2) incomplete nonprogressive spinal cord deficit; (3) incomplete, but progressive spinal cord deficit; and (4) injuries of the conus medullaris or cauda equina with neurologic deficit of varying severity. Among these groups, the

Table 35.8 Characteristics of spinal cord injury following gunshot vs. nonviolent trauma [46]

	GS SCI [%]	NT SCI [%]
Neurologic status		
Paraplegic	78.0	48.8
Tetraplegic	22.0	51.2
Level of injury		
C1-4	12.2	13.4
C5-8	9.8	37.8
T1-6	22.0	16.5
T7-12	36.5	18.1
L1-5	19.5	14.2
Frankel		
A	56.1	36.7
B	17.1	17.9
C	17.1	17.3
D	9.7	25.8
E	0.0	2.3

authors noted that groups 1 and 4 were the most common. The authors also observed that the initial neurologic level may ascend one or two levels several days following injury; however, a complete neurologic deficit did not improve regardless of the treatment regimen employed [89]. These findings were corroborated by Isiklar and Lindsey's [33] more recent review of spinal gunshot injury patients in whom no initially complete spinal cord injury improved a single Frankel grade.

Spinal Stability Following Gunshot Injury

Spinal instability secondary to low-energy gunshot injury is rare [20, 48]. Typically, the direct spine trauma associated with missile injury disrupts a limited portion of the motion segment, and most of the bone, and supplementary ligamentous and muscular constraints remain intact. In fact, most of the reported cases of instability secondary to spine gunshot injuries have been iatrogenic as a result of an ill-advised surgical decompression [72]. However, spine instability following gunshot injury has occasionally been documented in the literature. Stauffer et al. [72] identified four cervical spine gunshot injury patients with instability according to the criteria of White and Panjabi

and a lumbar spine gunshot injury patient who was unstable according to the Denis classification (Fig. 35.12). Subsequently, Isiklar and Lindsey [33] described several cases of gunshot-related cervical and lumbar instability. The cervical spine gunshot injury patients demonstrated frank instability with segment collapse and hypermobility despite application of a halo-vest or cervical orthoses. In each instance, the missile completely disrupted the cervical body and the otherwise intact posterior elements were insufficient to support the weight of the head and the subsequent flexion moment. These authors concluded that although spinal instability following gunshot injuries is typically uncommon, it should always be considered. This is especially valid for gunshots to the hypermobile cervical and thoracolumbar regions of the spine. Therefore, patients with spine gunshot injures should initially be placed in an appropriate orthotic support or brace, and closely monitored until spinal stability has been established. Significant comminution of the entire vertebral body poses a special concern as it increases the risk for spinal collapse and/or pronounced angular deformity. High-energy gunshot injuries to the spine carry increased risk for spinal instability and, therefore spinal precautions have to be maintained in these patients until instability has been ruled out. These injuries must be carefully analyzed and followed to detect potential malalignment and/or progression of neurologic symptoms.

Fig. 35.12 Examples of cervical (**a**) and lumbar spine (**b**) instability following low-energy gunshot injury. Cervical (C6) spine injury caused the destruction of the posterior elements, pedicle, and the facet joint rendering the spine unstable (>5 score) according to White and Panjabi criteria. Lumbar (L1) vertebra injury included bilateral pedicle fractures with middle column involvement and was classified as unstable injury following Denis criteria. Adapted from: [33]

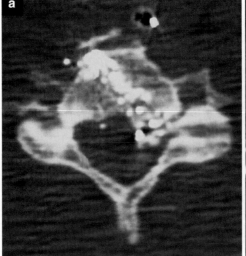
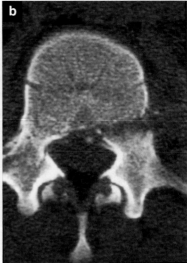

References

1. Adams BD (1982) Wound ballistics: a review. Milit Med 147:831–835
2. Annest JL, Mercy JA, Gibson DR et al (1995) National estimate of nonfatal firearm-related injuries: beyond the tip of the iceberg. JAMA 273:1749–1754
3. Arasil E, Tascioglu AO (1982) Spontaneous migration of an intracranial bullet to the cervical spinal canal causing Lhermitte's sign. A case report. J Neurosurg 56:158–159
4. Avci S, Acikgoz B, Gundogdu S (1995) Delayed neurological symptoms from the spontaneous migration of a bullet in the lumbosacral spinal canal. Case report. Paraplegia 33:541–542
5. Bashir EF, Cybulski GR, Chaudhri K, Choudhury AR (1993) Magnetic resonance imaging and computed tomography in the evaluation of penetrating gunshot injury of the spine. Case report. Spine 18:772–773
6. Belkin M (1978) Wound ballistics. Prog Surg 16:7–24
7. Benzel EC, Hadden TA, Coleman JE (1987) Civilian gunshot wounds to the spinal cord and cauda equina. Neurosurgery 20:281–285
8. Brywczynski JJ, Barrett TW, Lyon JA, Cotton BA (2008) Management of penetrating neck injury in the emergency department: a structured literature review. Emerg Med J 25:711–715
9. Burney RE, Maio RF, Maynard F, Karunas R (1993) Incidence, characteristics, and outcome of spinal cord injury at trauma centers in North America. Arch Surg 128: 596–599
10. Carrillo EH, Gonzalez JK, Carrillo LE, Chacon PM, Namias N, Kirton OC, Byers PM (1998) Spinal cord injuries in adolescents after gunshot wounds: an increasing phenomenon in urban North America. Injury 29:503–507
11. Conway JE, Crofford TW, Terry AF, Protzman RR (1993) Cauda equina syndrome occurring nine years after gunshot injury to the spine. J Bone Joint Surg 75A:760–763
12. Cook PJ, Lawrence BA, Ludwig J, Miller TR (1999) The medical costs of gunshot injuries in the United States. JAMA 282:447–454
13. Cybulski GR, Sone JL, Kant R (1989) Outcome of laminectomy for civilian gunshot injuries of the terminal spinal cord and cauda equina: review of 88 cases. Neurosurgery 24:392–397
14. Daniel EF, Smith GW (1960) Foreign body granuloma of intervertebral disc and spinal canal. J Neurosurg 17: 480–482
15. Delamarter RB, Sherman J, Carr JB (1995) Pathophysiology of spinal cord injury: recovery after immediate and delayed compression. J Bone Joint Surg 77A:1042–1049
16. DeMuth WE (1969) Bullet velocity and design and determinants of wounding capability: an experimental study. J Trauma 6:222–232
17. Denise F (1983) The three column spine and its significance in the classification of acute thoracolumbar spine injuries. Spine 8:817–831
18. De-Wen W, Zhun-Shan W, Xao-Gang Y, Yan-Ping L, Zhing-Ming N, Xao-Ming W, Bao-Zhen W, Yi Y, Wen-Hua H (1996) Histologic and utrastructural changes of the spinal cord after high-velocity missile injury to the back. J Trauma 40:90–93
19. Dillman RO, Crumb CK, Lidsky MJ (1979) Lead poisoning from a gunshot wound. Report of a case and review of the literature. Am J Med 66:509–514
20. Dubose J, Teixeira PG, Hadjizacharia P, Hannon M, Inaba K, Green DG, Plurad D, Demetriades D, Rhee P (2009) The role of routine spinal imaging and immobilisation in asymptomatic patients after gunshot wounds. Injury 40:860–863, Epub ahead of print
21. Ebraheim NA, Savolaine ER, Jackson WT, Andreshak TG, Rayport M (1989) Magnetic resonance imaging in the evaluation of a gunshot wound to the cervical spine. J Orthop Trauma 3:19–22
22. Eismont FJ (1998) Gunshot wounds to the spine. In: Levine AM, Eismont FJ, Garfin SR, Zigler JE (eds) Spine trauma. WB Saunders, Philadelphia PA, pp 525–543
23. Fackler ML (1988) Wound ballistic: a review of current misconceptions. JAMA 259:2730–2736
24. Fackler ML (1998) Civilian gunshot wounds and ballistics: dispelling the myths. Emerg Med Clin North Am 16:17–28
25. Frankel HL, Hancock DO, Hyslop G, Melzak J, Michaelis LS, Ungar GH, Vernon JD, Walsh JJ (1969) The value of postural reduction in the initial management of closed injuries of the spine with paraplegia and tetraplegia. Paraplegia 7:179–192
26. Golueke P, Scalfari S, Philips T, Goldstein A, Scalea T, Duncan A (1987) Vertebral artery injury diagnosis and management. J Trauma 27:856–865
27. Gotsch KE, Annest JL, Mercy JA, Ryan GW (2001) Surveillance for fatal and nonfatal firearm-related injuries: United States, 1993-1998. MMWR 50:1–31
28. Grogan DP, Bucholz RW (1981) Acute lead intoxication from a bullet in an intervertebral disc space: a case report. J Bone Joint Surg 63A:1180–1182
29. Gugala Z, Lindsey RW (2003) Classification of gunshot injuries in civilians. Clin Orthop 408:65–81
30. Heary RF, Vaccaro AR, Mesa JJ, Balderston RA (1996) Thoracolumbar infections in penetrating injuries to the spine. Orthop Clin North Am 27:69–81
31. Heary RF, Vaccaro AR, Mesa JJ, Northrup BE, Albert TJ, Balderston RA, Cotler JM (1997) Steroids and gunshot wounds to the spine. Neurosurgery 41:576–583
32. Insull P, Adams D, Segar A, Ng A, Civil I (2007) Is exploration mandatory in penetrating zone II neck injuries? ANZ J Surg 77:261–264
33. Isiklar ZU, Lindsey RW (1997) Low-velocity civilian gunshot wounds of the spine. Orthopedics 20:967–972
34. Isiklar ZU, Lindsey RW (1998) Gunshot wounds to the spine. Injury 29-S1:A7–A12
35. Kane T, Capen D, Waters R, Zigler JE, Adkins R (1991) Spinal cord injury from civilian gunshot wound: the Rancho experience 1980-88. J Spinal Disord 4:305–311
36. Karim NO, Nabors MW, Golocovsky M, Cooney FD (1986) Spontaneous migration of a bullet in the spinal subarachnoid space causing delayed radicular symptoms. Neurosurgery 18:97–100
37. Kihtir T, Ivatury RR, Simon R, Stahl WM (1991) Management of transperitoneal gunshot wounds of the spine. J Trauma 31:1579–1583
38. Klein Y, Cohn SM, Soffer D et al (2005) Spine injuries are common among asymptomatic patients after gunshot wounds. J Trauma 58:833–836
39. Kumar A, Wood GW 2nd, Whittle AP (1998) Low-velocity gunshot injuries of the spine with abdominal viscus trauma. J Orthop Trauma 12:514–517

40. Leonard MH (1969) Solution of the lead in synovial fluid. Clin Orthop 64:255–261

41. Levy ML, Gans W, Wijesinghe HS, SooHoo WE, Adkins RH, Stillerman CB (1996) Use of methylprednisolone as an adjunct in the management of patients with penetrating spinal cord injury: outcome analysis. Neurosurgery 39:1141–1148

42. Lin SS, Vaccaro AR, Reisch S, Devine M, Cotler JM (1995) Low-velocity gunshot wounds to the spine with an associated transperitoneal injury. J Spinal Disord 8:136–144

43. Linden MA, Manton WI, Stewart RM, Thal ER, Feit H (1969) Lead poisoning from retained bullets. Pathogenesis, diagnosis and management. Ann Surg 195:305–313

44. Lindsey D (1980) The idolatry, lies, damn lies, and ballistics. J Trauma 20:1068–1069

45. Lindsey RW, Gugala Z (1999) Spinal cord injury as a result of ballistic trauma. In: Chapman JR (ed) Spine: state of the art reviews spinal cord injuries, vol 13. Hanley & Belfus Inc, Philadelphia, pp 529–547

46. McKinley WO, Johns JS, Musgrove JJ (1999) Clinical presentations, medical complications, and functional outcomes of individuals with gunshot wound-induced spinal cord injury. Am J Phys Med Rehabil 78:102–107

47. Messer HD, Cerza PF (1976) Copper-jacketed bullets in the central nervous system. Neuroradiology 12:121–129

48. Meyer PR, Apple DF, Bohlman HH (1988) Symposium: management of fractures of the thoracolumbar spine. Contemp Orthop 16:57–86

49. Miller BR, Schiller WR (1989) Pyogenic vertebral osteomyelitis after transcolonic gunshot wound. Military Med 154:64–66

50. Moon E, Kondrashov D, Hannibal M, Hsu K, Zucherman J (2008) Gunshot wounds to the spine: literature review and report on a migratory intrathecal bullet. Am J Orthop 37:E47–E51

51. Oktem IS, Selcuklu A, Kurtsoy A, Kavuncu IA, Pasaoglu A (1995) Migration of bullet in the spinal canal: a case report. Surg Neurol 44:548–550

52. Ordog GJ, Wasserberger J, Balasubramaniam S (1988) Shotgun wound ballistics. J Trauma 28:624–631

53. Plumley TF, Kilcoyne RF, Mack LA (1983) Computed tomography in evaluation of gunshot wounds to the spine. J Comput Assist Tomogr 7:310–312

54. Prendergast MR, Saxe JM, Ledgerwood AM, Lucas CE, Lucas WF (1994) Massive steroids do not reduce the zone of injury after penetrating spinal cord injury. J Trauma 37:576–580

55. Primm DD (1984) Lead arthropathy: progressive destruction of the joint by a retained bullet. J Bone Joint Surg 66A:292–294

56. Quigley KJ, Place HM (2006) The role of debridement and antibiotics in gunshot wounds to the spine. J Trauma 60:814–819

57. Rajan DK, Alcantara AL, Michael DB (1997) Where's the bullet? A migration in two acts. J Trauma 43:716–718

58. Rhee P, Kuncir EJ, Johnson L et al (2006) Cervical spine injury is highly dependent on the mechanism of injury following blunt and penetrating injury. J Trauma 61:1166–1170

59. Rhee JM, Martin R (1997) The management of retained bullets in the limbs. Injury 28(S3):23–28

60. Robertson DP, Simpson RK (1992) Penetrating injuries restricted to the cauda equina: a retrospective review. Neurosurgery 31:265–270

61. Roffi RP, Waters RL, Adkins RH (1989) Gunshot wounds to the spine associated with a perforated viscus. Spine 14:808–811

62. Romanick PC, Smith TK, Kopaniky DR, Oldfield D (1985) Infection about the spine associated with low-velocity-missile injury to the abdomen. J Bone Joint Surg 67A:1195–1201

63. Roon AJ, Christensen N (1979) Evaluation and treatment of penetrating cervical injuries. J Trauma 19:391–394

64. Rosenfled JV (2002) Gunshot injury to the head and spine. J Clin Neurosci 9:9–16

65. Schwab CW, Members of the Violence Prevention Task Force of the Eastern Association for the Surgery of Trauma (1995) Violence in America: a public health crisis - the role of firearms. J Trauma 38:163–168

66. Schwab CW, Richmond T, Dunfey M (2002) Firearm injury in America. LDI Issue Brief 8:1–6

67. Shepard GH (1980) High-energy, low-velocity close range shotgun wounds. J Trauma 20:1065–1067

68. Sherman IJ (1960) Brass foreign body in the brain stem. J Neurosurg 17:483–485

69. Sherman RT, Parrish RA (1963) Management of shotgun injuries: a review of 152 cases. J Trauma 3:76–85

70. Shuman M, Wright RK (1999) Evaluation of clinician accuracy in describing the gunshot wound injuries. J Forensic Sci 44:339–352

71. Simpson R, Venger B, Narayan R (1989) Treatment of acute penetrating injuries of the spine: a retrospective analysis. J Trauma 29:42–46

72. Stauffer ES, Wood RW, Kelly EG (1979) Gunshot wounds of the spine: the effects of laminectomy. J Bone Joint Surg 61A:389–392

73. Tanguy A, Chabannes J, Deubelle A, Vanneuville G, Dalens B (1982) Intraspinal migration of a bullet with subsequent meningitis. J Bone Joint Surg 64A:1244–1245

74. Teitelbaum GP (1990) Metallic ballistic fragments: MR imaging safety and artifacts. Radiology 177:883

75. The US Department of Justice. Bureau of Justice Statistics. http://www.ojp.usdoj.gov/bjs/glance/firearmnonfatalno.htm. Accessed on Jul 15, 2009

76. The Violence Prevention Task Force of the Eastern Association for the Surgery of Trauma (1995) Violence in America: a public health crisis–the role of firearms. J Trauma 38:163–168

77. Thoresby FP, Darlow HM (1967) The mechanisms of primary infection of bullet wounds. Br J Surg 54:359–361

78. Tindel NL, Marcillo AE, Tay BK, Bunge RP, Eismont FJ (2001) The effect of surgically implanted bullet fragments on the spinal cord in a rabbit model. J Bone Joint Surg 83A:884–890

79. American College of Surgeons Committee on Trauma (2004) Spine and spinal cord trauma. In: Advanced trauma life support for doctors. The student manual, 7th edn. First Impression, Chicago, pp.177–189

80. Velmahos G, Demetriades D (1994) Gunshot wounds of the spine: should retained bullets be removed to prevent infection? Ann R Coll Surg Engl 76:85–87

81. Waters RL, Adkins RH (1991) The effects of removal of bullet fragments retained in the spinal canal: a collaborative

study by the National Spinal Cord Injury Model Systems. Spine 16:935–939

82. Waters RL, Adkins RH, Yakura J, Sie I (1991) Profiles of spinal cord injury and recovery after gunshot injury. Clin Orthop 267:14–21

83. Waters RL, Sie IH (2003) Spinal cord injuries from bunshot wounds to the spine. Clin Orthop 408:120–125

84. Bono CM, Heary RF (2004) Gunshot wounds to the spine. Spine J 4(2):230–240.

85. Waters RL, Sie IH, Adkins RH (1995) Rehabilitation of patient with a spinal cord injury. Orthop Clin North Am 26:117–122

86. Weinshel S, Maiman D (1989) Spinal subdural hematoma resenting as an epidural hematoma following gunshot: report of a case. J Spinal Disord 1:17–19

87. Wigle RL (1989) Treatment of asymptomatic gunshot injury to the spine. Am Surg 55:591–595

88. Wintemute GJ (1996) The relationship between firearm design and firearm violence, handguns in the 1999's. JAMA 275:1749–1753

89. Wolf AW, Benson DR, Shoji H, Hoeprich P, Gilmore A (1978) Autosterilization in low-velocity bullets. J Trauma 18:63

90. Yashon D, Jane JA, White RJ (1970) Prognosis and management of spinal cord and cauda equina bullet injuries in sixty-five civilians. J Neurosurg 32:163–170

91. Yoshida GM, Garland D, Waters RL (1995) Gunshot wounds to the spine. Orthop Clin North Am 26:109–116

Complications in Spine Surgery

Evalina Burger

36.1 Introduction

Complications pertaining to spine fracture fixation can be divided into preoperative, intraoperative, and postoperative complications. The specific complications, inherent to each procedure, are outlined in the text. However, complications pertaining to spine trauma surgery, in general, will be discussed in this chapter.

Most complications arise from poor planning or the lack of anticipation. This is a very common pitfall in trauma surgery as decisions sometimes have to be made quickly. Maintaining a good algorithm is vital to avoid most of these complications.

36.2 Preoperative Planning

36.2.1 Imaging and Clinical Impressions

Lack of appropriate testing, including inadequate X-rays or CT scans and/or MRI's, usually lies at the bottom of most complications. It is vital that the appropriate X-rays of the injured area be taken and that the patient's whole axial spine is imaged to view adjacent and nonadjacent level injuries. For the cervical area, X-rays should include the C7–T1 junction and specific attention should be paid to both the occiput-C1–C2 junction and the cervical-thoracic junction. CT scans must be obtained if these areas are not adequately visualized.

When patients have a neurological deficit, it is appropriate to order a MRI, but not to delay potential life saving measures to get the MRI.

Incorrect numbering on CT scans or mislabeling and miscounting are among the most common reasons for intraoperative mistakes starting with inadequate exposure and leading to wrong level surgery. CT scans and intraoperative X-rays should be compared, especially in the event of a cervical rib or lumbosacral variant.

Preoperative X-rays for the thoracic area not only should include the thoracic spine, but attention should also be paid to the sternum and the manubrium to judge the severity of the fractures. Often a "benign compression fracture" can be part of a thoracic dislocation, which can be missed when appropriate X-rays and examination are not performed.

In the lumbar spine, rare but devastating injury, such as traumatic spondylothesis, can be missed especially in high energy accidents and military blast accidents. The most common injury to be missed is the compression fracture, which is actually part of a flexion-distraction injury. These can only be diagnosed with an appropriate clinical exam and MRI to adjudicate the posterior elements and the soft tissue.

36.2.2 Equipment

Equipment is crucial to successful trauma surgery. It is important that the surgeon familiarize himself or herself with the equipment available in the OR. Appropriate beds, Mayfield tongs, neuromonitoring, radiology, lighting, and a microscope should all be available. It is often the case that the surgeon assumes that these things will be available, especially if the surgeon is taking call

E. Burger
Department of Orthopaedics, University of Colorado, Denver,
12631 East 17th Avenue, Aurora, CO 80045, USA
e-mail: evalina.burger@ucdenver.edu

V.V. Patel et al. (eds.), *Spine Trauma*,
DOI: 10.1007/978-3-642-03694-1_36, © Springer-Verlag Berlin Heidelberg 2010

in a hospital where he or she does not perform his or her daily routine. It is important to make sure that the equipment is available and in a working order. After-hour untrained staffing, can also be problematic staffing, It is important to communicate with the team to ensure that everyone from the anesthesiologist to the neuromonitoring personal, the circulator, radiology technician, and the scrub tech are on board with the surgical plan. It is important to inform the anesthesiologist of the goal of the surgery, whether muscle relaxation is appropriate, and for which part of the case. Baseline neuromonitoring should be coordinated to ensure that pre and postpositioning baseline values have remained the same, before the surgery starts. The appropriate fluid resuscitation and blood pressure maintenance should be discussed with the anesthesiologist to avoid disastrous neurological deteriorations.

36.2.3 Preoperative Evaluation of the Patient and Documentation is Extremely Important

It is important to have a detailed preoperative exam and correlate the findings with the X-rays and other appropriate imaging studies. If the findings do not correlate 100%, both the imaging and the patient should be reevaluated to make sure the deficit correlates with the appropriate X-rays. Common mistakes can be mislabeling of X-rays. In a busy trauma unit, X-rays might be labeled incorrectly not only for patient name, but also for left, right, and level. This cannot be overemphasized. This is vital to avoid wrong level surgery and has medical legal ramifications.

36.3 Intraoperative Complications

Intraoperative complications are usually related to the finding of unexpected trauma or underestimation of the trauma during the initial planning of the surgery. Interoperative complications may necessitate the surgeon to extend the incision, include more levels in the fusion, perform additional decompressions, deal with uncontrollable bleeding, and compromise on fixation.

36.3.1 Underestimation of Trauma

It is vital during the trauma situation to prep the skin wide. It is not advisable to prep a small area for a single level fusion in a trauma patient. The general advice is to prep the patient really wide. The incision should also be planned in such a manner that it would be easy to extend. There could be an argument made for using longitudinal excisions in the c-spine vs. horizontal, but the surgeon should be prepared to extend the incision all the way to the corner of jaw and down to the manubrium into the chest. Unexpected aneurysm or trauma of the jugular vein and artery can complicate anterior exposures. Since these injuries might not always be evident due to tampanade, they can lead to unpleasant surprises, especially if the surgical field is not well prepared.

Another unexpected finding can be extensive soft tissue trauma, such as unrecognized esophageal injury. Furthermore, the ALL may be ruptured on the level above or below, which is, at that point, a coincidental finding, but it may necessitate the inclusion of a potential unstable level on the fusion.

In the thoracic spine, dislocated rib heads are a common finding and can lead to tension pneumothorax during positive ventilation, necessitating the placement of an intercostal tube and water seal drain. In the lumbar spine, occult injury can be as little as a ruptured supraspinous ligament to as much as a compartment syndrome of the paraspinal muscles.

Draping the patient wide for all the above reasons cannot be overemphasized. Dural leaks should be anticipated, especially in burst fractures. Dural repair instruments should be readily available.

36.3.2 Bleeding

Bleeding in a trauma situation can be a massive problem. Coagulopathies can develop due to concomitant injuries. Extensive blood loss may also be inherent to the spine fracture pattern. This is most commonly seen with corpectomies performed in the acute setting. It is important in the preoperative planning to have hemostatic agents available and to make sure that enough blood components including fresh frozen plasma and platelets are available to resuscitate the patient appropriately. If bleeding cannot be controlled, it could lead to exsanguination. The surgeons should be prepared to pack the area with hemostatic agents and revert to temporary fixation to avoid damage to vital neural structures. The patient should be taken to the ICU, resuscitated, and the surgical approach could then be facilitated with IR ablation of the veins and arteries such as in tumor surgery. This is especially important in pathological fractures where the primary pathology might be overlooked or undiagnosed.

36.3.3 Soft Tissue Coverage

While placing internal fixation in areas with tenuous skin, it is important to make sure that the appropriate tissue coverage can be obtained. If this is not possible, it is not advisable to undermine flaps and compromise the paraspinal blood supply any further. Consultation with plastic surgeon should be obtained quickly and appropriately. Extensive soft tissue injury can lead to compartment syndrome, and just as in a limb, the vitality of the paraspinal muscles should be inspected. This is particularly important when patients have blunt trauma or have been involved in high energy blast injuries.

36.3.4 Fixation Failure

Failure to obtain adequate fixation of the fracture during surgery is not uncommon. This can be due to the underestimation of the injury and inadequate preoperative planning or because of a patient's unstable medical condition. It is, therefore, vital to not hesitate to extend the incision and incorporate more levels in cases where adequate fracture fixation cannot be obtained. The use of cement augmentation for pedicle screws should always be considered and augmentation of the fixation with an, either staged anterior or posterior approach, depending on the kind of procedure, should be decided at the time of surgery. It is also important to look at the patient's bone structure and stature and to make sure that appropriate instrumentation is ordered for the fracture. Most complications of fixation occur where pedicle screws are too big, cannot

be placed appropriately, or where fractures extend into the junction zone and the appropriate implant sets were not ordered in the preoperative planning. It is vital to have a full array of spine implants available before embarking on trauma fracture fixation.

36.4 Postoperative Complications

Postoperative complications can be divided into acute and long-term complications. The most devastating postoperative complication is the discovery of a neurological deficit. Acute complications stem from the original surgery and include massive blood loss, failure of fixation, and misplaced internal fixation. They can also include acute infection and failure to obtain soft tissue closure. Long-term complications include infections, failure of instrumentation, and pseudoarthrosis. In managing postoperative complications, it is important to reevaluate the patient directly after surgery to get the appropriate X-rays in a timely manner, to assess the fracture pattern with the appropriate fixation, and to anticipate possible failure.

36.4.1 Neurological Complications

Some of the most devastating postoperative complications are that of neurological paralysis. Neurological injury can vary from a nerve root paralysis to dysesthesia secondary to traction, which can be both due to the positioning as well as direct injury of the nerve root. The most serious complication is that of spinal cord injury. To avoid spinal cord injury is the ultimate goal of fracture fixation of the spine. However, this does occur and it is important to understand the mechanisms by which this can occur. Direct trauma of the spinal cord can occur when fracture dislocations are being reduced and herniated discs in the canal are undiagnosed. Most commonly, however, spinal cord injury is due to a vascular compromise, which can occur during the reduction maneuver and can also be a combination of direct injury of the cord in a patient with hemorrhagic shock and preexisting partial ischemia of the cord. Most spinal cord injuries can be avoided when there is collaboration between the surgeon and the anesthesiology team. It is important to maintain the perfusion pressure to avoid ischemia, and most of all, to have adequate equipment when delicate reduction maneuvers are made. The value of a good neuromonitoring team cannot be underestimated and this argument might be so strong that postponement of surgical procedures that are not life threatening can be argued. When the ultimate complication is spinal cord injury, it is important to rethink appropriateness of rushing a patient to the operating room in the middle of the night for a nonthreatening injury vs. waiting until a fresh team with appropriate anesthesiology coverage, neuromonitoring, and surgeon is available in the morning.

36.4.2 Postoperative Infection

Postoperative infection is a common problem in spine surgery and can mostly be avoided by appropriate antibiotics and maintaining the patient's nutrition. Trauma patients tend to be malnourished due to repeated surgeries and tend to lose their proteins quickly, which is the normal metabolic response to trauma. It is vital to make sure that the patient's nutrition is managed in an appropriate way to avoid disastrous infections in the unstable spine. Appropriate antibiotics should be administered in conjunction with the trauma team. Undiagnosed Urinary tract infections are a major cause of delayed infections as bacteria spread to the spine via the Batson Plexus.

36.4.3 Misplaced Instrumentation

This is one of the most common occurrences in Spine surgery and may be as high as 20% of all pedicle screws. When performing fixation of a fracture in the middle of the night without the regular team support, one may postulate that it would be even higher. Anticipating these types of complications by taking appropriate post-op X-rays and not hesitating to take the patient back for repositioning of instrumentation can avoid disastrous late outcomes.

36.4.4 Pseudoarthrosis

In the haste of obtaining adequate fracture fixation, the importance of appropriate biological augmentation might be overlooked. It is sometimes not possible to obtain adequate graft from the iliac crest, or the patient's general condition will only allow for stabilization. Many of the trauma patients might also include an undesirable lifestyle such as smoking and alcohol abuse. All of these factors combined may lead to pseudoarthrosis. It is important to assess this problem globally and ensure adequate addition of bone graft and biologics even as a staged procedure. Inappropriate bone grafting or poor biology will ultimately lead to instrumentation failure. Pseudoarthrosis should be anticipated and recognized early and appropriately treated before implant failure occurs as this leaves complicated bailout options.

36.5 Summary

Good judgment comes from experience and experience comes from poor judgment.

Most complications can be anticipated. It is crucially important that additional time be taken to plan fixation of fractures in the trauma patient. Due to the nature of the pathology, the scene is already set for disaster and the surgeon needs to be vigilant and aware of the pitfalls.

36.6 Pearls

- Correlate the clinical exam and the radiology findings.
- Plan the surgery and ensure appropriate equipment is available.
- Drape the surgical field for the possibility of additional surgical incisions.
- Anticipate complications and treat the patient holistically.
- Early appropriate intervention can diminish complications.

References

1. Cammisa FR Jr, Eismont FJ, Green BA (1989) Dural laceration occurring with burst fractures and associated laminar fractures. J Bone Joint Surg Am 71(7):1044–1052
2. Hill GL, Blackett RL, Pickford I et al (1977) Malnutrition in surgical patients. An unrecognized problem. Lancet 1(8013):689–692
3. Hu SS, Fontaine F, Kelly B et al (1998) Nutritional depletion in staged spinal reconstructive surgery. The effect of total parenteral nutrition. Spine 23(12):1401–1405
4. Jules-Elysee K, Urquhart BL et al (2004) Pulmonary complications in anterior-posterior thoracic lumbar fusions. Spine J 4(3):312–316
5. Klein JD, Hey LA, Yu CS et al (1996) Perioperative nutrition and postoperative complications in patients undergoing spinal surgery. Spine 21(22):2676–2682
6. Lapp MA, Bridwell KH, Lenke LG et al (2001) Prospective randomization of parenteral hyperalimentation for long fusions with spinal deformity: its effect on complications and recovery from postoperative malnutrition. Spine 26(7):809–817
7. Lenke LG, Bridwell KH, Blanke K et al (1995) Prospective analysis of nutritional status normalization after spinal reconstructive surgery. Spine 20(12):1359–1367
8. Mandelbaum BR, Tolo VT, McAfee PC et al (1988) Nutritional deficiencies after staged anterior and posterior spinal reconstructive surgery. Clin Orthop 234:5–11
9. Picada R, Winter RB, Lonstein JE et al (2000) Postoperative deep wound infection in adults after posterior lumbocosacral spine fusion with instrumentation: incidence and management. J Spinal Disord 13(1):42–45
10. Thalgott JS, Cotler HB, Sasso RC et al (1991) Postoperative infections in spinal implants. Classification and analysis – a multicenter study. Spine 16(8):981–984
11. Wukich DK, Van Dam BE, Graeber GM et al (1990) Serum creatine kinase and lactate dehydrogenase changes after anterior approaches to the thoracic and lumbar spine. Spine 15(3):187–190

Index